The Encyclopedia of
❧
Natural
PET CARE

Other Books by the Author

Herbs to Improve Digestion
Herbs for the Heart
Herbs for Men's Health
Herbs for Detoxification
Herbs to Relieve Arthritis
Herbs to Help You Breathe Freely
Herbal Teas
Nature's Antiseptics: Tea Tree Oil and
    Grapefruit Seed Extract

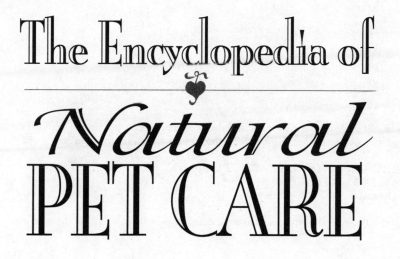

The Encyclopedia of
Natural PET CARE

CJ Puotinen

Foreword by Beverly Cappel-King, D.V.M.

 Keats Publishing, Inc. New Canaan, Connecticut

THE ENCYCLOPEDIA OF NATURAL PET CARE
Copyright © 1998 by CJ Puotinen
All Rights Reserved

Puotinen, C J
        The encyclopedia of natural pet care / C J Puotinen ; foreword by
Beverly Cappel-King.
        p.   cm.
        Includes bibliographical references (p.   ) and index.
        ISBN 0-87983-797-7
        1. Pets -- Diseases -- Alternative treatment. 2. Pets -- Health.
    I. Title.
    SF981.P86   1997
    636.089'55 -- dc21   97-43372
                                                              CIP

Printed in the United States of America

Keats Publishing, Inc.
27 Pine Street (Box 876)
New Canaan, Connecticut 06840-0876
Website Address: www.keats.com

In memory of Sari Louise Fennel
for Sophie Fennel Knot
and in memory of Marjorie A. Major
and Tiffany,
who together crossed Rainbow Bridge

Photo and Illustration Credits

Many people and animals helped with the photographs that illustrate this book. Special thanks go to Sarah Wilson, her cat, Lucy, and her German Shepherd, Star; Dolores Schaub and her Moluccan cockatoo, Gizmo; Mary Silversweig and Sirabi's five-week-old Labrador Retriever puppies; Hudson Valley Humane Society and its mascot rabbit, Tawny; Ken and Arlene Nadasdi and their cat, Sam; Joan Tortorello and her Golden Retriever, Indiana Jones; my own cat, Pumpkin; homeopathic pharmacist Ezzat Hanna at the Weleda Pharmacy, Chestnut Ridge, New York; photographer Harvey Salem at MotoPhoto, Pomona, New York; photographer Gwen Barba; and my husband, Joel Hollenberg.

Page 1, Chapter 1: Gizmo, Tawny and Sam, photo by Harvey Salem.

Page 59, Chapter 2: Pumpkin, photo by Joel Hollenberg.

Page 97, Chapter 3: Supplements, photo by Joel Hollenberg.

Page 113, Chapter 4: Tea Brewing, photo by Gwen Barba.

Pages 131 to 135 and 143: Line drawings of herbs from *Medicinal Plants Coloring Book*, published by Dover Publications, Inc., New York; used with permission.

Page 163, Chapter 5: Lavender, photo by Joel Hollenberg.

Page 189, Chapter 6: Homeopathic Remedies, photo by Joel Hollenberg.

Page 213, Chapter 7: Lucy, photo by Gwen Barba.

Page 220, Accupressure points in dogs and cats, adapted from a drawing by C. Stroh in *Canine Acupressure: A Treatment Workbook* by Nancy Zidonis and Marie Soderberg; used with permission.

Page 239, Chapter 8: Calendula Blossoms, photo by Gwen Barba.

Page 257, Chapter 9: Gizmo, photo by Harvey Salem.

Page 271, Chapter 10: Sirabi's Puppies, photo by Harvey Salem.

Page 287, Chapter 11: Sam, photo by Harvey Salem.

Page 309, Chapter 12: Star, photo by Gwen Barba.

Page 465, Chapter 14: Indiana Jones, Joan Tortorello and a Friend at Nyack Manor Nursing Home, Valley Cottage, New York, photo by Gwen Barba.

Page 471, Chapter 15: Pumpkin, photo by Joel Hollenberg.

Contents

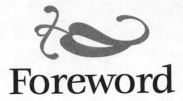

Foreword

by Beverly Cappel-King, D.V.M.

WELCOME TO THE EXCITING, controversial, rapidly growing and often confusing world of holistic pet care. No matter what your situation, now is the perfect time to read this book. If you're about to bring a companion animal into your life, it will show you how to avoid making common mistakes that may contribute to your pet's physical, mental and emotional problems. If you already have a dog, cat, bird, rabbit or other pet, it will help you understand the major trends in veterinary medicine while teaching you simple ways to improve your pet's health and behavior.

Today's interest in natural pet care is a logical extension of the changes taking place in human medicine. Growing numbers of Americans want to take control of their health and not just be told, "Take this cortisone and these antibiotics and you'll feel fine." When I had an adverse reaction to the penicillin I was given as a teenager for recurring strep throat infections, I decided there had to be a better way. Studying nutrition and herbs on my own, I took echinacea, vitamin C and garlic, and never had another strep throat. As a result, I've been fascinated by the body's ability to heal itself. There are many gentle, effective methods that don't have the adverse side effects of powerful drugs, and people are beginning to demand them for their pets as well as for themselves.

I chose a veterinary school in Italy because I like the European method of instruction and because Europe's medical training emphasizes herbs and homeopathy as well as conventional care. After graduation, I stayed in Italy to study homeopathy in depth, then returned to the U.S. and learned acupuncture. These disciplines, combined with improved nutrition and a natural diet, are the foundations of holistic health care for both pets and people.

The demand for natural pet care is growing fast. In 1990, I attended a national holistic veterinary conference and there were only 60 of us present. Today in 1998, the American Holistic Veterinary Medical Association has over 1,100 members, 650 of whom are veterinarians, and 300 attended last year's conference. Not only is interest growing on a national level, but locally even conventional veterinarians are becoming involved. That's because they see the good results that alternative methods have produced in their own patients. They'll call and say, "I don't quite understand it but it worked. Can I send you another case?"

The Cornell University School of Veterinary Medicine, which is the country's foremost conventional veterinary school, is now admitting that there may be more side effects than benefits to annual vaccinations. That's a conclusion I am amazed but thrilled to see. The American Veterinary Medical Association has published journal articles documenting problems with vaccines and showing that dogs vaccinated as puppies still have antibodies produced by the vaccination five years later. At our clinic we run antibody titers and find that most dogs maintain their antibodies year after year without being revaccinated. In addition to the trend away from annual vaccinations, there is growing interest in herbs and nutrition. In fact, the AVMA has recently adopted guidelines embracing alternative and complementary medicine.

When I opened my holistic clinic five years ago, we had just a receptionist, a technician and myself. Today we have four doctors, three receptionists and two technicians, there is a three-week wait for appointments, patients are coming from all over, we're on the Internet and we get phone calls from people all across the country. It's amazing.

About half of the clients who come here for the first time already know about holistic medicine and it's their preferred method of treatment. The other half were recommended by a friend or they're seeking a second or third opinion for a serious illness that conventional therapy hasn't been able to improve, such as liver failure, kidney failure, cancer, heart disease or diabetes. We try to keep our treatments as simple and gentle as possible, for example, by improving the diet, mixing a few herbs into the animals' food, using supplements that are easy to take and removing toxic chemicals from their environment, such as pesticides, herbicides, lawn fertilizers, flea collars, sprays and foods full of additives and preservatives. Whenever possible, we attempt to wean animals off any pharmaceutical drugs. Until recently, conventional doctors never said anything hopeful about kidney or liver failure; the only recommendation anyone ever made was to euthanize the animal. Now some conventional doctors are telling their clients that kidney failure is not necessarily fatal, and they're willing to recommend alternative methods because they've seen some of their own worst cases turn around. With herbs, natural diet, acupuncture and homeopathy, many hopeless cases do well. We have quite a few cancer patients who are in total remission and leading normal lives years after they were given only three months to live.

The fundamental driving force behind holistic health care is Mother Nature. The methods we use don't heal our patients as much as they stimulate our patients to heal themselves. In the wild, animals know what herbs and grasses to eat, what prey to kill, when to rest and when to go without food. I've seen it with my own animals and on farms. If you keep animals in their natural environment and let them live the way nature made them instead of filling them with drugs, they'll figure out exactly what they need to do to stay healthy. In the wild, you don't see the cancers or the chronic diseases so common among pets. We feed our animals the wrong foods, overvaccinate them, stuff them with heartworm pills, treat them with flea preventives, spray them with chemicals, put pesticides on the lawn, use chemical floor cleaners, get asphalt, tar and oil all over their feet and expose them to cigarette smoke and car exhaust, and then we wonder why they die at age six from cancer or kidney failure or liver disease.

The other day I saw a cartoon that showed a prehistoric boy groaning with a stomachache while his mother pulled bark off a tree to make him well. In the next panel, a few thousand years later, the boy had a stomachache and his mother gave him mixed herbs. Three more panels focused on modern approaches. In the mid-20th century, the boy was treated with antibiotics and other wonder drugs and a few years later with new antibiotics and even more powerful drugs. But in the 1990s, the boy had a stomachache and his mother said, "Forget the antibiotics," and pulled some bark off a tree. We've come full circle.

Of course, if you stand back and look at the world, it's really the United States and Canada that have been out of synch. The rest of the planet has used natural remedies all along. Despite what some conventional minds believe, holistic medicine is not off-the-wall alternative weirdness or untested, unproven, anecdotal nonsense. It isn't even new. Homeopathy was a proven medical science 200 years ago, herbal medicine has been used without interruption for thousands of years, acupuncture is truly ancient and the only thing new in animal nutrition is the bizarre and unnatural food that comes out of cans and packages labeled for dogs, cats, birds, rabbits and other pets.

Any rapidly changing field can be confusing and controversial, and that's certainly true of veterinary medicine in America today. CJ Puotinen has focused on the most helpful, effective and widely practiced therapies in holistic pet care, interviewed leading practitioners and organized a handbook that will be useful to everyone who cares about their companion animals.

If some of these procedures sound complicated at first, that's only because they are unfamiliar. As you grow accustomed to using them, they will become a comfortable part of your daily routine. At first, they may also seem expensive. While an appropriate, well-balanced, raw, whole-food diet can cost more than supermarket pet food, it isn't when you factor in the animal's medical bills. After ten years of veterinary practice, I can assure you that every investment you make in the careful selection, training, feeding and health of your pets will save hundreds or thousands of dollars in medical expenses, not to mention anxiety and heartbreak. At the same time, you will improve the quality and length of your pets' lives as well as your own. Researchers are repeatedly finding that people who live with pets have longer, happier, calmer, healthier lives than those who don't, and if your companion animals are themselves the picture of health and not shedding dander all over everything or adding stress to your life, the health benefits increase.

I hope *The Encyclopedia of Natural Pet Care* will inspire you to become more involved in your pets' care, to improve their diet, to question and learn about every medical procedure that anyone, including a holistic veterinarian, recommends for them, to become actively involved in their care and to expect a lifetime of good health, glossy coats, bright eyes, strong bones, alert intelligence and calm dispositions in your furred and feathered companions.

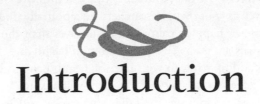

Introduction

ONE DAY YEARS AGO I was talking with a health food store sales clerk and the conversation turned to cats. She told me a long and complicated story about an infant kitten her roommate found abandoned in a storm. They rushed the kitty to a veterinarian who recommended that she be put to sleep, for she probably wouldn't live through the night and, if she did, she would never be healthy. The roommates refused and took their tiny pet home, where they fed her raw milk and supplements. When she was ready to eat solid food, they gave her raw chicken, bones and all. The cat was now three years old, the clerk told me proudly, and in addition to never eating a bite of commercial cat food, she had never been back to the veterinarian.

I was shocked. I thought these women were completely irresponsible to neglect the vaccinations their cat obviously needed, and feeding her human food rather than something designed especially for cats and giving her everything raw, including bones, which everyone knows not to feed their pets, only made it worse. I went home patting myself on the back for being a far more responsible pet owner and probably picked up a bag of cat chow on the way.

But in the months that followed, the kitten's story tumbled around in my mind. I had dismissed the clerk's description of her cat's glossy coat, bright eyes and excellent health because it sounded so improbable, but maybe she really was healthy. And how was this pet's diet any different from the mice and shrews my cats had dined on in their youth? After all, as friends reminded me, cats in the wild don't walk around with frying pans and can openers in their pockets. Maybe feeding raw meat wasn't such a bizarre notion after all.

Then the books began to appear. There were actually veterinarians with impressive credentials advocating home-prepared diets and raw meat for dogs and cats. Some of them blamed vaccinations for a host of medical problems, and they advocated therapies I'd never heard of.

I began subscribing to health magazines and newsletters. Our home library expanded with books on nutrition and healing. A friend decided to study herbal medicine and encouraged me to do the same. In 1988 I began a two-year course of study with Rosemary Gladstar, one of America's foremost herbalists, and later apprenticed with Dora Gerber at the Swissette Herb Farm in Salisbury Mills, New York. When Rosemary helped found the Northeast Herbal Association, I was invited to write its journal's question and answer column. Goldie Oatstraw (my pen name came with the column) has provided answers to many questions about pet nutrition and herbal therapies, and this book is their logical extension.

When Keats Publishing launched a new series of books about herbs, writing about medicinal plants became my full-time job. All the while, I shared what I learned about natural pet care with workshop audiences and journal readers, and my file cabinet filled with questions, answers and information.

This guide is an introduction to several but by no means all of the therapies available to America's pet owners. It is impossible to cover everything in just one book, so I focused on what I hope will prove most helpful to most people. Every chapter emphasizes simple, practical things we can do to improve and enhance the lives of our animal companions.

Even though the world of veterinary medicine is changing rapidly, holistic practitioners are still a small minority. Fortunately, when we need help making informed decisions about veterinary care, we can usually find it, either in books, by phone or, if there's a holistic veterinarian in the neighborhood, in person. Increasingly, conventional veterinarians are referring patients to practitioners of alternative therapies or accepting their clients' refusal of standard procedures with good grace.

An informed owner is a pet's best medical insurance. I hope you will keep on hand not only this book but others recommended here, for each offers a different perspective. I am not a veterinarian, scientist, healthcare worker, breeder, trainer, groomer or pet store employee, nor do I make or sell pet-related products. Although I've studied and written about medicinal plants, I am not a practicing herbalist. I have no financial interest in any of the books, magazines, products, services or procedures recommended here. My perspective is that of a writer who lives with and loves animals. In order to learn what I wanted to know, I read everything I could find and interviewed every expert who would talk to me.

In the field of holistic pet care, these experts are not only well-informed and articulate, they're very nice people. I owe special thanks to animal trainers Sarah Wilson, Brian

Kilcommons, Diane Bauman, Nancy Strouss and Elizabeth Teal, veterinarians Richard Pitcairn, Allen Schoen, Susan Wynn, Joanne Stefanatos, Larry Bernstein and Beverly Cappel-King, herbalists James Green, Jean Argus and Deb Soule, veterinary chiropractor Marc Sommer, animal nutritionists Celeste Yarnall, Pat McKay and Marina Zacharias, shelter manager Cathy McGrath, bird experts Doreen Gluck and Fred Bauer, hands-on therapists Margie Amster-Herr, Nancy Zidonis, Carol Robin and Christiane Wolski, flower essence authority Patricia Kaminski, essential oils importer Jim Dierking, Price-Pottenger Nutrition Foundation curator Pat Connolly, the staff at the AHVMA and color expert Darius Dinshah for their patience in answering my endless questions. My editor Phyllis Herman, copy editor Anne Harris and the staff at Keats Publishing worked tirelessly to produce this book and they have my sincere appreciation. I am especially grateful to my teacher, Rosemary Gladstar, and Dora Gerber, who taught me the European traditions of herbal medicine and gave me two years of practical, hands-on experience.

A note on language. The term "allopathic" refers to medical procedures that treat symptoms. These procedures are usually surgical or pharmaceutical and they seldom address or treat the symptoms' cause. Allopathic medicine is only one approach to healing, but it is the only form endorsed by most states, the U.S. Food and Drug Administration and major insurance companies, and it is the only approach practiced by most physicians and veterinarians. For this reason, allopathic medicine is also called conventional or orthodox medicine.

The term "holistic," which is sometimes spelled "wholistic," refers to the entire human or animal patient, not just his or her most affected parts. A condition in one part of the body always relates to activity in other parts as well as in the mind and spirit. Holistic practitioners look beyond obvious symptoms in an effort to understand and involve the whole being.

"Alternative" therapies are treatments that can be used in place of the orthodox, conventional, allopathic treatments usually prescribed for acute and chronic conditions. Recently the term "complementary" was coined to describe unconventional treatments that work well in conjunction with allopathic medicine. The evolution of these terms reflects the shift taking place. Veterinarians and pet owners are so rapidly adopting alternative and complementary methods that some of the people I interviewed, such as Dr. Susan Wynn, believe the terms alternative and complementary will soon become obsolete because everything they represent will be part of mainstream veterinary medicine.

Whenever people talk about animals, the pronouns shift from "it" to "he" or "she" and back again. Nearly everyone I interviewed refers to an animal in the abstract as "it" or "he" while specific animals have names and genders. Some refer to animals *that* do things; others talk of animals *who* do things. I found the same grammatical inconsistencies in my own words and eventually gave up trying to correct them.

Many of the people I interviewed spoke of "traditional" medicine when they meant orthodox, conventional or allopathic medicine. I reserve the word traditional for older methods, such as those practiced by native tribes and folk healers. In that context there is nothing traditional about modern allopathic medicine, so I changed this term whenever it was used. Otherwise, the words of the people I've quoted are their own.

Some readers will object to the term "owner," when a better term would be "human companion," "caregiver" or "caretaker." References to the buying or selling of animals offends those who prefer the term "adoption," even when substantial sums of money change hands. No one can really own a cat or dog or other animal, but in the eyes of the law, my husband and I own Samantha, whom we bought (paid money for) from a breeder, and Pepper, whom we adopted (received as a gift) from a farm stand. I offer a blanket apology to anyone whose sensibilities are disturbed by the word owner, references to animals as "it" and what some may see as the excessive use of masculine pronouns, for they appear throughout and are not meant in any disrespectful sense.

Because I want this book to be a useful tool, I have included as many resources as possible, with names, addresses, phone numbers, fax numbers, e-mail addresses and websites. Of these, e-mail addresses and websites tend to change least often. To find a company that has moved since this book went to press, check current issues of pet magazines, the referral services of national organizations, newsletter editors or public library reference desks.

Please remember that this book's purpose is to define, explain and demonstrate drug-free methods and techniques that many pet owners have used with good results. Nothing in this book is meant to diagnose a specific illness or prescribe a specific treatment for your pet. No alternative or complementary treatment is a cure-all that will work in every case or for every animal. However, the more knowledgeable you are about your pet and its species, the more you understand its digestive processes and nutritional requirements, the more you learn about common illnesses and how to prevent them and the more time you spend with your pet using effective training methods and appropriate equipment, the happier, healthier and longer your animal's life is likely to be.

Chapter 1

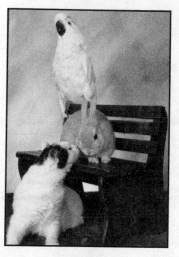

Peace in the House:
Finding, Training and Living with Your Perfect Pet

FOR A STRESS-FREE LIFE with a happy, healthy companion animal, no single step is so important as finding the right companion in the first place. Many pet-related problems stem from the impulsive, uninformed way in which most of us acquire our dogs, cats and other pets. People who fall in love with an animal's appearance often know nothing about its needs or personality. As a result, they have unrealistic expectations for their new puppy or they don't understand how a cat thinks, how fragile a rabbit can be or how much attention a parrot requires. If prospective pet owners did their homework, they might not join the unhappy millions who abandon their animals every year.

With more luck than brains, as the saying goes, my husband and I decided to share our home with a Labrador Retriever. We'd find a puppy, name her Samantha and live happily ever after. How complicated or time consuming could that be? Enough, as it turned out, to fill a magazine article. "Our Search for Samantha, or How Two People Who Knew Nothing About Dogs Set Out to Find the Perfect Puppy and Accidentally Did Everything Right" was published in the February 1995 *Dog World*.

We knew we wanted a black female, but when we started our search, that's literally all we knew. The first newspaper ad I saw mentioned black and yellow puppies and I assumed they came from different litters. The breeder patiently explained that a single litter of Labrador Retrievers can include not only black or yellow puppies but chocolate pups as well. "I think we'd better learn some things about Labs," I said, and to fill the alarming gaps in our knowledge, we bought and borrowed books about Labradors, subscribed to dog magazines, introduced ourselves to every Lab we saw and talked to owners and trainers for hours.

At about this time neighbors across the parking lot came home with a Golden Retriever puppy. Hobbes was alone during the week while his owners worked so I volunteered to puppy sit and, with the help of training books and video tapes, we worked on basic commands.

Armed with both practical experience (thank you, Hobbes) and information, I began to enjoy conversations with breeders. Some were families whose bitch had a litter with the dog down the road. Some were field trial competitors. A few were professional breeders. Most were helpful, sympathetic, honest and informative.

Still, there were moments. One man's puppies were four weeks old when he sent their leased mother home. "They didn't need her after that," he told me. "I come home on my lunch break every day to feed them." Another explained that his breeding schedule (one bitch, ten pups a litter, two litters a year since her first birthday) produced happy, healthy offspring. When I told one man that I wanted a dog with a calm disposition, he announced, "The parents of this litter are so laid back I even let them in the house. You can't do that with Labs, you know." When I asked a woman if I could test her puppies' personalities, she lost her temper. "I don't think you want a normal dog. You want a fancy dog," she fumed. "Didn't it ever occur to you that all a puppy needs is love?"

And that was before we met a single litter. By December of 1991, we understood what we wanted — a healthy, happy, calm, intelligent, responsive, affectionate, lively girl with a spark in her eye. Joel, my husband, had a hunch that we'd find Samantha north of New York City, so we asked a friend in Albany to check his local paper, where he found plenty to choose from. I made an appointment with the most promising lead and, props and checklist in hand, we set out to meet our first puppies.

The test we planned to follow was adapted from the comprehensive examinations given to prospective seeing eye dogs. When knowledgeable and experienced trainers test young puppies, they see far more than adorable expressions and exuberant energy. They are able to predict with impressive accuracy the puppies' adult personalities, everything from social interaction and dominance to sound and sight sensitivity, stability, energy level and trainability.

We were far from experienced testers, but by now we had a basic understanding of retrievers and a wish list. We hoped that with perseverance, a detached attitude and the puppy test, we would recognize our dream dog.

Between December and March we met over 20 sweet, serene, glossy, happy, calm and docile black females in seven litters, not to mention their tumbling, teething, tail-wagging black, yellow and chocolate siblings. All were adorable; none was Samantha. We looked in vain for the alert intelligence we hoped to find, and the test often revealed traits that would make training, especially for novices like us, a serious challenge.

We were beginning to despair of ever finding Samantha when I found an ad for an upstate referral service. Hoping for a lead, I called all three numbers and talked with helpful breeders who consulted their directories. I wrote down every name they offered and put a star beside the one all three singled out. "Do call Linda Oldham," they said. "She's absolutely the best and she's expecting puppies."

Sure enough, when I reached Mrs. Oldham, she verified the news. "However," she said, "all the puppies in this litter have been reserved for some time. If you tell me what you're looking for, I may be able to refer you to someone."

I told her about Sam, the elderly Lab who had inspired our search and for whom we would name Samantha, then about Hobbes and our puppy auditions. Slowly the conversation changed and she asked more pointed questions. Did we know how much exercise a Lab needs? About as much as a Golden Retriever, I guessed, an hour or more of exuberant play every day. Did we have a big back yard? No, but the woods just down the street offered miles of sheltered trails. What had I taught Hobbes, then six months old? How to heel, sit, lie down, stay, come, shake hands, jump over a broomstick and go down a playground slide. Did we have any other pets? Yes, and I gave our cats' life stories. Did we want a show dog? We didn't care what she looked like as long as she was sweet and smart. We'd take obedience classes, but we weren't likely to compete. Did we plan to breed Samantha? No, we'd have her spayed. We wanted a pet, a best friend, a companion for life.

"Well," said Linda after half an hour of quizzing, "you sound exactly like the kind of people I want my dogs to live with. If you like, I'll put you on the waiting list for a black female."

Now it was my turn to ask questions. A hobby breeder, Linda produced a litter every one or two years from a resident population of eight to ten Labs rich in obedience titles and show ribbons. Some of her pups have become field trial competitors or trained as therapy or assistance dogs. An occasional show judge, perfectionist breeder and Lab Rescue volunteer, she sounded ideal. When we realized that both of us are Finnish, that settled it. Onto the waiting list we went.

As we discussed her health guarantee, I began to appreciate the problems we might have encountered with a backyard breeding. Labradors had recently become the most popular dogs in America, and to Linda this was tragic news because no breed is immune to the deterioration caused by increased demand. With no special care our first cats had lived to be 19 and 20 and we took their good health for granted. But we had just lost Joel's three-year-old Pumpkin, a red tabby, to lymphosarcoma. Suddenly health was a top priority and guarantees about hips and eyes and evidence of the dogs' sound medical histories took on special significance.

The next week, Linda called to announce a delay. Tara (Barbaree Tampbrae Salute, UD) had had a false pregnancy. Well, these things happen. We'd wait. Meanwhile, we went for a visit and fell head over heels in love with her Labs — they were exactly what we hoped Samantha would be. Unbeknown to us, we passed a crucial test when Pilgrim, (Ch. Barbee's Dark Command, UD, WC) the 12-year-old patriarch and Tara's father, inspected us and approved. Later we met Duke('Appylands Marm-a-Duke), the yellow Texan we hoped would be Samantha's sire. This time, instead of sending Tara to Texas, Duke was on loan for a more relaxed summer breeding.

The puppies were born September 1, and when we saw them for the first time five-and-a-half weeks later, we were completely confused. We'd been looking at eight-week-old Labs and these were altogether different. I'd never seen puppies wiggle so much. We could only marvel at the way they climbed into our laps, gnawed on our fingers with incredibly sharp teeth, untied our shoelaces and pounced on plastic milk bottles. Fortunately, Linda was understanding. Yes, we could wait until they were eight weeks old before making a decision. We had recently made friends with dog trainers Brian Kilcommons and Sarah Wilson, and, yes, they were welcome to come with us.

The minute we saw the puppies on our return visit, we were reassured. The girl Linda hoped would be our Samantha had grown up. We ran through the tests, which she passed with flying colors. She came when I called, followed at a happy trot, wriggled on her back when I rolled her over, then sighed and settled down, ran to investigate my keys when they landed behind her and even fetched her soccer ball, bringing it back like a trained retriever.

I was holding the puppy when Brian and Sarah arrived. Sarah took one close look and nodded. "Yes, that's definitely Samantha," she said and walked away. Brian's inspection was only a minute longer and just as positive. Later they explained that the way she held her ears, the alert look in her eyes, her response to having her paw held and her sweet disposition told them volumes at a glance. "She's perfect for you," they agreed.

And she was. We put her red collar with its red bone tag around her neck, and she looked adorable. Whenever we called, she came running. Her ears were velvet, she smelled wonderful, she loved to be petted and she untied my shoelaces just as fast as I could tie them. When it was time to leave. Samantha picked up her soccer ball, raced to the puppy pen to show it to her siblings, then turned away and never looked back. She ran straight to our open arms and into our life, which she promptly turned upside down.

We're proof that anyone who wants a perfect puppy can find one, even if you start out not knowing a thing. All you need are patience and a willingness to learn, which are by themselves sensible prerequisites for life with a puppy — and with any other pet, for that matter.

Your Puppy Search

Good dogs have come from every imaginable background. Most went to their owners from humane society shelters, pet stores, friends or responsible hobby breeders, and some simply showed up in the back yard and stayed. Unfortunately, problem dogs come from these backgrounds, too, and only one of them offers a secure safety net for dog and owner.

If you purchase a puppy from a pet store, the puppy was probably bred as a commodity, as an item to be sold for profit and not as the result of an organized attempt to strengthen the breed, prevent genetic defects or improve a line's temperament or health. If your puppy comes from a well-intentioned backyard breeder, that person may not have had the expertise to research the parents' lines to prevent common problems, such as hip dysplasia or eye defects. Puppy mills, pet stores and shelters are seldom able to guarantee a puppy's health or provide a home and appropriate care for a puppy who develops a serious illness or behavioral problems. Nor can they provide for dogs whose owners die or are no longer able to care for them.

However, responsible hobby breeders do all of these things. This is why, if you are interested in a specific breed, it is worth searching for a good hobby breeder instead of buying your puppy from a pet store or from someone who has casually bred the family dog. Don't be shy about asking questions. If you are interested in providing a home for a puppy or older dog from an animal shelter, newspaper ad, breed rescue organization, trainer or breeder, the same common sense applies. Find out as much as you can about the dog and its background, from breed to personal history and health records. An educated pet owner always has a head start.

1. Don't buy or adopt on impulse. Be sure you understand the breed, its personality and the demands it will make. Read books and magazines, watch puppy training videos, attend a dog show and seek advice from veterinarians, kennel clubs, trainers, groomers and breeders. Make friends with someone who already has the type of dog you want and get to know it. Is the breed considered easy for a novice to train, good with small children or appropriate for apartment living? Does it require extensive grooming or does its high energy level require active outdoor exercise? Many puppies are abandoned every year because their owners expected something entirely different from what they brought home. Do your homework. Take your time. Don't let anyone pressure you into getting a puppy for Christmas, a birthday or any other occasion. Wait until you have narrowed your search to a single litter of sound puppies of the breed you want to live with before bringing your family to see them. Even then, consider leaving small children and people who are not dog experts (including friends and relatives who will not be living with or caring for the dog) out of the selection process.

2. If you're looking for a purebred puppy, contact breeders through magazine or newspaper ads, kennel clubs, trainers, veterinarians and referral services. Look for someone who works to improve the line. That person should interview you as carefully as you do him or her. Some prospective puppy buyers are taken aback or insulted when breeders ask about their knowledge of the breed or their lifestyle and living conditions, but you should be suspicious of any breeder who doesn't want to know where you live, how much space you have, how much exercise you get, how much time you spend at home and what you know or don't know about the type of dog you think you want.

When you talk with breeders, look for honest answers, caring advice, open invitations to visit, a willingness to let you bring experts such as trainers into the selection process, and, depending on the breed, documentation of factors such as the condition of the parents' hips, eyes or other health concerns.

Be sure you understand the breed's most common health problems. Congenital defects in dogs include hernias, cataracts, glaucoma, epilepsy, hemophilia, spinal deformities, kidney disease, liver disease, deafness, diabetes, circulatory problems, excessive or missing teeth, nerve defects, obstructed breathing, weak skin, abnormal aggression, heart defects, malformed elbows, dwarfism, susceptibility to distemper, retinal atrophy, joint problems and hip dysplasia. Some problems can be improved with a well-balanced natural diet or controlled with medicinal herbs or other holistic therapies, but serious genetic defects cannot.

To become familiar with common problems in a breed, get in touch with breed clubs, kennel clubs and veterinarians. Check the breeder ads in dog magazines for references to medical tests, such as "heart tested, "eyes clear" or "OFA hips and elbows." Any condition mentioned in ads is likely to be common in the breed. Individual breeders may not be forthcoming and may not even have this information, but responsible breeders know the complete medical histories of their own dogs and their dogs' close relatives. They research the medical histories of potential mates, spay or neuter any dogs that carry genetic defects and work hard to prevent inherited problems in their puppies. Knowing about your favorite breed's most common problems will help you ask the right questions. Have the parents' hips and eyes been checked? What about other close relatives? Ask what the breeder has done to prevent problems in the line. The more knowledgeable and responsible the breeder, the more information and documentation he or she will be able to provide.

3. Can you meet the puppies' parents? Other puppies from the same parents? Are these relatives calm, intelligent, friendly, energetic, gorgeous or whatever matters to you?

Is the mother two years of age or older and has it been at least 18 months or two years since her last litter? Are the pups raised from birth with plenty of handling for socialization? Are they raised with children, cats or other animals? Are they still with their mother? Does the breeder refuse to let the pups go before seven to eight weeks? Can you talk to owners of other pups from this breeder? If the sire is not in residence, can you see photos or a video?

4. Does the breeder show his or her dogs, compete for obedience titles, participate in a kennel club, train dogs and their owners, judge shows, etc.? The more activities of this kind, the more knowledgeable he or she is likely to be.

5. A good pedigree does not guarantee a good puppy, but a variety of show ribbons, obedience titles and working titles among parents, grandparents and close relatives improves the odds of well-rounded offspring. The TT (Temperament Test) title from the American Temperament Test Society demonstrates that a dog's temperament is appropriate for the breed. Some breeds have developed their own version of the Temperament Test. This credential on the parents, their older offspring and other relatives suggests that the puppies are unlikely to have aberrant personalities.

While you're checking the puppy's pedigree, look for family relationships. Inbreeding is the mating of two very closely related animals (brother and sister, father and daughter or mother and son), while line breeding is the mating of more distantly related animals, ideally focusing on one particular dog of proven outstanding quality. Breeders use both line breeding and inbreeding to emphasize desired traits, but the practice reinforces negative traits as well, such as genetic medical problems and personality defects. "I would consider any father-daughter, mother-son or brother-sister breeding a red flag," says Linda Oldham. "Also, if the same dog appears more than three times in a four-generation pedigree, which lists 14 names and goes from parents to great-grandparents, question the breeder closely. Unless that person has 20 or 30 years of experience and 10 or more dogs on hand to show the results of the breeding program, I would be suspicious."

6. Has the breeder prepared a contract? Are the pups guaranteed? What will happen if your pup's health is defective? Will the breeder pay for medical treatment? What if you can't keep the dog? Good hobby breeders stand by their dogs with health and lifetime placement guarantees. If something goes wrong, these people want their puppies back.

The best way to use a contract is as a vehicle for communication between buyer and seller. Discuss all of the contract's clauses with the breeder so you know what's expected of you and what you can expect in return. For example, if you purchase a pet-quality puppy from a responsible breeder, you will be required to spay or neuter the animal. Some breeders offer a refund of part of the purchase price when this is done. On the other hand, if you buy a show-quality dog, the contract may require you to produce one or two litters of puppies. You may not even be the dog's registered owner.

Discuss your puppy's registration with the breeder. You may have a limited registration, the breeder may withhold registration papers until the dog has been spayed or neutered or full registration may require certain health tests.

By itself, a high price tag isn't a guarantee of anything, but breeders who perform medical tests, travel to find the right mates for their dogs and make other efforts to improve their lines must charge higher-than-average fees in order to break even financially. A popular-breed puppy costing $800 is more likely to have the advantages of careful breeding and health guarantees than one costing $200.

7. Trust your intuition. Does the breeder offer excuses instead of straight answers? Do you feel pressured to make a decision? Do you dislike the pup's mother, father or other relatives? Is there anything you don't like about the breeder, the puppies, the parents or anything else? Even if your intuition is difficult to articulate, walk away. All the breeders and trainers I talked with agreed on this. Never buy a puppy if you have misgivings, and never buy a pup you feel sorry for. There is plenty of time, there are plenty of puppies, and this takes us back to rule #1: Don't buy or adopt on impulse.

Testing the Puppies

For most people, puppy selection is something that just happens. You take the pup who runs to you first or who looks most adorable, or you let the breeder, your children or someone else decide.

Well, that's one way to do it. But in the 1950s, trainers at Guide Dogs for the Blind, Inc., began testing puppies in hopes of predicting which would do well as adult guide dogs. The result of their efforts, a comprehensive examination of which there are now several versions, has saved guide dog organizations substantial time and money by identifying most-likely-to-succeed candidates before they leave their mothers. In addition, it has given trainers, breeders and buyers a way to preview the adult personalities of young puppies.

Puppy testing is most accurate when conducted by trainers who have years of experience with different breeds and who thoroughly understand the test's purpose, techniques and scoring procedures, which are well described in the booklet *Understanding Puppy Testing* by Suzanne Clothier. Clothier, who began testing puppies 20 years ago when she worked at Guiding Eyes for the Blind, cautions that a single test, especially when given by someone who doesn't have sufficient experience with the breed and with puppy testing, can produce meaningless results. For scientific accuracy, each litter should be tested several times in different locations by a knowledgeable tester.

Scientific accuracy may be the ideal, but most pet buyers want simplified guidelines that will help them screen out hard-to-train or hard-to-live-with puppies. If you want a dog for a specific purpose, such as for hunting, obedience trials, the show ring or other activities, it's worth hiring an expert to help you. If you're looking for a good family pet, the criteria are different, but a good trainer can verify your decision after you find what you believe is the right litter or the right puppy. In either case, a basic understanding of puppy testing is an asset.

Before testing anyone, become familiar with the breed. If you don't know how the breed's "normal" or most desirable puppies act, you may not recognize bizarre behavior.

When you talk with breeders who have pups for sale, ask for permission to conduct the test. If the breeder refuses, be suspicious. If the breeder assures you that the pups were already tested, ask for details. If they were tested by the breeder and all are perfect, be skeptical. Most breeders are emotionally attached to their puppies and many have limited experience or knowledge.

The following are simplified guidelines. Please remember that the test as described here is not the detailed, comprehensive examination given to guide dog candidates, but it will help even novice buyers identify puppies who are sociable, stable, well-adjusted and appropriate as family pets.

Test puppies between seven and ten weeks of age, not earlier or later.

Tie a different color ribbon or yarn around the neck of each puppy to keep identities separate, and take notes. Make your own score sheet or use the checklists in Clothier's booklet.

Test the puppies separately, one at a time, in a location that is not familiar to the pups. This location should be quiet and free of distractions.

Do not try to test a puppy in the company of other dogs, littermates or anyone the puppy knows.

Before testing a puppy, gently run your hands all over him or her, peer into the ears, open the mouth and inspect every part of the body. The pup's nose should be cool with no crusty deposits around the nostrils; the eyes should be clear of discharge; the ears should be clean and sweet, not malodorous, red or sensitive to your touch; the gums should be pink and healthy around clean, smooth, white teeth; the skin should be free of scabs, growths or red, irritated patches, just as the coat should shine, smell sweet and look healthy, not dull and drab or with bare patches; and when you comb the fur with a flea comb or run your hand back across the grain of hair growth, you shouldn't see fleas, dark specks of flea excreta, flaky skin or any sign of skin or coat problems. If the pup dislikes this handling and attempts to get away, yelps in pain, growls or bites (a mild, gentle, inquisitive mouthing is normal; biting hard enough to cause you pain is not), the pup is not a good house pet candidate. If the pup has medical problems, think long and hard before making them your problems.

1. Following. Set the puppy down, step back and call while clapping softly, hands at puppy level. A pup who comes at once will be people-oriented and should be easy to train; one who wanders away and shows no interest in you will be independent; one who runs from you in fear will always be fearful. Repeat this test while moving backward, away from the puppy. The best family pets start life as sociable puppies who are used to physical handling and want to be with people.

2. Restraint. Gently roll the pup on his back and hold him there for 30 seconds; have someone time you and give a signal at the end of 30 seconds or silently count the seconds to yourself. Use both hands, wear a neutral expression, keep your head above the pup, don't speak and don't allow him to brace his feet against you. Clothier recommends wearing a long-sleeved shirt to protect against bites and scratches. A docile pup will relax and lie still; a frightened pup will lie still without relaxing (watch for stiff, frozen muscles and a rapid pulse); an easy-to-train pup will struggle briefly, then lie still; a willful pup will struggle without stopping; a dominant, willful pup will bite. Polite puppies look away; be careful of a dominant, willful pup who makes direct eye contact.

While still crouching beside him, let the puppy roll over and stand or sit in front of you. Gently place one hand on his chest and lightly stroke him from head to tail with the other. If the pup is calm and relaxed, bend your face close to him. A well-adjusted pup will recover quickly from being rolled over and may wag his tail, kiss your face or try to climb into your lap. A frightened pup will take several minutes to recover and may be hesitant, with ears and tail down, freeze in place or avoid you. Don't try to restrain a pup who jumps at your face, growls or tries to bite. Don't take him home to your children, either.

With both hands cradling the puppy's chest, lift the pup a foot off the ground and hold him there for 30 seconds. A docile pup will relax and lie still; a dominant pup will struggle the entire time; a dominant, willful pup will bite in order to escape; a stressed or frightened puppy will freeze and you'll feel his elevated heartbeat.

3. Touch sensitivity. Firmly press between the puppy's toes and hold the pressure until she reacts by whining or trying to pull her paw away. Don't use your fingernails, and release the pressure as soon as the pup responds. A physically sensitive pup will react at once and won't be appropriate for a household with children, especially if she yells and bites your hand; an easy-to-train pup will respond after several seconds and may gently mouth your hand; an insensitive pup won't react at all, making her difficult to train using physical corrections. This does not make the pup untrainable, but you will have to emphasize alternative methods, such as operant conditioning or positive reinforcement, which are less familiar to most trainers. Breeds that are known for being good with small children, such as retrievers, usually have a high pain threshold.

4. Noise sensitivity. Throw something noisy, such as a set of keys, on the floor behind the pup, or have someone hit an empty metal pan with a spoon. A pup who runs away, cowers or is frightened by unexpected sounds will be hard to train and even harder to live with; you want a pup who turns to investigate the sound or simply ignores it. If the pup shows no response, check his hearing by repeating this exercise with other noise distractions. Some dogs are born deaf, and while they can be wonderful pets, they require special care and training.

5. Curiosity and retrieving. Bending close to the floor, toss a ball or throw a wadded piece of crinkly paper (use a separate prop for each puppy so the only scent on the object is yours) and see whether the pup goes after it. If so, does she bring it back at least part way? Retrievers are most likely to return it, but any pup with curiosity and at least some retrieving instinct will be easier for most novice owners to train than one without these traits.

Tie a small towel, dishcloth, rag or handkerchief to a long piece of string and, while the pup is distracted, gently toss it three to six feet in front of her and to the side so that when you begin to drag the cloth toward you, it moves away from her. Slowly pull on the string and watch her reaction. If she follows the cloth, wait until she touches it with her foot or mouth and let go of the string. A puppy who immediately chases, attacks, bites and shakes the rag has a strong prey drive; one who continues to do so while growling, snarling and playing with the rag for several minutes is an extreme example. Depending on the breed, these behaviors may be appropriate for a working dog owned by an expert trainer, but they're not desirable in a household pet. Well-adjusted pups who are good family pet candidates usually follow with their tails up, then quickly satisfy their curiosity after the rag stops moving. A pup who runs away with a tucked tail, tries to hide or actively avoids the moving cloth will always be fearful.

6. Energy level. Observe the puppy. Is he constantly on the move, running everywhere? Tense, nervous or frightened? Calm and relaxed? Different breeds have different energy levels, but a calm puppy will be easier to live with than one who's extremely active or extremely shy.

7. Other tests. If you want your dog to compete or participate in specific activities, you or your trainer can develop further tests to determine which puppy is most suitable. *Understanding Puppy Testing* is an excellent guide and offers suggestions and examples.

Adopting the Perfect Adult Dog

Every year, millions of dogs are abandoned by the people who took them home when they were puppies. Many are still puppies (seven or eight or nine months old) who have grown larger or more lively than their owners expected. Some dogs become homeless when their owners divorce, die, move to "no pet" apartments or nursing homes, marry or lose their homes themselves. Millions of homeless dogs are ideal pets, or will be as soon as they move into a stable home with nutritious food, a predictable schedule, praise, affection, appropriate exercise and effective training.

If you are interested in adopting an adult purebred dog or older puppy who needs a home, ask local trainers, your humane society, veterinarians, individual breeders, local breed clubs or kennel clubs to refer you to breed rescue volunteers. These are hobby breeders or enthusiasts who take purebred dogs from owners who can't keep them and from animal shelters, give them appropriate veterinary care, pay for their spaying or neutering, provide temporary foster homes, test their personalities and place them with appropriate families. The American Kennel Club maintains a list of U.S. rescue groups by breed; see the notes for this chapter in the Appendix.

Rescue is such a heartwarming activity that everyone involved with it sounds saintly, but beware of unscrupulous rescue organizations. "Just as prospective owners must do their homework in investigating a breeder, so too must they do their investigating when planning on dealing with a rescue group," wrote Kathy DeWees in the January 1996 *Dog World*. DeWees listed as potential problems irresponsible breeders who call themselves "rescue" in order to sell unwanted dogs, unsold litters or retired dogs they no longer wish to maintain; people who sell lists of dogs available for "adoption" when the dogs are still with owners who are trying to place their pets; "rescues" who place a dog with known problems in one home after another, charging a fee each time and refusing to return the fee when the dog is brought back or charging an additional fee for accepting the returned dog; and people who call themselves "rescue" when they do nothing more than take purebred animals from shelters and place them without knowing anything about their health or temperament.

You can guard against these deceptions by dealing with reputable rescue groups that follow such ethical guidelines as having the dog checked by a veterinarian and either spayed or neutered, preparing an appropriate contract that protects both you and the dog, checking your references before allowing you to adopt a dog and requiring you to have enough knowledge of the breed to provide an appropriate home and training.

A homeless dog may have been abused, has certainly experienced stress and is probably malnourished. If he or she was given away because of a behavior problem, it might have resulted from ineffective training on the owner's part, in which case correcting it will require patience and education on your part. On the other hand, it might have resulted from defective breeding or congenital problems that can't be solved no matter what training classes you attend. Ask an expert to evaluate the dog if you need help deciding whether you can give the animal the attention he or she will require.

Finding the Perfect Cat or Kitten
A Conversation with Celeste Yarnall

Although puppies and kittens are different animals, you can apply many of the same guidelines to both. If you're in love with Siamese cats or Persians or another breed and want a sound, healthy kitten, look for responsible breeders and interview them. Inspect the parents and other relatives. Do these cats have the personality and disposition you're looking for? Do they glow with good health? Are they friendly? Are the kittens handled from birth, raised underfoot and used to human attention? Does the breeder provide a contract?

Whether you look in an animal shelter, visit a family cat who had kittens or go to a breeder, check for healthy-looking coats, shining eyes, alert curiosity and good reflexes. Play with the kittens, tossing a ball of paper or other cat toy. If you want a lap cat, see who climbs into your lap and falls asleep.

Always trust your intuition. We may have been systematic in our search for Samantha, but logic flew out the window when Pumpkin adopted Joel. One day at a pet supply store that took in homeless cats as space allowed, a red tabby sauntered across the room, walked straight to my husband, climbed up his leg, wrapped his arms around his neck and fell asleep purring. I thought Pumpkin was the homeliest cat I'd ever seen, gawky and gangly at four months, infected with fleas and ear mites, with crossed orange eyes and an unruly cowlick that made him look like Dennis the Menace. "Isn't he beautiful?" Joel exclaimed. "I think I've been adopted."

The moral of that story is simple. Educate yourself, yes, but when it's time to make a final decision, listen to what the animal tells you and trust your feelings. My husband was right, by the way. Pumpkin grew into a gorgeous, handsome cat — regal, mischievous and in charge of everything.

For more rational cat selection guidelines, I turned to Celeste Yarnall, author of the popular book *Cat Care, Naturally*. Yarnall, who recently earned a Ph.D. in nutrition, breeds exceptionally healthy Tonkinese and Oriental shorthairs. The following is a transcript of our converstion.

What advice would you offer someone who is looking for the right cat?

YARNALL: If they're already familiar with cats, they may know exactly what type they want. If they're not, one thing they should consider is all the bathing and brushing long-haired cats require. To look really gorgeous, a Persian has to be groomed twice a day, and you have to be prepared to deal with all that hair. For a person who's busy or who doesn't enjoy this activity, a short-haired cat is more practical.

The Siamese has a penetrating yowl, and all the breeds related to the Siamese are talkative, vocal companions. Most people get used to it and enjoy the conversation, but if you want a really quiet cat, you have to look elsewhere. Once you decide how much grooming you want to do and the noise level you want to live with, the world of pedigreed cats contains fewer extremes of size and behavior than the dog world. Most cats, if they're fed correctly, handled and socialized as kittens, not vaccinated to death and given a stable, caring home, can be perfect companions almost anywhere.

If you're interested in a particular breed, I would try to steer you toward responsible breeders, and of course if you were interested in Tonkinese or Oriental shorthair cats, I would discuss my own kittens. Responsible cat breeders want to know all kinds of things about prospective buyers, just the way responsible dog breeders do. For example, I'd want to know who you are, where you live, how much time you spend at home, whether there are children, who else lives in the house and whether both you and your spouse want a cat. I would ask about the other pets you have now and have had in the past and whether they lived indoors or outside. I'd also want to be sure that I'm talking to the primary caregiver. For example, if you're planning to give the kitten as a surprise gift to someone, I'm talking with the wrong person. These are only a few of the questions I would ask, and I would expect any responsible breeder to do the same.

A good way to see cats up close is at cat shows. There are about 50 cat breeds recognized by the major Cat Fancy associations, and shows provide information about their personalities and care requirements. For cat show calendars, check with breeders in your area or the listings in cat magazines. Also, take advantage of the many books, magazines and videotapes that describe breeds of cats; look in your local library, bookstore or pet supply store.

What are the most common health problems in America's cats today?

YARNALL: The list is practically identical to the problems in dogs: poor skin and coat, arthritis, tooth and gum problems, upper-respiratory infections, allergies and of course scary diseases like cancer. There is no denying that the health of America's cats has declined in the last 30 years. Twenty-year-old cats are unusual today, and among pedigreed cats they are practically unheard of. In fact, it's getting hard to find cats who live to be nine or ten. I believe most feline health problems stem from poor diet and overvaccination, and these are conditions a cat owner can control. While natural diet and holistic therapies can't cure everything, they can improve or prevent most of the common health disorders and help the animal live to a healthy old age.

In addition to learning how to prepare a natural diet, what should people do to prepare for a new cat?

YARNALL: You need to cat-proof your house, just the way you would child-proof it if you had toddlers running around. This means getting rid of any poisonous plant that the cat might eat and putting away loose paper clips, rubber bands, pieces of string, tin foil and other things he might swallow. Check your lighting. Your kitty could curl up for a cozy nap under a halogen lamp and get a severe burn on his eyes or the back of his head. Check your windows. If the screens aren't attached properly, your cat could fall out. These are not made-up examples; all of these things have happened to one or more of my kitten buyers.

What about cat litter?

YARNALL: I have tried every cat litter in the world, I promise, along with every type of litter box that exists. I have tried every scooping litter, every clumping litter, every pelletized litter and every organic litter, and at long last I've found one I really like. It's called Feline Pine, and it's made of little pellets that smell good, like wood, and the pellets break down into a powder when they get wet. You scoop out the solid waste once or twice a day, and when you dump the box out, it looks clean because nothing has stuck to it. It doesn't track like other litters and it isn't dusty. Feline Pine is sold at cat shows and it's showing up in supermarkets, so it's easy to find.

For those who prefer clumping litter, I highly recommend Better Way, which is manufactured by the man who invented clumping litter. However, it should not be used for young kittens because the clay it contains can clump in the intestinal tract and cause fatal obstructions. I use a product called Flush It for kittens instead.

How can you tell if a cat or kitten is healthy?

YARNALL: A visit to your holistic veterinarian will tell you for sure, but there are many signs to watch for, both in your own cats and in cats or kittens you may be interested in adopting. In my book I published a list of specific symptoms, but the most obvious ones are things you can see, feel or smell. If the cat or kitten is excessively timid or standoffish, bites when petted or for no reason, is hysterical when restrained, irritable, indolent, clumsy, uncoordinated or perching up high all the time, those are warning signs. So are freckles that develop on an aging cat's nose or around the face, a coat that is dry, oily, dull or thin, a failure to groom well, fleas, distorted or fragile claws, whiskers that fall out, discharges in the eyes or ears, frequently recurring ear mites, bad breath, loss of teeth, red gumlines, pale or red gums, vomiting or gagging on hairballs and other obvious symptoms like constipation or diarrhea.

How do you feel about declawing a cat?

YARNALL: As far as I'm concerned, it's just like amputating a person's fingertips and I think it's a terrible thing to do, just like the "de-meowing" procedure that involves cutting the cat's vocal cords. If you don't like the noise of a yowling cat, don't adopt a vocal breed. Spaying or neutering eliminates the vocalization associated with hormone cycles, and unless your cat is an exceptional example of its breed, there's no reason to leave it intact. Sometimes people ask me how I can recommend spaying and neutering when I advocate everything natural, and my answer is that in addition to preventing even worse overpopulation problems than we already have, these procedures have significant health benefits. There is nothing more stressful for a female cat or dog than going through repeated heat cycles without conceiving, and stress, as you know, lowers the animal's immune system. Spaying and neutering makes household pets much easier to live with, so there's less stress on the owners as well.

As for teaching a cat to use his scratching post, that's simply a matter of training. Cats are intelligent animals and they love to learn. Teaching cats where to scratch is easy, and so is trimming their claws to keep them short and blunt.

Any final word of advice for America's cat lovers?

YARNALL: Yes. Please keep your cats indoors. And love them with all your heart and soul, like they love you.

Your New Pet Is Home!
What Do You Do Next?
A Conversation with Brian Kilcommons and Sarah Wilson

When the reality of a pet doesn't match its owner's expectations, the result can be disastrous for the animal involved. Not only is the situation extremely stressful, which in itself is bad for health, but it can be fatal, for death is the fate of most animals taken to shelters. Brian Kilcommons and Sarah Wilson, authors of the best-selling *Good Owners, Great Dogs, Good Owners, Great Cats, Childproofing Your Dog* and other books, have worked with dogs, cats and owners for over 40 collective years. Kilcommons hosts the weekly "Pet News" program on cable television's Fox News Network.

About Dogs

What are the most serious problems facing new pets and their owners?

KILCOMMONS: The number one reason people give their dogs away is housebreaking. Part of the problem stems from the owner's desire to give a puppy freedom when what the dog really wants isn't freedom at all, it's structure. Dogs are happiest and most easily housetrained when they go out on a consistent schedule, eat a consistent diet and in general have a routine in their environment.

Many owners simply don't realize how much work a puppy is, how often it needs to go out or how much time and attention it requires. Good housebreaking is based on prevention, not correction. Most eight-week-old puppies need to go out every two hours during the day. If their last walk is at ten o'clock at night, and if their fluid intake is restricted after dinner, they can probably sleep until five or six in the morning.

In the case of adopted adult dogs, the more secure you make the dog, the faster and easier the transition. If the dog makes a mistake and all of a sudden you're correcting or punishing him, you're probably going to exacerbate the problem. Getting upset increases anxiety levels terribly. Most people get excited about the things a dog does wrong while ignoring whatever the dog does right, and that's the exact opposite of effective training. Dogs and cats respond to praise and rewards, which is what you should provide whenever your pet does what you want it to do. Twenty or thirty years ago, physical correction was the only way to train a dog. Today, that approach is old-fashioned and ineffective.

The best trainers teach their clients how to encourage good behavior by rewarding it, and in housebreaking, like everything else, this approach gives the best results.

WILSON: We estimate that 75 percent of the problems new owners face can be prevented or resolved by following a few simple guidelines. Be organized, have a routine, plan ahead, buy the right products and equipment and, from day one, reward the behaviors you want to see more of. The reward can be a treat, petting, a toy or enthusiastic praise. In fact, praise is one of your most important tools, for it encourages good behavior and strengthens the bond between you and your puppy. When you praise, you can say anything as long as it's in an enthusiastic, upbeat tone of voice. Commands, on the other hand, should be delivered in a straightforward, businesslike tone, and you should say the command only once. As soon as the dog responds, make a cheerful fuss, praise and give her the treat.

I certainly would include herbs like valerian, hops, skullcap and other relaxing nervines for the first couple of weeks just to help the animal calm down. I have several boarding kennel owners who are now using them routinely when animals first come in, and it really helps reduce stress.

KILCOMMONS: Another way to provide structure for your puppy is to get a crate. Most people don't know how to use crates, which are wire or plastic cages. They look like jails and people think it's cruel to lock the dog up. But for the dog, a crate is a refuge, especially if there are children in the house. I compare the crate to a playpen or crib. It's a way of keeping a dog or puppy safe and contained when you're out or not able to supervise it. It's a wonderful training tool. It isn't meant for permanent use, but some dogs like their crates so much that their owners leave them set up.

The owners come home with their eight-week-old puppy, where the puppy's crate is waiting. What else should they do?

KILCOMMONS: If you're going to have a baby, you spend months reading books, talking to experts, buying equipment and making plans. If you're getting a puppy, you should do the same. Most people don't. Then, when they have problems, they blame the puppy.

The main reason people fail at housebreaking is a lack of information. Follow a consistent schedule, one that's set up to help the puppy succeed, not fail. Never punish a puppy for having an accident. Doing things like rubbing the puppy's nose in the mess, yelling or whacking him with a newspaper, that all went out 20 years ago. Use an odor-neutralizing product to clean up after the puppy; anything else will leave the odor intact, and that encourages repeat mistakes at the same location. Most pet supply stores carry several brands that work by digesting or chemically changing the organic material in urine, vomit and fecal matter.

Give water freely in the daytime but withhold it after dinner, which makes it easier for the puppy to sleep through the night. Teach the puppy to go on command by saying, "Hurry up," or whatever command you want to use, as the puppy relieves himself. Then pet and reward him.

All this information is available from trainers and from books, but few people plan that far ahead. Most owners wait until they have a problem, then they look for help. And how do they describe the problem? "He's a very stubborn puppy." "The puppy knows better." "She's doing this to annoy me." None of which is true. You can correct problems after they develop, but it's easier and more rewarding, not to mention less stressful, to plan ahead, get the information you need and prevent problems from happening in the first place.

What about a destructive puppy?

WILSON: A lack of adequate exercise is a major contributory factor to problem behavior in dogs of all ages. Remember the motto, "A tired puppy is a good puppy." Exercise is especially important to retrievers, hounds, terriers and other active breeds. During the first two or three years, these breeds need a vast amount of exercise, and if you don't give it to them, they'll make up their own. Take a puppy who's lonely, underexercised and bored, and that puppy may unstuff the sofa or rip up the carpet.

Nutrition is another factor. Behavior problems of all kinds can stem from an unbalanced diet so correct feeding is essential.

It's important to structure your attention so that you don't overwhelm the dog. Sometimes if the dog is adopted or had an unhappy past, people coddle and indulge it. While people intend this as loving, the dog feels confused and over-whelmed. From a dog's perspective, that kind of behavior from a person puts the dog in charge. Its stress level goes up, bad behavior starts and then the people feel let down because they've been giving the animal all this love and attention and it's responding badly.

Instead of showering the dog with attention all day, schedule your interactions. Feed, exercise and play on a regular schedule, and in between, let the dog sleep and spend time alone.

What causes aggressive behavior, and how can it be prevented?

WILSON: It's important that everyone in the family be involved in responsible pet care. Don't accept behavior from your children toward a dog that you wouldn't accept from an older child toward a younger one. Children should not be allowed to chase or hit a puppy or jump on a sleeping dog or any other disrespectful activity. It's not good training for the kids and it sets the pet up for some kind of bad reaction. If the dog has retreated and a child pursues it, the dog has no other option but to become aggressive. It's already stated its desire to be left alone, and that desire has to be respected.

KILCOMMONS: Sometimes the cause is a lack of socialization, which is why everyone who gets a puppy should plan to enroll in a puppy kindergarten and obedience class, so that the dog is exposed to a variety of other dogs and people under a trainer's supervision. Sometimes the cause is a bad temperament, which may be inherited. Either way, you have a problem, and if the dog is left alone most of the day, either locked in a kennel, tied to a chain or left in a fenced yard, it's going to get worse.

When a dog is growling with a tense body and making direct eye contact, that dog is sending out a very clear signal, and it's a mistake to dismiss or ignore its behavior, especially if it happens in your house over things like food or toys. This is not something you want to tolerate. Ignore it and the behavior will escalate until someone gets bit.

What's the solution?

KILCOMMONS: Obedience training with an effective instructor is a good first step, preferably one-on-one in your home. A good instructor can show owners how to read their dogs so they become more observant and recognize the messages the dog is sending, then interrupt the behavior and redirect it. Whenever I'm working with a dog that's aggressive or misbehaving, I don't only look at the dog, I look at the other end of the lead. Who's there? It's usually an owner who is confused, misinformed or just uneducated. It takes time and effort to find the right trainer and then apply the trainer's advice, but in our society, we can't afford to own dogs that are dangerous to the community.

WILSON: Another factor is hormones. Although in an ideal world it would be lovely not to have to neuter animals, the fact is that dogs and cats should be neutered for a variety of reasons. From a behavioral standpoint, neutering a male dog prevents certain types of undesirable behavior from developing, such as dog-fighting, territorial behavior and pushiness. Anyone familiar with horses knows that the most reliable riding animals are the geldings, which are neutered males. Very few people have the capability of handling a stallion, which is an intact male.

I would say that that goes for pet dogs as well. It is the rare intact male dog that can be integrated successfully into novice households.

As far as female dogs are concerned, the advantage of spaying is that it stops the cyclical mood changes that cause some female animals to become quite, shall we say, "bitchy." Spaying early, before the first heat cycle, also greatly reduces the risk of mammary tumors. Intact males can develop certain types of hernias, which are painful, and testicular cancer is clearly prevented by removing the testicles. The risk of fights and resulting injury is far lower in neutered males.

From a moral and ethical perspective, neutering is necessary because of our pet overpopulation crisis. The lowest figure I ever hear is an estimated 10 million domestic pets killed every year because there are not enough homes for them. That is horrific, and it supersedes any belief one might have that pets should be allowed to reproduce at will. Neutering is morally and ethically the thing to do unless you have a specific animal that is genetically and temperamentally so superior that he or she deserves to perpetuate the breed. I think the only valid reason to continue a breed is to perform some kind of useful work. I have very little patience for people who breed animals simply for aesthetics; that is a human amusement in which I find very little value.

About Cats

What are the most common problems people have with cats?

KILCOMMONS: Again, it's housebreaking. Cats are normally so easy to housetrain that I won't consult on a cat case unless the owner first takes the cat to the vet. The owner usually thinks the cat is fine, it just has a behavior problem, but then the vet may diagnose a urinary tract infection or some other condition that interferes with normal behavior.

Cats are fastidious, and if they don't have a clean litter box, they aren't likely to use it. If you live in a big house, a kitten may have trouble reaching the litter box so it makes sense to have more than one. If it's a multi-cat household, with two or three cats sharing the same box, one of them may rebel and use the flower pots instead. The easiest way to solve that situation is provide a separate box for each cat.

Whenever there's a change in behavior, you want to look not at what the animal is doing, but why it's doing it. For example, scratching is a natural behavior and a necessary one. You're never going to stop a cat from scratching, but you can teach the cat where to scratch. A lot of the scratching posts sold in pet stores are way too short or they're not stable, and cats hate surprises. Make sure you get a solid, stable scratching post that's high enough; just measure your couch, that will give you a good idea. And get one that has a good, scratchable surface. I like sisal best, impregnated with catnip to make it even more attractive. Get more than one, placing one near the cat's favorite nap spot and one in the living area or wherever the cat will be spending time. Then play with the cat, praising and rewarding whenever it scratches where you want it to. Another important thing to do is trim your kitten's claws on a regular basis, keeping them short. Last, learn how to correct your kitten humanely, so you can discourage it from scratching on furniture. Squirt guns work well and so do shake cans. A shake can is an empty aluminum can taped shut with several pennies inside. When it's dropped on the floor, especially behind an animal, it makes a startling sound that discourages whatever behavior the pet is engaged in. Strong fragrances are cat repellents, so you can discourage scratching by putting a scent on the furniture. A lot of cats really hate the smell of Jean Naté or anything citrus.

WILSON: Cats can't be rushed. When you bring a cat or kitten into your home, she may hide under the bed or in a closet. Let her. The cat will emerge in her own good time. If there are children in the house, they need special instruction and supervision so that the cat isn't stressed or mistreated.

What if a cat becomes aggressive?

KILCOMMONS: People often don't know how to read a cat's body language; either they aren't observant or they don't understand what the signals mean. Cats do their best to inform you if they're becoming upset, and if you don't give them space, you show disrespect. If you're playing with a cat whose tail is swishing back and forth and whose ears are flat, back off. That cat needs a time out, not close handling. Some cat aggression problems result from the owner's insensitive or rough handling.

Remember, too, that cats have their own individual personalities, and they're going to do things on their own time line. You can boss them all you want, but you won't get any cooperation. The way to live happily with a cat is to provide food, shelter, regular exercise and play, a clean litter box, good scratching places, regular grooming, immediate praise and rewards for things done well and a relaxed attitude about everything else.

Summary

In a nutshell, what can an owner do to make life pleasant for both the pet and family?

KILCOMMONS: Make a wish list. If you want to wear your dog like a muff, that's fine with me, just know what you want. Remember that whatever behavior you get as a puppy or kitten will be carried into adulthood. Do you want her to jump on people? Do you want her on your furniture? Should he be fed from the table? Do you want to be able to handle his feet, ears, eyes and anything else in case he gets hurt? Do you want the dog or cat to get along with children? Do you want to travel with your dog or cat? Knowing what you want makes planning your pet's education a lot easier.

WILSON: Along with a good dose of common sense and responsibility, information is the greatest asset an owner can have, and if you open your mind to the wealth of information in books, magazines and videos about dogs, your particular breed, puppies, cats, kittens and training methods, you and your pet can live together happily.

Abandoning Fido and Fluffy
A Conversation with Cathy McGrath

Cathy McGrath manages the animal shelter of the Hudson Valley Humane Society in Spring Valley, N.Y., which takes in about 1,000 animals annually and has an unusually high adoption rate (over 75 percent compared to the national average of about 20 percent), thanks to the untiring efforts of its staff and volunteers.

What are the main reasons people give when they bring animals to the shelter and say they can no longer keep them?

MCGRATH: They usually tell us that someone in the family has allergies, but the real reason is often that the pet's not trained and the owners just don't want it any more. Between allergies and moving to Florida, which is the second most common excuse, it's a wonder there's anyone still living and breathing in the state of New York.

Another thing we hear a lot is that the family works, no one is home and the dog is alone too much. No one was home before the dog arrived, so that's not a big surprise, but people act amazed to discover that a dog needs company, supervision and training. Bored dogs are often destructive, and that's what usually brings them to us. Sometimes people get divorced in a messy way. We have two dogs here now who got kicked out of the house along with the husband. Once in a while someone dies or goes into a nursing home and we take their pets, but that doesn't happen often. Sometimes a dog or cat requires medical care that the owner can't provide or doesn't want to be involved with, so the animal comes to us.

But nine times out of ten, it's a simple behavior problem. The cat's not using the litter pan, the dog's having accidents in the house, the dog is destructive or jumps on people or barks too much or all of the above. With dogs, it's almost always a combination of problems, not a single issue. Only seldom do we see an actual temperament problem, like a truly aggressive, mean dog. The reasons people abandon their pets are almost always behavioral; the animals are simply untrained.

Are there any breeds that tend to be given up more than others because of aggression problems?

MCGRATH: Yes. I hate to be breed-specific, but we do have some problem breeds. A really high percentage of the Chows, Shar-peis and Dalmatians that are brought to our shelter come in because of aggression. Poor breeding and poor temperament are part of the problem, but it's always made worse by people buying these dogs without knowing what they're doing.

What is your largest incoming population?

MCGRATH: Aside from kittens in the spring, the majority are dogs in the 18-month range. An untrained 18-month-old dog is as big, strong, undisciplined and uncooperative as he's ever going to be. These dogs are difficult to place because when they reach the 18-month mark and they've never had a correction or been given any direction, it's very hard for them to become sufficiently socialized or calm or obedient to be attractive to people who are looking to adopt. Or they've been overcorrected, improperly corrected or physically punished by people who didn't know what they were doing, and then you've got a high-energy, bouncing-off-the-wall, uneducated adolescent who, whenever he perceives any anger, hits the floor in four. These dogs are hand-shy, voice-shy, afraid of men, easily startled and in general nervous wrecks.

Do you take in more dogs than cats?

MCGRATH: No, we get more cats than dogs, and that's a reflection of our population problem. People bring kittens in by the bucketful. If I can share one recommendation with your readers, it's this one: spay and neuter, spay and neuter, spay and neuter. And if you live in the suburbs or city, keep your cats inside. Every year we take in 200 absolutely lovely, healthy, spayed, declawed adult cats who are brought in by people who find them on the street, assume they're lost and bring them here. They wandered away from home and they aren't wearing ID tags or weren't implanted with a microchip, so we have no way to contact the owners. They're always in marvelous condition, with no fleas, no ear mites, no eye infections, well-fed, with great personalities, and they're here in the shelter because someone thought they were doing a good deed. I beg people all the time, please don't pick the cat up, it probably lives not far away and will wander home if left on its own.

What's a declawed cat doing outside, anyway?

MCGRATH: Exactly. It has no natural defenses. People have no common sense. Cats enjoy being outside and they like to roam, but it's dangerous for so many reasons. Keep your cats indoors.

People bring dogs in because of behavior problems. Why do they abandon their cats?

MCGRATH: I think the number-one reason is inappropriate elimination, and that's often just a housecleaning matter. If people would understand how clean cats want to be and keep their litter boxes that way, they wouldn't have this problem.

As far as dogs and puppies are concerned, I'm convinced that if everyone who took a dog or puppy home from us would take one six- or eight-week course with a good trainer, the world would be a better place. We give people information, recommendations, things to read and trainers to call, but most people don't pay any attention. They just take the puppy home. I tell all the people who adopt puppies from us, don't call me in a year and complain that this puppy is wild or untrained or impossible to live with. I've given you the book, I've given you the phone numbers, now do this for the dog. Fortunately our return rate on puppies is very low, but we do occasionally get them back, usually at 16 or 18 months, and the poor dog is just bonkers because its owners haven't lifted a finger to provide the structure, direction, training and support that dogs have to have.

What other animals do people bring you?

MCGRATH: We get occasional birds, for varied reasons, and we take in a lot of rabbits, usually because of biting. Raise a baby rabbit the right way and you have a sensational pet, but people often don't hold them enough. Hold, play with and pet your bunny, don't keep him locked in a cage where he gets no exercise and never gets socialized. Rabbits can be trained to do wonderful things. They're bright little creatures, they play with toys and they're easy to housebreak. I think rabbits are great.

They have real personalities if you take the time to develop them, and they're so easy to take care of and such low-maintenance pets that they're ideal for busy, overstressed households and families with kids. Give them a litter pan and put them in it whenever they defecate, and within a week they're litter-trained. Rabbits are safe, neat, clean little pets that can run loose in the house. I can't say enough good things about them, they're wonderful. You just need to start when they're small and give them a safe home with enough handling and play to make them comfortable around people.

Bunnies are often Easter presents. People get them spontaneously, just the way they take it into their heads to get a kitten or puppy, with no research or preparation, just bring it home and hope for the best. That often leads to disaster.

The only responsible way to bring a pet into your home is to prepare for its arrival by learning everything you can about its nature, its needs and the demands it will make on you. If you aren't prepared to provide whatever it requires, don't take it home.

Finding the Right Trainer and Training Methods for Your Dog
A Conversation with Diane Bauman

When it comes to obedience training, most owners are happy if Fido sits. Fine points, like Fido's posture, alignment, reliability and response time, don't matter. They do to Diane Bauman, who has spent over 22 years teaching novice owners, professional trainers and thousands of dogs how to do it right.

The author of *Beyond Basic Dog Training* and other books and training videos, Bauman, who lives in Sussex, New Jersey, has achieved 16 perfect scores of 200 at obedience trials with a Golden Retriever, Belgian Tervuren, Keeshond and Pomeranian, four very different breeds. She has earned scent tracking titles with a Golden Retriever, Keeshond and Papillon as well as six agility titles on three different breeds. Bauman specializes in working with breeds considered difficult to train, and some of her champions were rescued from shelters.

What is your approach to training?

BAUMAN: I believe that dogs learn by trial and error. If you agree with this premise, there has to be room for error without penalty. If the emphasis is on penalty, you get a dog who's afraid to be wrong and afraid to try. I don't penalize a dog for being wrong, but I reward him for being right and I stack the deck in his favor so he's more likely to succeed.

How do you do that?

BAUMAN: Let's take something simple, like a sit-stay. Some trainers will put a leash and collar on the dog, position him in a sit and then hold him there. The dog can't make a mistake because he can't move, but he also doesn't learn much. My approach is to tell him to sit and tell him to stay, which he does not understand at this point, then get in front of him with a loose lead and let him make a mistake. Sometimes I even encourage him to make a mistake by supplying a distraction. When he moves, I gently reposition him to show him that what he did was not the desired response, but he wouldn't have known that if he hadn't tried it. Dogs learn by experience, and this is a painless way to provide it.

In a recall, where I call the dog back to me, I don't force him to come by pulling his leash; instead, I call him and when he turns his head or starts moving toward me, he gets praise or a treat. As soon as he understands that "come" means I want him here by me, which usually takes about 10 minutes, I offer him a choice. He can go to someone else who's holding a cookie when I call him, or he can come to me. If he stays out there or goes to someone else, he gets a quick pop on the leash on his buckle collar; if he comes to me, he gets the cookie I'm holding.

I believe that dogs are thinking animals, they're capable of solving simple problems, and you can get better results by encouraging your dog to make decisions rather than by training for unthinking, automatic responses. You can train a mouse or a chicken with a sound or light in a straightforward stimulus-response manner, but I believe dogs are of a higher order. That's why we entrust them with the lives of blind people and train them to assist the handicapped. They have the ability to reason and, if you give them a command, they can size up the situation and decide what is the wise thing to do.

A dog will always do whatever is to his advantage, and it's the job of the trainer to set up each lesson so the dog clearly understands that the behavior the trainer wants him to perform is to his advantage. The dog responds not because the trainer is larger, meaner, stronger or more forceful, which only sets up resistance, but because the dog has learned to make an intelligent decision.

What advice do you have for dog owners who want professional help?

BAUMAN: The first thing to do is some research. Find out who is teaching obedience classes, where they are and what methods they use. For example, you'll probably find some who are still using the punitive approach. Typically, in these cases, the dog is in a choke collar on a loosely held six-foot leather leash. The dog is given a command and he has no idea what the command means, but if he doesn't do it, he's going to get corrected, either by a hard pop on the leash, a loud "No!" or forceful physical positioning. The dog is motivated to avoid unpleasant corrections, but this is an entirely negative way to teach him. The emphasis is always on what he does wrong. After World War II, a number of military trainers came out of the service and started dog training schools using this approach, which was most popular in the 1940s, '50s and '60s. It's been dying out ever since, but there are still some old-timers around who believe in it.

At the opposite extreme we have trainers who use no collars, no leashes, just treats, and the dogs are led around by a cookie or other food lure. It's questionable whether the dogs understand what they're doing, but they'll do their best to get the cookie. They might make certain connections in the classroom, but this approach doesn't hold up very well in real life, where there are distractions more interesting than cookies and where the handler might not always have a food treat. But the puppies are happy, none of them are depressed or frightened, they're having a great time, and somewhere along the line they usually memorize a pattern or a specific behavior. Of course, as soon as you take the food away, you have nothing left.

Then we have combinations that are somewhere in between. For example, there are some trainers who use both a lot of food rewards and a lot of heavy corrections. They want instant, immediate responses, no thought, just action, and they get this response by giving a command, correcting quickly, sometimes harshly, and then feeding quickly and profusely.

Almost everyone else uses a different combination of these basic ingredients.

How can the dog owner find the right instructor?

BAUMAN: It always used to amaze me that people would call and say they wanted to take lessons from me, and they never asked for my credentials. They never wanted to know where I'd been trained, what I'd done, what breeds I worked with, what methods I used, what I'd accomplished with my own dogs, nothing. People assume that someone who claims to be a dog trainer knows everything.

Here is a checklist for your readers. When you hear of a trainer or see an ad, call the trainer up and ask the following questions:

1. Where, how and from whom did you get your training?
2. What methods do you use?
3. What kinds of dogs do you have and to what degree have you trained them?

Finally, ask if you can meet the trainer's dogs. If someone called me and said, "Can I come see your dogs work? I'm thinking of taking lessons and I'd like to see how your dogs perform," I'd be thrilled. If the trainer's dog is always walking with his head down and his tail tucked, you have to ask yourself whether this is how you want your dog to act. If the trainer's dog is happy, active, confident, head up, tail wagging, intelligent and attentive, you're more likely to think that this might be the right place to take your pet.

For those who are interested in competition, I always tell people who move to a new area to go to all the local dog shows for a few weeks and watch. See who's winning and find out whom they're training with.

How can someone who is not familiar with training make sense of a trainer's background or credentials?

BAUMAN: It's amazing how many people call themselves trainers and even write books about training or consider themselves authorities, and they've trained only one dog, or they don't even have a dog or they took one weekend course.

It helps to understand how good trainers get their experience. Over the years I've trained many students, 10 of whom have opened their own schools and become full-time trainers. They did this by taking classes, then working as apprentices, all the while gaining experience with different breeds.

It takes a number of years and exposure to all different kinds of dogs and situations, as well as experience with different training methods, before someone is really qualified to take on the public. You might have a trainer who's only worked with German Shepherds, Rottweilers and Doberman Pinschers. This person has a very different perspective on training from someone who has only trained Toy Poodles. You definitely want a trainer who has experience with your breed of dog or your type of dog. Unless someone has worked with dogs of all different sizes, types and temperaments, that person's approach may be inappropriate for your situation.

When I meet a new dog, I'm constantly evaluating him, checking for whether he has a hard or soft temperament, whether he's under stress and what his response to stress is, how he thinks, what motivates him and how he's typical of his breed or different. All kinds of information gets processed really fast so that I can demonstrate and teach a training method that will work for this particular dog. Trainers who don't have this kind of experience really don't know what approach will work best. I always recommend that dog owners do their homework, interview trainers, watch trainers work, meet the trainers' dogs, talk with people who have studied with the trainer and meet their dogs, all the while looking for an effective combination of experience, knowledge and teaching skill that will help them work with the dogs they live with.

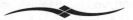

In addition, pet owners can contact their local Better Business Bureau or Consumer Affairs office to learn whether anyone has filed complaints against the instructor for unsavory or illegal business practices, fraud, injuring dogs or any other reason. Look for trainers whose methods work immediately and are easy to understand and implement. If a training program is so complicated or unwieldy that you will never follow it, keep looking. Effective dog training works right away, within minutes; you don't have to wait weeks or months to see improvement in most common problems. Of course, it's one thing to watch your dog's miraculous response to a good trainer and another to be the miracle-maker yourself, which leads us to our next conversation on how to get the most out of classes.

Getting the Most from Obedience Training
A Conversation with Nancy Strouss

Since 1977, Nancy Strouss has been teaching people how to raise and train their dogs humanely and successfully, using up-to-date motivational techniques. Her training center, People Training for Dogs in Valley Cottage, N.Y., offers classes in basic and advanced obedience, show handling, beginning agility and puppy kindergarten. Nancy has received national awards for her training skills and has worked as an instructor for humane societies and obedience training clubs. In addition to teaching owners and their dogs, which over the years have included all shapes, sizes, breeds and levels of training, she and her own Golden Retrievers, Standard Poodle and Fox Terrier compete in obedience trials and the show ring.

What steps can dog owners take to be sure they get the most from obedience class?

STROUSS: It helps if the owner has a good idea of what he or she wants to accomplish. Do you want a home companion who doesn't jump on people, sits on command and is easy to live with? Do you want to train your dog for a particular sport or activity, like obedience competition, field trial work or making therapy visits to hospitals? A basic obedience class prepares the groundwork for all of this, but the instructor can tailor parts of the lesson for people with specific goals, and a person who has a well-defined end result in mind always does better than one who doesn't.

Most people who come to puppy kindergarten or basic obedience sign up for an eight-week course, and that's all they think they want. But eight weeks is usually not enough. It takes time for the handler to learn basic techniques, for the dog to get used to this new activity, for the necessary teamwork to develop and for a puppy to go through the different stages of development that puppies go through. The first eight weeks are preparation, following which the dog and handler are usually ready to really learn obedience.

People should realize that the purpose of a group class is to train dogs to work around distractions; a group obedience class is not the place to deal with unusual behavior problems. Normal out-of-control behavior like jumping, pulling on the leash, excessive barking, gnawing on the furniture, nibbling at your hand or not being consistently housebroken can be dealt with in a group because solving them is a matter of simple advice. But if you have an older dog who becomes hysterical and rips the paintings off the wall whenever you leave the house, that's not something that can be dealt with in a group.

Does your dog have a serious problem? If so, don't hide it from the instructor! I'm a good screener on the phone, but occasionally someone with an aggressive dog slips by me. Some of these dogs are people-aggressive; they're fine around other dogs but they attack people. Others are dog-aggressive; they're fine around people but they go after other dogs. Neither of these problems is going to be solved in a group class; they should only be dealt with in private training, away from other dogs and people. Sometimes we can eventually work aggressive dogs into a group class for socialization, but never at the beginning.

Would you call aggression an increasingly common problem?

STROUSS: Looking back over 21 years of training, I'd say aggression has always been a problem. What I have seen is a general improvement in the temperament of certain breeds and a decline in the temperament of others. If you're talking about German Shepherds, I'd say yes, aggressiveness is more of a problem. Jack Russell Terriers and Rottweilers, because of all the backyard breeding resulting from their overwhelming popularity, have increasingly common temperament and aggression problems. Pit Bulls seem the same as I've always seen them, with some who are nice and some who aren't. But some breeds have actually improved, at least in my experience. The breeders of Portuguese Water Dogs have done a good job, I think, as have some of the unusual breeds, like Great Pyrenees and others that you don't see often. An aggressive temperament is really characteristic of some working breeds, so it may be that breeding them for a calmer disposition results in their not being good working dogs, but the improved temperament helps them fit into society and live as pets in someone's home.

What should people do when they arrive for their first lesson?

STROUSS: They should be on time. In fact, they should arrive early enough to take the dog for a walk before they come into the building. Even if the dog went to the bathroom before leaving home, the excitement of travel and arrival may cause a young dog to go again. Owners should always have plastic bags or paper towels handy for cleaning up after their dogs.

When they walk in, even if they haven't had any training, they should physically control the dog. This means keeping the dog close and not letting it run to other dogs.

Once the class starts, students should be prepared to watch, listen and focus on the instructor. This is not the time to act in a distracting manner, engage in conversation with other people or let your dog play with other dogs.

What are the common mistakes people make that interfere with learning and training?

STROUSS: Obedience class is not a playtime or recess, but some people act as though its only purpose is to let the dogs play with each other. These people don't think of themselves as students who are here to learn how to train their dogs, and if they're going to get anything out of the class, they really need to focus on what they're being taught.

Also, they need to be patient. It's impossible to get everything right away and it takes time to practice, learn and absorb all this new information. Going to a beginning-level dog training class is hard work. You're not only teaching your dog, you're learning yourself, so you're in the position of being both student and teacher. Beginning students sometimes get discouraged or drop out because they can't make sense of everything right away, and that's a shame.

What can students do between classes to improve their performance?

STROUSS: Practice the exercises you learn in class, and do them correctly. Every lesson you take teaches a new technique, an exercise or something you can do for a few minutes a day to perfect and reinforce what you did in class. This practice time is vital because it's your one opportunity to work with your dog and practice on yourself without a lot of distractions. Many instructors distribute handout material that gives homework assignments, training tips and background information. Students should read and digest this information because it will help them make sense of what they're learning. What people are taught in class, they may not get in class, but they should get it during the week while practicing. If the instructor doesn't give handouts, bring a small notebook and write in it while you're there so you remember what to practice and so you can take notes on things that come up in class. Beginners forget a lot, I think they suffer from information overload, and they can't process or make sense of everything they're told until they gain some experience.

How much time should students schedule for practice?

STROUSS: Depending on the dog and handler, anywhere from 15 minutes to half an hour a day, broken into two sessions or even more, depending on your schedule. Some adult dogs can work longer, but for puppies, young dogs and dogs who are new to obedience, short sessions are better. You don't want to tire your dog or make training unpleasant or boring; you want your dog to look forward to practice and leave each session with a sense of accomplishment, praise and a well-earned reward.

Here's some important advice. If you're working with your dog and have a problem, don't try to train around it, call the instructor for help. People don't do that enough. It's a mistake to keep working when a phone call may clear up the difficulty right away. Another thing students can do if they're really confused is take a private class during the week.

Private classes can be taught in the home or at the facility. Which is best?

STROUSS: If the problem has to do with learning the skill, a lesson at the facility will work well. If the problem relates to behavior in the home, such as housebreaking, stealing food from the counter and things of this nature, home is the best place. The more specific the owner can be in describing the problems he or she wants to solve, the easier it is for the trainer to help resolve them.

The main advantage of working with an instructor one-on-one is that you're free of all the distractions that come with group lessons, and the trainer can focus on your individual situation in detail rather than addressing it in a general way.

What about people who think that you're going to fix the dog and the problem and they won't have to be involved?

STROUSS: This happens sometimes, or a family will send the husband to class hoping that once he trains the dog, then the dog will listen to everyone. But most people realize that classes and private consultations are not about the trainer training the dog, but rather the trainer training the owner to train the dog.

Is it appropriate for whole families to attend classes?

STROUSS: If small children come, the family needs both parents there, one to work with the dog and the other to manage the kids. All too often we have young kids running through the store or along the sidelines, distracting their parents and everyone else. If a parent is trying to train the dog and keep an eye on children at the same time, that person won't be focused enough to learn anything.

When children are older, we try to involve them in the training, and that usually works pretty well. Children who are under nine or ten years of age are not going to be able to participate fully in an adult class; they need to be supervised themselves, but ages ten and up can do very well.

Sometimes a parent shows up with a child who's ten or eleven years old, turns the dog over to the child, then sits on the sidelines chatting. Children of that age can do a lot of the lesson, but not the whole thing. It can be overwhelming, and they need their parents for support or they need a break. I often have to go over and get the parent, who has been paying no attention and doesn't know what's going on, and that doesn't help the dog, the child or the parent.

What do the people who get the most out of class have in common?

STROUSS: They show up on time, don't carry on conversations after the lesson begins, pay attention, practice every day, call the instructor for help between lessons if help is needed and study the handout material.

If the trainer suggests a change of equipment and explains why it would be helpful, the motivated student at least tries it. If it doesn't work for you, don't use it, but you won't know unless you try. I've had classes with dogs that were overpowering, but their owners refused to try a different training collar. Week after week they stayed with a collar that didn't give them any control, one in fact that harmed and stressed the dog, and they didn't progress because of it.

Motivated handlers accept other advice, such as when and how to exercise the dog. One dog might need more exercise before coming to class, another might need less, and an experienced trainer can see at a glance who's overstressed from a lack of physical release and who's exhausted. A common problem in group lessons is people who let their dogs play with other dogs before the class starts so that by the time the lesson begins, the dog is panting, stressed, in a mental state that interferes with learning and more difficult for the owner to control.

Any other advice?

STROUSS: Yes. When people aren't happy with what they're getting, they should tell the instructor. If they feel they're not getting enough individual attention or they don't understand the lesson or something bothers them, they should stay after class or call the next day and let the instructor know. I'm always willing to change things or give extra help, and so are most instructors.

Also, when a student has to miss a class, it's helpful to try to do a makeup. There may be another session that the dog and student can attend, or the student might want to schedule a half-hour private lesson.

Holistic pet care always includes good training. By finding the right trainer and by following these common sense suggestions, even novice owners can help their dogs lead a safe, happy, stress-free life.

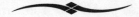

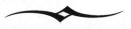

Finding and Living with the Perfect Bird
A Conversation with Doreen Tamara Gluck

When Doreen Gluck adopted her first parakeet, she never imagined that 20 years later, she would be finding homes for over 70 birds a year, living with even more and educating the public about avian care. No bird has ever been refused by this one-woman adoption agency. She has taken in birds with only a few hours to live, baby birds whose inexperienced parents attacked them, even birds with contagious diseases. If she is able to place the bird with an appropriate family or individual, she does so with the understanding that if the placement isn't successful, she will provide a permanent home for the bird. Doreen Gluck is named in the wills of owners who know she will provide a home for their birds when they die. She also cares for birds with special needs.

How many birds do you live with?

GLUCK: Over a hundred. I don't keep normal, "nice" birds any more, because they are easy to place with good familes, or wild birds, which go to live with other birds in breeding environments. I keep the birds that really need help, whether it's because of a handicap, physical injury or other reason.

The birds that come in are everything from little finches to endangered species macaws and large cockatoos. Most of these birds are given away because the owners made poor choices or their lifestyle changed. People might have a bird that they realize is too small because the children might hurt it, or it's too noisy or it's way too big and destructive. A lot of birds are displaced when a single owner marries or when a married couple has a child. Parrots and other birds can be very possessive, and if you have a bird that doesn't like your spouse or resents the arrival of a new family member, that bird can make everyone miserable. Safety is another concern, with small children sticking their fingers into the cage of a bird that could bite them off.

How time consuming is responsible bird-keeping?

GLUCK: Not as much as some people think. You don't have to stay home 14 hours a day. As long as you have a comfortable routine and interact with the bird on a regular basis, you can have a loving, mutually satisfying relationship. A stable, predictable routine is important, and so is the security of a stable location.

Most birds can amuse themselves in their cages. I have birds that hang upside down, play with their toys or roll around on their backs; they can amuse themselves for hours.

Some birds need more attention than others. Cockatoos, for example, are very demanding. They bond with people and they're physical. They like to be sitting on, petted by or at least near the person or people they live with, and if you don't provide the companionship they need, they'll let you know. An unhappy cockatoo might scream, pull its feathers out or just become nasty.

Budgies and cockatiels, on the other hand, are excellent first birds. They can amuse themselves and they aren't so physically or emotionally demanding and are often overlooked because of their size and availability. A cockatiel can be happy on your shoulder while you do homework or watch TV and will sit quietly without interrupting.

Then there are other birds who act the same way, they're just noisier about it. Domestic Nanday conures are great companion birds. They're a nice size, about the size of a robin and they love to talk, love to be petted and have their heads and feathers scratched, but like most of their conure relatives, they make an incredible racket. Most people who buy them have no idea how much noise these birds make.

What is the most common mistake people make when buying a bird?

GLUCK: They buy on impulse. When the TV program *Baretta* was popular, everyone wanted a cockatoo. Here's this smart bird that answers the telephone, plays with Robert Blake and does neat tricks. What the program never showed was how demanding these birds are, or what they sound like when they're screaming. Also, cockatoos are an impressive size. They don't weigh much, but they're big enough to be intimidating. A lot of people ran out to buy cockatoos thinking they would act exactly like the bird on *Baretta,* and they were disappointed.

Or someone spends $10,000 on a hyacinth macaw because it's gorgeous, but there are three young children in the family. A macaw can bite through a Brazil nut or a broom handle as easily as it can bite off a finger.

What bird would you recommend for a suburban family with small children, one or two other pets and no experience with birds?

GLUCK: I would get something non-threatening, such as a cockatiel. If the bird is going to be handled by the children, it shouldn't be so small that they might accidentally injure it. If it's going to be an environmental bird, like finches and canaries that live in cages and don't require hands-on attention, then size is not an issue.

When there are cats in the house, it's often easier if the bird is there first, before the kitten arrives. Cats who grow up with birds are more likely to see them as companions and less like dinner. However, don't leave your cat or dog alone with your bird; keep them separate. I've known several instances where dogs killed birds, especially terriers or other working breeds. They weren't being malicious; they were just responding to something bred into them. Even if a dog or cat can't reach a bird, its presence can be stressful.

What would be the perfect bird for a couple living in an apartment in the city, assuming they have older children, lead a quiet life and don't have a lot of room?

GLUCK: There are many birds that are great for couples, but not for apartments in the city. I'm always amazed at the number of pet shops in cities that sell macaws and cockatoos to people who live there. Because of the noise volume, that's something I would never recommend. Even if you have a loft or live on the top floor, their sound will carry. Cockatoos in the wild can be heard half a mile away, and it's no different in the city. There are birds like Senegals or Meyer's or Jardines that are not noisy, and they're all-around, good family birds. Another bird that isn't noisy is the pionus, but it tends to be a one-person bird. So a lot depends on who in the family wants the bird. Birds are pretty outgoing about letting people know whom they like and don't like. They're not like most dogs. A dog might not like you, but it probably won't bite you. A bird that doesn't like you can do a lot of damage.

Whenever I place a bird, even if it's for one person and no one else in the family has an interest, I still want to be sure that no one in the family really dislikes this particular bird or dislikes birds in general or is afraid of them. If that's the situation, it's set up for disaster. I wouldn't want to place a bird in a situation where its arrival made someone really unhappy. That's bad for the people involved and for the bird as well.

I'm fortunate to have a family that loves animals, and they always keep an eye out for a water bowl that gets knocked over or a food bowl that needs refilling. If you have to go away for a few days, is the person who's looking after the bird going to be attentive, careful and not afraid of it? Bird owners have to think along these lines.

African greys are known for their intelligence. What kind of pets do they make?

GLUCK: African greys are excellent talkers and they're very smart. They tend to be single-person birds, although some are more well-rounded and will accept other people. I have 15 of them, and most are single-person birds. They're not comfortable with other people, but they'll let me do anything, scratch them, turn them upside down, things like that. This is a real sign of trust because an upside-down bird is in an extremely vulnerable position. These birds are not as physically affectionate as cockatoos, they're more stoic, but they enjoy having their heads scratched and they will sit on your shoulder for hours.

They're enthusiastic mimics. They're also devilish. Norman, one of my African greys, knows how to open his cage. I think it's a mistake to get an African grey just because you think it's going to talk and that's your main motivation. It might talk or it might not. I have several that never talk at all.

Another popular bird is the Amazon but it has its limitations. Amazons can talk, and those that do are extremely verbal, but when they become sexually mature, they can be downright dangerous. I've had a mature male Amazon fly off the perch and attack my face. It usually happens when the bird is around five years old, and in some cases, if the people maintain a detached attitude and don't try to fight it, the bird works through this in two or three years and becomes a reasonable companion again. But most of the people who sell them will never tell you about this problem.

What if someone has an Amazon or African grey and wants to encourage it to talk?

GLUCK: There are tapes you can play that say things like "Hello" over and over, but I tried that method only once. The bird listened without saying a word for several sessions and then, as I carried the tape player in one day, he spoke his first word: "Stop!" I never said it and the tape never said it, but the bird did. So I stopped.

I think it's better just to talk to the bird yourself. Say whatever's appropriate. Every morning I say "Hello" or "Good morning" or "Hi, everybody," and at night I say "Goodbye" or "Good night." I sing the same song to them at night and a few of them have learned it. One of my birds says "Bye" and lifts both wings as though he's waving. My family all say "Hi, guys!" when they walk into the bird room, so about half of the talking birds automatically say "Hi, guys!" when anyone walks in, or "Hi, sweetheart!" or "Hello, everybody!"

When you hand a bird an apple, say "apple." When you hand him a peanut, say "peanut." Talk to them the way you would a small child. They'll catch on.

What are the most common health problems in pet birds?

GLUCK: Accidents happen all the time. Birds fly into walls, or they get caught on things or injured by poorly made toys. Birds fed a poor diet can suffer from weight loss, or they pull their feathers out, or their resistance to disease declines and they suffer from bacterial problems. I think it's important to wash all the fruits and vegetables you feed a bird so that you don't introduce chemicals or bacteria that might harm them.

There are some diseases that are common in certain species. Rose-breasted cockatoos are prone to fatty tumors as well as obesity. People who have them often feed them a general parrot diet, which tends to be high in fat because of its sunflower seeds and peanuts. These birds would be less likely to gain weight or develop fatty tumors on a diet that emphasized raw vegetables, fruits and legumes instead of just seeds and nuts.

Any bird can develop problems that we have no control over, like feather cysts or preening gland cysts, which are kind of like ingrown hairs. There are some highly contagious avian viruses, some of them from imported birds, like polyomavirus, parvoviruses and cloacal papilloma, which is a wart-like virus. These viruses are mostly found in wild, imported birds and, since many birds have multiple homes, these viruses have infected domestic birds along the way.

If you bring me a bird you can no longer keep and you've had the bird since it was a baby 12 or 15 years ago, I can be reasonably sure it doesn't have any unusual diseases, but I would still have it checked by a veterinarian. There is an illness called psittacine beak and feather disease, which was originally called cockatoo beak and feather because it was only seen in Australian and island birds. But then it began to show up in South American and African birds. It's extremely contagious and can be passed on through feather dust, saliva, airborne flakes of dried fecal matter and from parents to eggs. If you petted a bird with beak and feather, then went home and petted your own bird, you could transfer the disease.

I'm very careful whenever I go out not to bring anything home to my birds. If I've been handling birds at a bird club meeting or pet store, I take a shower and change clothes before going into my bird room.

The only zoonotic disease that can be transferred from birds to people is psittacosis or parrot fever, which is caused by a Chlamydia bacteria, and it's pretty uncommon. A bird showing no symptoms can be a carrier, and infected humans develop flu-like symptoms. I have an autoimmune disease, and I've handled many birds that have psittacosis, so whenever I've been hospitalized, that's the first thing they check for. I've never been infected with it, and I know people who have owned bird stores for 20 or 30 years and have never had it. I'm not saying it never happens, but some people refuse to consider a bird as a pet because they're afraid of parrot fever, and I think their concerns are misplaced.

What can a prospective bird owner do to obtain the necessary information, education and equipment to find the right bird and provide a good home for it?

GLUCK: There are many avenues, but you have to be willing to look for them. They're not going to fall into your lap. There are books and magazines sold in bookstores and pet supply stores, some of which are available in libraries, that provide information and advice such as descriptions of specific species, how noisy they are, how much attention they need, what their dietary requirements are, what kind of cages they need, what their personalities are like, what to expect when they first come to live with you and how to interact with them. Illustrated books are helpful because they show photos of different birds, so you see what colors they are and what they look like. Also, there are seminars you can attend about how to select your first bird and what to do with it once it's home. Bird clubs, bird shows, seminars and other events are listed in every issue of *Bird Talk* and some other magazines.

One of the best ways to learn about birds is to go look at them. Go to pet stores, see if you can find someone who has a large collection and will let you into their home, find a bird club and go to bird fairs or bird shows. More than anything else, talk to people. Some private breeders and pet shops have educational programs to inform people about birds before they buy. Keep in mind that everyone will have opinions; remember that breeders have a financial interest in selling you their type of bird, and often their experience with other types may be limited. If you have a dream bird, a particular kind of bird that you really want after you've found out all about its needs, personality and requirements, don't let anyone talk you into settling for anything else. If you have your heart set on an African grey and you know it will fit into your home well and you can provide for it, then don't take a pionus or a cockatoo just because someone offers you one or because someone wants you to have it.

Secondhand birds can make wonderful pets. There's often nothing wrong with a bird that's being given up for adoption; it's just a matchmaking problem — wrong family, wrong lifestyle, wrong owner expectations.

Keep in mind that birds live a long time. It's unusual to have a 20-year-old dog or cat, but birds can live to be 40 or 70 or more. They often outlive their owners. You have to consider your future plans. There are circumstances we don't have control over. But if your goal is to marry and have children, a bird known for being possessive, demanding and devoted to one person is not a good choice. If a bird is known for being difficult or dangerous around children, that's not a good choice, either.

Birds can be wonderful companions for people of all ages, but they are also a responsibility.

Finding the Perfect Rabbit

Rabbits, with their continually growing front teeth, were once considered rodents, but they are now considered part of the *Lagomorph* family. More than 40 breeds are recognized in the United States. Although the names rabbit and hare are often used interchangeably, rabbits are characterized by giving birth to blind, naked, helpless offspring and by their tendency to live in gregarious colonies underground. Hares are born with fur and the ability to see; they live more solitary lives and construct simple nests above ground.

Baby rabbits are so adorable and cuddly that they are often impulse purchases, especially at Easter. While rabbits can make exceptional house pets, their success depends on caring owners who educate themselves before buying or adopting. Your best local source for information and referrals may be your county extension agent or 4-H club; check your phone book or contact the National 4-H Council (see the Resources for this chapter in the Appendix). Fancy Publications (see *Critters USA*) maintains a directory of American organizations dedicated to small animals, including rabbit specialty clubs and breeder associations. In addition, check your public library for books about rabbit selection and care.

As with cats and dogs, fur length and maintenance requirements vary. Some breeds have short, dense coats that require little grooming while others, like Angoras, have long, silky hair that needs regular brushing. Rabbits have either long and "loppy" or erect ears, and they come in a variety of colors and sizes ranging from dwarf to giant, or about two to fifteen pounds.

Rabbits' teeth grow all their lives, and they need items to chew on to keep them from growing too long. Untreated wood, hardwood tree prunings, hard hay cubes, chew toys and some bird toys are appropriate for gnawing. Assuming the rabbit is healthy when young, it can be expected to live for six to eight years or longer with few if any health problems. Rabbits sometimes get ear mites, ringworm, digestive disturbances or a lackluster coat. Indoor rabbits are sensitive to cold and easily chilled when taken outside, and they are highly sensitive to noise. Rabbits have died from being too close to stereo speakers, and loud sounds stress them. So do disruptions of their normal schedule; therefore, a comfortable routine of feeding, play and exercise is important.

If you want more than one rabbit, provide a separate cage or hutch for each as rabbits of the same sex may fight if housed together and rabbits of the opposite sex reproduce. Rabbits reach sexual maturity at three to six months of age, and they don't go through heat cycles the way dogs and cats do. Ovulation is triggered by mating, which can occur whenever the opportunity presents itself.

In mild weather, house rabbits can be taken outdoors and, for safety if the yard isn't fenced, fitted with a harness attached to a leash. They can't be walked like dogs, but an accommodating owner can allow a curious rabbit to explore the backyard or a sheltered grassy park in safety.

When moving to a new home, a rabbit should be left in peace for a few days in order to adjust. Its introduction to children and other pets should be made gradually and gently. Most rabbit breeds are sociable and enjoy handling; however, these animals are fragile and too much handling can kill them. Keep your new rabbit in a quiet room and protect him from stress.

A rabbit's moods, once you learn to decipher them, are clearly communicated by foot stomping or thumping (a threat or warning), chirping sounds when held (the rabbit would like to be set down), tooth grinding (a sign of contentment) and, if the pet is a male, gifts of leaves, twigs or small pieces of paper accompanied by a soft, humming noise (a nesting behavior). Beware of any rabbit that makes short, barking growls, as this is a sign of aggression, often accompanied by ears held flat against the body and followed by a biting or scratching attack.

Scent glands on the chin mark the rabbit's territory with a substance noticeable to other rabbits but indiscernible to people.

When selecting a rabbit, look for one that's at least eight weeks old. Hold it in your lap to be sure it enjoys being handled. Stroke it gently down its back and along its sides; you should not be able to feel the spine or ribs. The rabbit should look alert and well-fed, with bright eyes, a dry nose and upper and lower teeth that come together. Don't take a rabbit that has malocclusion, or buck teeth. Check inside the ears to be sure they are clear and don't contain the crusty brown scales that indicate ear mites. For the most pleasant, affectionate house pet, many authorities suggest a male or buck rather than the female or doe.

Training and Caring for Your Pet at Home

Positive Reinforcement

When Karen Pryor became a dolphin trainer, she worked with animals that can't be punished, hit or yanked around on a choke chain. They just swim away. As Pryor wrote in *Don't Shoot the Dog: The New Art of Training and Teaching,* "Positive reinforcement, primarily a bucket of fish, was the only tool we had."

What exactly is positive reinforcement? It's anything, says Pryor, which, occurring in conjunction with an act, tends to increase the probability that the act will occur again. Memorize that statement, she instructs, for it is the secret of training not only dolphins but all animals, including our pets, ourselves and other people.

At the supermarket one day I heard a woman exclaim, "Samantha! Sit!" Having said those words myself, I turned around and saw a bright-eyed toddler lean precariously over the edge of the shopping cart. "Sit!" said the mother. "Sit, sit, sit, sit down. Please sit down." She sounded just like most puppy owners. I'll bet I know what happens next, I thought. Sure enough, the daughter sat and the woman sighed, turned away, checked her list and reached for a can of soup. As soon as she did, her daughter, who watched her intently, stood and waved her arms. "I told you to sit down! Sit!" Sound familiar?

American parents tend to ignore their children's good behavior, as though it should happen automatically and doesn't deserve recognition, while they spend incredible amounts of energy and emotion on whatever upsets them. As effective trainers point out, that's the exact opposite of good training. The mother could have said, "Sit down, Samantha," in a calm voice and patiently waited for her daughter to do so. Then she could have kissed her, given her a hug and told her what a good girl she was or how grown up she was acting. Reaching for the can of soup, she could have glanced back to be sure Samantha was still sitting, immediately smiled and nodded, then come back to reinforce her good behavior by repeating the praise.

To be effective, a positive reinforcement must be something that the subject wants, and its delivery must be well-timed. Dolphins eat fish, so fish are an appropriate reward for their trainers to use in motivating them to jump higher, dive deeper or learn new behaviors. Delivering the fish in the right place at the right moment is what matters, and that's usually impossible. So the trainers taught their charges a simple equation: a blow on the whistle equals fish. It didn't take long for the dolphins to consider the whistle itself a reward, and when occasionally reinforced by more fish, the well-timed whistle became a powerful motivator.

Whistles and other signals associated with the arrival of a reward are called conditioned reinforcers. The best reinforcers are signals the animals can perceive instantly.

Trainers have used everything from words and other sounds to gestures, flashing lights and facial expressions to communicate with animals. One of the easiest tools for novice trainers to master is the inexpensive, hand-held clicker noisemaker sold at party stores and toy shops. Today's training clickers are more solidly built, but they deliver the same distinctive sound. Using their dolphin-training techniques, Pryor and her disciples have taught people of every description how to shape the behavior of nearly any animal, from zoo residents and animals in the wild to domestic pets.

To try it yourself, choose a time when your pet is hungry, alert and responsive. Using a small piece of a favorite food, give a treat. For best results, use something special or unusual that the animal really likes. As your puppy, kitten, dog, cat, bird or rabbit takes it, click the clicker. Repeat this enjoyable exercise several times. Do it again, substituting praise and petting for the treat, assuming that your pet enjoys praise and petting. Do it again while tossing a ball, dragging a kitty toy or dangling a shiny new bell. It won't take long for your pet to associate the clicker's sound with something he or she really enjoys.

Then click when your pet does something you want to encourage, like sitting, lying down, coming to you, turning his head or whatever you want him to do. I taught Samantha to bow by waiting for her to yawn and stretch, then saying the word "Bow" and clicking just as she reached perfect position.

Click to reward any voluntary or involuntary movement toward the desired position or action, without waiting for it to be complete. The next time I said "Bow," Samantha stood still, watched, cocked her head, looked to the right, then slowly locked her front legs and began to lean back. This earned an immediate click. It also stopped her in her tracks, but that's to be expected because the click is a logical end marker. The next time I said "Bow," she repeated her performance, but this time the click came later, after she stretched further. Waiting for an additional effort before giving the reward is called shaping the behavior. After a few more tries, Samantha caught on and gave a complete bow, which earned a click and a special treat; Pryor suggests expressing special enthusiasm by increasing the number of treats, not the number of clicks.

In the sessions that followed, Samantha occasionally looked bored, responded slowly and barely bowed before lying down with legs stretched in front of her. This would have earned enthusiastic praise, a click and treats at the beginning, but now it didn't earn anything. I put the clicker in my pocket and walked away to do something else for a few hours. These no-reward bows were always followed in our next session by an enthusiastic, maximum extension with wagging tail held high, earning a click plus an extra treat. Altogether, Samantha and I spent four short (two- or three-minute) training sessions, or about ten minutes, learning to bow.

According to Pryor's guidelines, when you are building toward a desired behavior, wait until the animal learns the complete pattern and performs it spontaneously in hopes of receiving more clicks before giving it a name or identifying cue. Because I began with the finished behavior, I named Samantha's bow when we started. You can do it either way; just don't use a command or cue until the animal completes the pattern. The cue can be a word or other sound or a gesture or other visual prompt.

Clicker training is not command-based, so if your pet doesn't respond to the cue you are using, it's incorrect to assume the pet is disobeying. He just hasn't learned the cue yet.

Over time, your pet will work harder and perform better for fewer clicks, and you will learn to time them precisely. A clicker is faster than verbal praise or any physical reward, so it helps the animal understand exactly what he or she did correctly. Of course, everything depends on your timing, your understanding of how to shape behavior, a sharp eye and alert responses. The novice and professional trainers who share their experiences in *The Clicker Journal* have taught intricate behaviors to a variety of animals in record time, such as the cockatiel who learned to retrieve a Q-tip in six five- to seven-minute sessions and the dangerously uncooperative horse who now willingly enters a trailer after six five- to ten-minute training sessions, all without physical or verbal corrections of any kind. Their stories are entertaining and informative, for the writers explain what they did right and did wrong, and their experiences have direct application to the work we can do at home with all our pets. Like any effective training device, the clicker is a tool that can strengthen the bond of communication between handler and animal. By using several conditioned reinforcers and not just one, the novice trainer and his or her pet can work well together in any circumstances, including those in which clickers are not appropriate or not allowed.

The system of using well-timed rewards to shape behavior is nothing new. Its fundamental laws were defined by Harvard professor B.F. Skinner in the 1930s and '40s and are variously known as behavior modification, reinforcement theory, operant conditioning, behaviorism and behavioral psychology.

Labels always produce controversy, misunderstanding and misrepresentation, and the concept of operant conditioning is sometimes dismissed or denounced by dog trainers who don't understand what it is or how it works, or because of behavioral research conducted by heavy-handed, unimaginative psychologists in laboratories. Clicker training is the latest trend in animal training and it excites all kinds of passions, from the enthusiastic acceptance of any activity that involves a clicker to the denunciation of clickers as the dumbest thing that ever happened. Before dismissing or embracing clicker training, let Karen Pryor's books or videos introduce you to this new training strategy.

Collars, Leashes, Halters and Harnesses

The most basic item in a dog's wardrobe is his or her collar, and next comes the leash.

Collars

The appropriate collar for young puppies and dogs of all ages is a flat buckle collar made of canvas webbing, which fastens like a belt around the dog's neck. The correct size is important; the collar should be loose enough for you to insert your fingers underneath and not so loose that it slides over the puppy's head. Smaller, thinner, narrower collars are appropriate for small dogs and puppies; larger, wider, thicker collars are suitable for large dogs. Periodically check a growing puppy's collar to be sure it still fits. As soon as it begins to feel snug, move to the next notch or buy a larger collar.

A similar flat collar fastens with a parachute clasp, a quick-release mechanism that opens the collar in an instant, instead of a buckle fastener. Two on-leash dogs can tangle their leashes faster than the eye can follow and, if a fight ensues, a quick-release collar can prevent injury to both.

Another type of fabric collar is the half-choke, which consists of two webbing strips, one of which is a small loop attached to either side of the larger piece by metal rings. A third metal ring attaches the leash to the fabric loop. This arrangement, which slips on over the dog's head, gives the handler more control than a buckle collar and is safer than slip or choke collars.

Should a dog or puppy wear a flat collar at all times? Letters to dog magazines reflect both sides of this debate. Some dogs have been injured by buckle collars caught on fences, shrubs, industrial equipment and other hazards. One woman wrote that her dog had caught his front paw in his buckle collar while swimming and nearly drowned. Are dogs safer without a collar? Because collars provide the most obvious form of identification, a collarless dog who runs away or gets lost is less likely to be returned to his or her owner than one wearing an ID tag.

Many dogs are tattooed on the inner thigh, but tattoos are not always visible under fur, and not everyone who finds a lost dog has ever heard of tattoos or knows what to do with that information. Microchips embedded beneath the dog's skin are even more esoteric, both because the technology is still so new that it's unfamiliar to most Americans and because the scanning equipment needed to read microchips is not widely available. There is also a question of standardization, for different types of microchip require different scanners. While most breeders and veterinarians recommend tattooing and/or microchip identification because they are permanent, easy-to-read ID tags on a dog's collar remain the most visible, conspicuous and informative method of identification in most situations.

There is also debate about how much information should be attached to a collar. Some people give the dog's name, owner's name, street address and phone number. Others use phone number alone, with or without a "Reward if found" notice. The phone number doesn't have to be the owner's; it can be that of a pet registry service that will contact the owner if the dog is reported found. My husband and I, trusting the good intentions of most people, have everything on Samantha's collar from a riveted flat brass tag giving her name, the National Dog Registry's 24-hour phone number and the registration number tattooed on her inner thigh to her New York State dog license tag, a rabies tag showing her veterinarian's address and phone number, a tag with our name, address and phone number and her therapy dog registration tag. If she should ever disappear from our lives, we want her to be easy to identify not only as our pet but as a dog who has been vaccinated for rabies as well as one who is tame and safe around people.

The next item on the accessory shopping list is a training collar. Choke chains, which are made of metal, and slip collars, their fabric equivalent, are by far the most popular choice. They may also be the most dangerous. Choke chains got their name for a good reason: when the dog lunges ahead or pulls against the leash, this collar tightens around his neck. Trainers who recommend them argue that a properly used choke chain is both safe and effective and that problems arise when owners who have no control over their dogs use them incorrectly. Tracheal damage is more common among dogs who wear choke chains than any other training collar.

Diane Bauman never uses choke chains or slip collars. "I don't believe that choking the dog or giving him the sensation that he can't breathe in any way contributes to a state of mind that encourages learning," she explains.

Most owners leave the choke chain or slip collar on their dog at all times, a practice that can be fatal. Dog magazines routinely publish heart-wrenching accounts by grieving owners describing the many ways dogs have strangled themselves while wearing choke chains and slip collars, and their common plea, "If this letter saves one dog's life, it will at least serve a purpose," is a reminder for all. If you must use a choke chain or slip collar, put it on when you need it and take it off when you don't, and this includes whenever your dog is running off-leash in the woods or backyard (hazards include everything from other dogs to anything that might snag them, including fence parts), riding in the car (dogs have been killed in minor accidents not from injuries but from strangling after their collars caught on door or window handles) and even lying in their kennels (if there's a way to catch a collar on a metal part, a dog will find it). Sometimes a happy, playful dog gets a paw or tooth caught in another dog's collar. Choke collar tragedies happen every day.

The pinch or prong collar is the most controversial inexpensive training collar. Electric training collars, which deliver an adjustable shock and are used on hunting dogs and dogs who work off-lead, may be more controversial, but their use is outside the scope of this book and is best addressed by competent trainers in that field.

Prong or pinch collars are studded with short, long, thin or thick, rounded (not sharp) bent metal prongs that point toward the dog's neck and resemble items used in the Spanish

Inquisition. The lightweight small ones look like torture devices for tiny dogs, and the heavy models for large dogs look worse.

"They do have an unfavorable appearance," says Diane Bauman, "but prong collars are actually very safe if used correctly. People fear that their dogs will be injured or that the prongs will puncture the dog's skin, but this doesn't happen. The prong collar, which must be fitted properly, is designed to pinch the skin evenly and not puncture it. There are rubber tip covers available for overly sensitive dogs and dogs without thick coats. I use only buckle collars and prong collars in my training. Choke chains and slip collars can't help but injure dogs. Give a hard correction and you injure the trachea; resist a pulling dog and you choke him. The pinch collar may look awful, but it gives a much safer, gentler correction."

Because a dog won't usually lunge or pull while wearing a prong collar, it is often recommended for large, strong or unruly dogs or dogs who don't feel other types of correction. If you're always yanking at your dog's collar without much effect, your dog probably doesn't even notice. This is why choke chains are so hazardous. A strong, sturdy dog who really wants to get where she's going will huff, puff and wheeze while pulling her owner, who's dragging like an anchor behind her, up hill and down dale. To give her a correction she pays attention to, the owner has to give a powerful yank, maybe one that knocks her over. There is nothing healthy about a training device that deprives your dog of oxygen every time you use it or one that injures her neck. In the hands of most American dog owners, the choke chain does both.

Pinch collars have neither of these disadvantages. In addition, they can be safer for the handler. Any strong dog, even a small one, can pull the person at the other end of the leash off his or her feet if the circumstances are right, and the use of a properly fitted pinch or prong collar can reduce the risk of injury.

If my conversations with dog owners are anything to judge by, prong collars excite even more passionate debate than crates. I've seen people approach strangers and begin the conversation with, "Take that thing off!" I've heard trainers denounce them as ineffective and dangerous.

"People who claim that prong collars are ineffective have simply never used them," says Sarah Wilson. "The same people who criticize an owner for holding the leash of a well-behaved dog that isn't pulling or being obnoxious but is wearing a prong would think it's perfectly OK for the same dog to be lunging around on a choke chain, asphyxiating himself. European studies have shown that tracheal damage is far more likely to be caused by choke chains than by pinch collars, so claims that they are innately more dangerous simply aren't true. Sure, in the wrong hands they can be brutal, but the same can be said about many pieces of training equipment. Effective training with a pinch collar can break dangerous habits without harming or hurting the dog, and they make some dogs a lot safer to walk with. It's a mistake to condemn their use just because of their appearance."

The best way to select a training collar is to consult an expert trainer who can help you decide which equipment to use, what size your dog needs and what to do with it.

Leashes

Leashes come in so many colors, materials, shapes, sizes and lengths that the novice owner can only be bewildered. Obedience instructors usually sell a variety of leashes and make appropriate suggestions, depending on the size and type of dog as well as the activity involved. Another consideration is the handler's size, for people with large hands are comfortable holding thick, wide leashes and those who have small hands aren't.

The spring-loaded Flexi lead was an instant best-seller when it arrived in the U.S. from Germany. What could be more convenient? This brightly colored leash extends automatically when the dog pulls, retracts slack line when the handler presses a button on the handle and locks, preventing extension, when desired. Flexi leads give on-lead dogs freedom to run and play and give a privacy-seeking dog room to maneuver when seeking the right place to eliminate. They also make untrained dogs and handlers even more of a menace than they would be otherwise. Any inattentive handler can be dangerous, but if the dog is trailing behind her owner at the end of an extended Flexi, that danger increases. Small dogs crossing the street in this position have been run over by drivers who never saw them. Inattentive handlers holding Flexi leads are a threat to other dogs and people because they have so little control over their animals' behavior.

"We usually hear these things coming before we see them," says Sarah Wilson. "ZZZzziipppp! They sound like a tuna spinning the line out. The dog is thrilled to see another dog and charges straight in our direction with the owner desperately trying to keep up, or maybe he sees a squirrel to chase or some trees to inspect. For all the interaction I see between these owners and their dogs, they might as well have a raccoon at the end of the leash."

Halters and Harnesses

Another training device for dogs is the head halter, which looks like a cross between a collar and a muzzle, for its fabric loop slips over the dog's nose. The leash attaches to the halter and prevents lunging or pulling without choking the dog. Wilson says, "These are wonderful management tools, especially for people whose dogs are much stronger than they are. Since some halters are designed to close a dog's mouth when pulled on, they can be especially helpful for dogs who are aggressive toward other dogs and for dogs that eat off the sidewalk. Not all dogs can be fitted with head halters; Boxers, Pugs, Pekingese and Bulldogs are obvious examples of short-nosed breeds that a head halter won't properly fit. They should never be used with a Flexi lead, nor do they take the place of good, solid practice and behavioral training."

Small animals such as cats and rabbits can be taken outdoors on a leash but it should be attached to a body harness, not a collar. A retractable Flexi lead designed for small animals or a leash that can be tied around the waist or attached to a nearby stake is ideal for someone whose kitten or rabbit is exploring the outdoors while they read, relax or work in the garden.

In your car, use a seat belt harness or portable carrier that can be attached to a seatbelt or otherwise secured for safe travel. Seat belt harnesses for dogs have a loop on the back for insertion of the seat belt. If your car is equipped with passenger-side air bags, keep your dog in the back seat. Rapidly inflating air bags have killed small children in minor traffic accidents and they're just as dangerous to pets.

Clean Up After Your Pet

Unless your backyard is a large field in the country, cleaning up after your dog is not only a healthy practice, it's responsible pet ownership. Dog waste is extremely disagreeable stuff to step on and, because it's slippery, it can be dangerous. People have skidded on dog droppings in streets, on sidewalks and at dog shows, badly injuring themselves. What an unpleasant and unnecessary way to break a leg!

Unfortunately, dog and cat waste, unlike cow or horse manure, has no commercial value, so no one collects it for fertilizer or other commercial applications. It doesn't compost well, so it's of no interest to gardeners. It's unsightly and offensive, and it often carries disease. Pets and children can pick up worms and other infections from canine or feline fecal matter, and when it dries and becomes airborne, which happens whenever the wind blows, small particles can cause respiratory problems in people.

The easiest way to clean up after your dog is to pick up the droppings with a paper towel or plastic bag. Place your hand inside the plastic bag and after collecting the waste, invert the bag so the droppings are inside it. Pet supply stores sell all kinds of pet waste collection bags and related equipment.

While collecting your dog's feces, cleaning the cat box or changing the paper in your bird's cage, notice what's there. Are the stools firm and well-shaped, loose or runny, covered with mucus or an odd color? Is there blood? Do you see long, stringy pieces of grass, household objects, carrot bits, twigs or candy wrappers? The art of stool watching is an important health monitor.

If your dog or cat has an accident in the house, don't use household cleaning products or anything containing ammonia. Instead, lift what you can with paper towels and apply an enzyme stain and odor remover sold in pet supply stores for this purpose. Treat stains from bird droppings the same way. Enzymes literally digest the proteins in the stain, removing the scent completely.

Cats are tidy by nature and rarely urinate or defecate outside a clean, convenient, well-maintained litter box, assuming one is available. Any kitten, cat or even dog that is otherwise in good health and makes large or frequent deposits in inappropriate places may simply be overfed. Reducing the pet's rations will often cure this problem.

Birds, like rabbits, can be housetrained. Gizmo, a Moluccan cockatoo, delights everyone who meets him by defecating whenever he is held over a waste basket. House-training is usually fast and easy if you're observant, set things up so your pet is likely to succeed, then praise and reward the desired response.

If You're Allergic

Because animal dander triggers so many adverse reactions, allergists often recommend that if anyone in the family has trouble breathing, the pets be given away. In 20 years of doctor appointments for the treatment of hay fever and asthma, I was usually told by the second office visit to get rid of my cats. Like many pet lovers who receive this prescription, I refused. None of my dozen doctors in five states offered alternative solutions; all announced in authoritative voices that there was no way to remove the problem without removing the pets, and all but one expressed annoyance at patients who refuse to cooperate.

But for every study that links pet dander to respiratory problems, others show that pet owners live longer, have happier lives, have lower stress levels and enjoy more meaningful relationships than those who don't share their lives with pets. For many Americans, pets are members of the family. Getting rid of them, even on a doctor's orders, is as traumatic as losing a relative.

Pet dander is more of a problem in carpeted homes than in homes with bare floors, although any rug or fabric can harbor dander. The source of the problem isn't hair that the animals shed but proteins in their saliva and flakes of skin. Young kittens and puppies don't usually trigger allergic reactions; they have no old skin to shed and therefore no dander. This explains how someone can develop a sudden allergy to a pet that was for weeks a comfortable roommate.

Years ago my husband and I lived in a carpeted house and, a few days after washing the carpets with steam-cleaning equipment, we had a house guest who was ordinarily violently allergic to cats. He kept looking at Kanga and Hang 12 and wondered why he wasn't sneezing. We had only wanted to remove old stains but, as a bonus, we had a dander-free home.

Removing dander from rugs, carpets and furniture is only part of the solution. Washing the pets themselves is just as important. Research has shown airborne allergens are reduced dramatically if a cat is washed once a week; the same is no doubt true for other animals. Full baths were traumatic for our elderly cats, but we found they would tolerate sponge baths. Pet stores and pet magazines sell equipment to make cat bathing easier and there are products just for allergy grooming, solutions you can apply with a damp cloth or spray onto dogs, cats and birds. They contain enzymes that digest the proteins in dander, rendering them harmless. Some effective nonchemical shampoos that don't require rinsing are sold for rabbits and other small pets; they are safe for cats and kittens, too. Or simply use plain water or chamomile tea to rinse the dander away. Don't use soap for weekly cleanings; it's too harsh, strips away protective oils and is difficult to rinse out. The secret to success in using any of these methods is reaching the skin. Look for dander removal products in pet supply catalogs or check with your veterinarian, groomer or pet store. If you start when a kitten is tiny, you can even convince a cat to enjoy baths.

Pet owners who give their animals a well-balanced natural diet of raw food and nutritional supplements usually notice a rapid improvement in their animal's coat: glossy fur, healthy skin and a substantial reduction in flaking or dandruff. This is as true for birds and rabbits as it is for cats and dogs. It makes sense to reduce dander at the source, and the source is always affected by diet.

Air filters make a big difference in bird rooms and living areas occupied by pets. Human hair can vary between 75 and 100 microns in thickness; animal dander is about 15 microns thick. High-efficiency particulate air (HEPA) filters, which were developed for use in laboratories and manufacturing plants, remove 99.97 percent of particles 0.3 microns in size and larger. Position air filters above, not directly on, carpets.

Brush pets outdoors or wear a pollen mask while brushing inside near an air filter and follow with immediate vacuuming to reduce the accumulation of new dander. Remember that pet dander is so light that most vacuum cleaners merely redistribute it; if you're serious about controlling dander and dust mites, you need a vacuum cleaner equipped with special high filtration bags and carpet steam-cleaning equipment.

Many people who are allergic to pet dander become less so when they change their own diets. This is how I finally solved my allergy problems. As long as I stay away from wheat and dairy products, I'm fine around dogs, cats, birds, rabbits and even ragweed pollen. When I don't, I'm sneezing within the hour. Some of the herbs recommended in Chapter 4 for dogs and cats are also useful for their allergic owners, such as stinging nettle and mullein. Drinking these teas or taking the herbs in capsules has helped many people with hay fever, pet allergies and asthma. For more about natural methods of allergy control, see my book *Herbs to Help You Breathe Freely* (Keats Publishing, 1996). ⊱

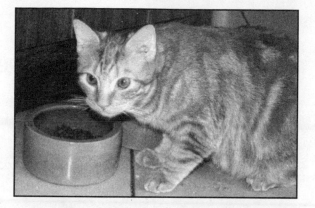

Food Is Everything:

Natural Diet for Dogs, Cats, Birds and Rabbits

PET FOOD MANUFACTURERS and the veterinarians courted by their sales representatives have convinced most Americans that because commercial pet foods are designed in laboratories by people with academic credentials and because their labels contain long lists of nutrients and claims of being "scientifically balanced" and "nutritionally complete," they are superior to anything an animal might otherwise consume. Table scraps, raw food, "people food" and any supplements that might disrupt the commercial food's precisely controlled distribution of vitamins and minerals are particularly frowned on.

There is no doubt that commercial pet foods sustain life. Dogs, cats and other animals live for years on foods that come out of bags, cans and boxes. But do these foods promote health? If they did, our companion animals would enjoy long, happy lives free of arthritis, hip dysplasia, eye problems, ear problems, fleas and other parasites, gum disease, lick granulomas, thyroid imbalances, skin and coat problems, personality disorders, birth defects, breeding problems, diabetes, cancer and other major and minor illnesses.

Before World War II, most Americans fed their pets raw bones and table scraps. Today, everyone uses convenience foods, and pet food companies are industry giants. Diet isn't the only thing that has changed. So has life expectancy, with the life span of many breeds now less than half what it was two or three decades ago. Skin and coat problems are so common that we accept them as unavoidable, and today's veterinarians routinely treat conditions that used to be unusual or even rare.

Of course, more has changed in the last 50 years than our pets' diets. Environmental pollution, toxic chemicals and stress take their toll on companion animals as much as they do on people. But a growing number of experts attribute the epidemic of modern animal illnesses in large part to diet.

Dr. Pottenger's Experiment

One of the most impressive experiments demonstrating the connection between animal health and diet was conducted from 1932 to 1942 by Francis M. Pottenger, Jr., M.D., at his clinic in Monrovia, California. Pottenger was a mainstream physician: he wrote articles for medical and scientific journals and served as president of the Los Angeles County Medical Association, the American Academy of Applied Nutrition, the American Therapeutic Society and other organizations. His research is described in the book *Pottenger's Cats: A Study in Nutrition* and in reports compiled by Pat Connolly, curator of the Price-Pottenger Nutrition Foundation.

Pottenger noticed that the health of the clinic's resident cats, which appeared to be well fed on a diet of raw milk, cod liver oil and cooked meat scraps, in fact declined. This observation inspired him to embark on a 10-year study conducted according to the most rigorous scientific standards of the day, during which 900 cats were studied and complete records were kept on 600. The cats, which were kept in outdoor pens, were routinely weighed, numbered and examined. Whenever a cat was donated, its owner was interviewed about the animal's medical history and the type of food it had been fed. Whenever kittens were born, complete records were kept regarding the mother's behavior during birth, the kittens' weight on the day of birth and their individual descriptions; clinical notes were kept on each kitten as it grew and developed.

All of the cats were fed scraps of the meat served at the sanatorium, which included beef, lamb and poultry muscle meats, bones and organs such as liver, tripe, sweetbreads, brains and heart. All of the meat was organically raised and of the highest quality.

In one experiment, cats were divided into two groups and fed an identical diet of two-thirds meat, one-third milk and cod liver oil. All of the cats received raw milk, but the meat was cooked for one group and served raw for the other. The group fed raw meat was healthy, alert, calm, well tempered, physically coordinated and resistant to fleas, infections, worms and other parasites. They reproduced easily and had healthy kittens.

In contrast, the cats fed cooked meat suffered from dental and vision problems, arthritis, heart disease, thyroid problems, skin lesions, allergies, fleas, intestinal parasites, poor coordination, miscarriages and personality disorders. Adults often died of pneumonia, kittens of pneumonia and diarrhea.

While the raw meat/raw milk cats produced generation after healthy generation, there was no fourth generation of cats fed cooked meat because none of its third generation's kittens lived to six months.

Other experiments used four groups of cats, all of which were fed one-third of their diet as raw meat and cod liver oil. The cats received the other two-thirds of their diet as either raw milk, pasteurized milk, evaporated milk or sweetened condensed milk. All but the group fed raw meat and raw milk suffered from infections, reproductive problems and diseases, and cats fed evaporated or sweetened condensed milk were irritable, nervous and physically deformed.

Describing the cats receiving either cooked meat or pasteurized milk, Pottenger wrote that they developed all kinds of allergies. "They sneeze, wheeze and scratch," he reported. "They are irritable, nervous and do not purr." One allergic cat developed an intense itching around the anus that caused it to rub most of the fur off its buttocks. When milk was removed from the cat's diet, the allergic symptoms immediately cleared.

Vermin and parasites abounded. Skin diseases and allergies increased from an incidence of five percent in normal cats to over 90 percent in the third generation of cats fed cooked meat or milk. The cats fed cooked food suffered from frequent infections; severe osteoporosis was universal and mortality rates were high. "These cats suffered from most of the degenerative diseases encountered in human medicine," wrote Pottenger, "including endocrine dyscrasias. Their autopsy findings were revealing."

Those findings included measurements of the intestinal tracts of allergic cats, which measured as long as 72 to 80 inches (48 inches is normal) and lacked tissue tone and elasticity. Hypothyroidism (underactive thyroid) verified at autopsy was common in females eating cooked food and Pottenger associated this hormonal disorder with deformities in their kittens' skulls, small teeth and lower jaws. The typical kitten born to parents eating raw meat and raw milk had a large skull, large bones, large thorax, long body, relatively short legs, broad dental arches and excellent teeth which were regular and well-spaced. None of the cats fed raw food had kittens with thyroid imbalances, but a significant number of kittens born to mothers on cooked food had thyroid deficiencies, and the use of supplementary thyroid in the diet of a nursing mother sometimes produced symptoms of hyperthyroidism (overactive thyroid) in her young.

Of the second generation male cats fed cooked food, 83 percent proved to be functionally sterile, exhibiting no spermatozoa; 53 percent of the second generation of females fed cooked food showed underdeveloped and infantile ova.

Could the health of deficient cats be restored by changing from cooked food to raw? It took Pottenger's cats three and sometimes four generations of an all-raw diet to recover their perfect tooth and jaw formation, skeletal structure and health, but interrupting their cooked food regimen slowed and to some extent reversed the deterioration of individual cats. This was especially true for kittens born to parents fed raw food. "The deficiency produced in a nursing kitten with a healthy lineage cannot match the deficiency produced in a kitten born of a deficient mother during the nursing period," wrote Pottenger. "Milk produced by a deficient mother lacks the nutrients necessary for her kittens' normal growth and development." Deficiencies in the mother's milk reinforced deficiencies already present in her kittens at birth, resulting in the serious and irreversible problems experienced by the second and third generation of cats fed cooked food.

After the feeding experiments concluded, weeds began to sprout in the pens that had housed Pottenger's cats for 10 years. Their dramatic growth differences inspired another experiment, this one involving navy beans. The noncomposted excreta of cats from the different pens was used to fertilize navy beans in identical, adjacent plots; a control plot was not fertilized.

Pen 15, which had housed males fed raw meat and raw milk, produced deep green plants with exceptionally thick stems that produced 2000 blossoms over 70 days resulting in 1,142 beans. Pen 19, which housed females fed pasteurized milk, produced weak beans of poor color that produced 500 blossoms over 42 days, resulting in 615 beans. Pen 22, which housed males fed evaporated milk, produced weak, sprawling plants of fair color that set 300 blossoms over 49 days, producing 329 beans. Pen 23, which housed females fed sweetened condensed milk, produced poor plants of fair color that produced 350 blossoms over 49 days, resulting in 190 beans.

One month after planting, when the beans were transplanted to larger plots, the roots of the beans fertilized with excreta from the pens of cats fed raw food were at least twice as numerous, tougher and longer than those of the others; roots of the unfertilized plants were intermediate; roots of the plants fertilized with excreta from the pens of cats fed cooked meat were few, soft and mushy.

When the beans' ash, calcium and phosphorous contents were compared, the beans from the pens of cats fed raw meat had substantially higher percentages than those from the pens of cats fed cooked meat.

In additional experiments, Pottenger found that cattle that grazed on fresh grass had far richer milk for their calves than cattle fed on dried feed, and the latter group had high infant mortality rates. Farm chickens allowed outdoors to scratch for worms and eat green grasses and weeds (today we call them free-range chickens) produced eggs with hard shells and deep yellow yolks that, when fertilized, hatched husky, healthy chicks. The chickens themselves had supple skin, firm muscles and nearly twice as much calcium for a given weight of bone as mass-produced, hatchery chickens. Hatchery chickens, housed in wire pens and fed grains and other dry feeds, laid eggs with thin shells and pale yolks that, when fertilized, often failed to germinate. These chickens had thick skin, lax muscles, pale fat, soft flesh and much smaller bones than the farm chickens.

Pottenger and his staff compared the diets of both groups of cattle and both groups of chickens and found that all contained adequate amounts of fat, protein, carbohydrates and minerals. "It is the fresh, raw factors in feed," Pottenger concluded, "that appear to hold the balance between a healthy animal capable of reproducing healthy offspring and one that is unhealthy and has poor reproductive efficiency." In addition, he observed, the nutritional value of animal products such as milk and eggs depends on the nutritional value of the diet fed to the animals producing those products.

In another experiment, Pottenger fed guinea pigs a diet of rolled and cracked grain with supplements of cod liver oil and field-dried alfalfa. These animals soon suffered hair loss, paralysis, high infant mortality, diarrhea, pneumonia and other deficiency symptoms. When fresh cut green grass was introduced into their diet, the guinea pigs showed remarkable improvement. Infant mortality decreased, the animals gained weight, no new cases of paralysis developed and their hair loss decreased, although it did not disappear. Instead of being fed cut grass, some of the guinea pigs were allowed to run in outdoor pens and feed on weeds and growing grass. In less than a month, the foraging animals showed greater improvement than those eating fresh cut grass indoors. Their diarrhea stopped, their hair returned to a healthy condition and their overall health returned to normal.

Pottenger was not the only scientist to test the difference that cooking makes. When Sir Robert McCarrison fed monkeys in India their usual diet cooked rather than raw, he discovered that all of the animals developed colitis and their autopsies revealed gastric and intestinal ulcers. O. Stiner in Switzerland cooked the food his healthy guinea pigs had been eating raw and they developed anemia, scurvy, goiter, dental cavities and malfunctions of the salivary glands. When he added pasteurized milk to their daily fare, they developed arthritis as well. In Finland, Dr. Rakel Kurkela at the University of Helsinki fed safflower oil to laboratory animals eating a standard laboratory diet. One group received raw, unheated oil, which is rich in unsaturated fatty acids; the second group's oil was heated in the presence of oxygen, the same thing we do when frying food. The group fed raw oil thrived and gained weight; the health of the group fed heated oil deteriorated and the animals died prematurely. Feeding experiments in zoos always show that cooked food causes serious deficiencies and deterioration while fresh, raw food improves health.

Why Raw Is Best

Cooking destroys heat-sensitive vitamins, trace elements and amino acids, deforms proteins and enzymes and changes the molecular structure of fats. Foods can be warmed to a few degrees above body temperature without destroying heat-sensitive vitamins, amino acids, trace elements and enzymes, but the temperatures required for pasteurization (131° to 158° Fahrenheit) or for baking, boiling, frying or poaching have a deleterious effect. Microwaves may pose a special threat. Holistic veterinarians and physicians have for years warned their clients and patients not to use microwave ovens. Now some clinical studies seem to support that warning.

Assuming that the health of dogs, cats and other animals improves on raw food, what should that food be? Everything about the anatomy of domestic dogs and cats points to a meat-based diet: like the fox, coyote, wolf, hyena, puma, lynx, lion, tiger, leopard and other canine and feline relatives, they have sharp teeth for tearing flesh and gnawing bones, their digestive secretions are highly concentrated and their intestines are short, all of which makes them well suited for processing freshly killed animals. Ruminants and humans, on the other hand, have flat molars for grinding grain or fibrous plants and long digestive tracts that absorb the slowly released nutrients they contain.

There is some debate over whether cats and dogs are true carnivores. Cats in the wild are almost exclusively meat-eaters, preying on rodents, birds and their eggs, small fish and other animals. Occasionally cats seek plant foods, like melon, cucumber or corn, and they are well-known for chewing grass, but these are occasional treats, not staple fare. Cats that catch live animals ingest small amounts of grain or whatever the prey has been eating, most of it broken down by digestion. Dogs evolved on a more varied diet, making them versatile opportunists who supplement meat with a variety of fruits, roots and other vegetation.

Learning to Feed Like Mother Nature

In *The New Natural Cat*, Anitra Frazier recounts her experiences as a cat groomer visiting owners who wanted to improve their pets' coats. The veterinarian she worked for suggested that they try to duplicate Mother Nature as much as possible with the same kinds of food the cats' ancestors ate and feed it on a similar schedule. Animals in the wild don't spend all day lounging around food dispensers; their digestive systems are stimulated only when food is available. By feeding their pets only once or twice a day and removing uneaten food after 15 or 20 minutes, Frazier's clients saw rapid improvement in their cats' coats.

If using food as a reward while training, try giving food treats in short practice sessions rather than scattering them through the day. In *Don't Shoot the Dog!*, Karen Pryor recommends using the smallest treat that will motivate the animal, such as a small piece of cheese for a dog. Pryor wrote, "A trainer's rule of thumb is that if you are going to have only one training session a day, you can count on the animal working well for about a quarter of its rations; you then give it the rest for free." Pryor has found that 80 reinforcements delivered in three or four training sessions is a good maximum for most animals, with larger or more favorite treats rewarding more difficult tasks. As an experiment, I cut a one-ounce slice of cheese into 40 small pieces, each of which Samantha considered a motivating reward. If your dog is sufficiently food-oriented, a large number of treats doesn't require dietary adjustments. Otherwise, wait until the animal is hungry enough to be interested and divide a portion of his daily rations into training treats.

Many experts on feline and canine nutrition recommend occasional fasting, such as one day without solid food per week or month, to simulate the natural conditions in which these animals evolved. Fasting gives the digestive organs an opportunity to rest and helps the body repair itself. In the wild, predators alternate between gorging themselves and going for one or several days without food, so a once-a-week or once-a-month fast is both beneficial and easy for most dogs and cats to adjust to.

The Basics

Water

The purity of your pet's drinking water is a serious consideration. In his book *Pet Allergies,* Alfred Plechner lists contaminated drinking water as a common cause of health problems. The simple act of replacing tap water with distilled, bottled or filtered water can bring surprising, dramatic improvements.

Water is the one thing to which your pet should have unlimited access. Animals know when they're thirsty and they should have free access to clean containers of pure, healthy water.

Municipal water contamination has become a national concern now that chemical pesticides, fertilizers, industrial solvents, road salt, bacteria, parasites and heavy metals have found their way into kitchen faucets. One result is a rapidly growing water purification industry in which contradictory claims about charcoal filters, reverse osmosis, ultraviolet ozone generation and distillation abound. Another expanding business is bottled water. A few lucky people have access to pure, clean well water or an uncontaminated stream, but the rest of us do well to consider tap water alternatives.

Some nutritionists swear by distilled water, while others condemn it for its lack of minerals. Some say that charcoal filters are all you need and others say they're worse than useless. Everyone has something bad to say about plastic containers, but some spring water is sold in clear (not cloudy) plastic jugs, which are more stable and prevent the plastic taste that often migrates into water from opaque bottles.

Whatever you can do to improve your drinking water is worth the effort. If you use a charcoal filter on your kitchen faucet, change it more often than the instructions indicate. Health magazines often report on water safety and home treatment methods; look for these themes wherever magazines are sold or check your local library. Your own health as well as your pet's health will improve.

Basic Foods

Ingredients should be raw, fresh and, as much as possible, grown or raised organically, without exposure to pesticides, chemicals, antibiotics, synthetic hormones and other drugs.

Bones: Raw, meaty bones from beef, chicken, turkey, lamb, venison and other healthy animals. For cats and small dogs, use poultry necks, breasts, thighs and drumsticks or cut bones such as from center-cut chuck steak. For additional bone nutrients, remove the marrow from beef marrow bones for cats and small dogs.

Protein: Raw beef, lamb, chicken, turkey, small amounts of organ meats (beef heart, chicken giblets, chicken liver, calves liver, lamb kidneys, sweetbreads). Raw (if very fresh and free of parasites) or lightly cooked fish or shellfish. In a pinch, canned sardines or baby food (lamb, beef, turkey, chicken, veal) containing only meat and water; check labels and serve with digestive enzymes. Raw organic eggs. Raw milk, raw milk cheese, yogurt, milk or cottage cheese treated with lactase enzymes.

Grain and Legumes: Fresh, raw sprouted grains such as wheat or rye; raw flaked oats or other grains soaked in raw milk, yogurt, raw vegetable juice or water; lightly cooked beans, rice or other grains or legumes in small quantities. Serve with enzyme powder containing amylase, which digests carbohydrates.

Vegetables: Finely grated or puréed raw carrots, parsnips, zucchini, cucumbers, sweet peppers, celery, peas, sweet potatoes, sprouts, wheat grass, finely minced herbs. Lactic acid fermented vegetables from a Japanese salad press. Lightly cooked broccoli, corn, peas, potatoes, green beans and similar vegetables, served with enzyme supplement. Fresh raw vegetable juice.

Fruits: Grapes, apples, blueberries, mangos, bananas, watermelon, cantaloupe, peaches, plums, pears, raisins, dates, avocado. Fresh raw fruit juice.

Seeds and Nuts: Sunflower seeds, chia seeds, Brazil nuts, walnuts, pecans, almonds, hazelnuts. Grind or purée. Make seeds (like sunflower seeds) more digestible by sprouting before grinding.

Forget It! My Fluffy Won't Eat That!

Sure she will. She just needs time to get used to the change. You can help her by introducing new foods slowly, in tiny quantities, adding them to what she already eats. Don't leave food lying out; remove whatever she hasn't eaten after 20 minutes, and don't feed between meals. Fluffy won't die of starvation if she skips dinner. Yes, you can try something else, but don't turn your life upside down preparing five different dinners to tempt her. Fluffy is a creature of habit (aren't we all?) and the unfamiliar disrupts her comfortable routine. If Fluffy's been living on treats that come in foil packages and that's all she'll eat, go slowly. Put unfamiliar supplements on hold; focus on raw meat or poultry and add a little at a time until she's used to the new foods; then, just as slowly, add new supplements.

Convenience Foods

What if you're in a hurry? Or you didn't have time to stop at the store? Or your husband/wife/parents/friends/neighbors/children insist on giving Fido or Fluffy a dog biscuit, cat treat or other not-raw, not-at-all-natural tidbit?

Relax. A few deviations here and there won't derail your feeding plan. Both Pepper and Samantha have had their share of baby food and other emergency rations. The next day we're back on track and so will you be. I think of minced wheat grass, garlic and enzyme powders as antidotes to processed convenience foods.

You can create your own convenience dinners by preparing more than one meal at a time and storing single servings in self-sealing plastic bags in the refrigerator. Gently warm refrigerated food by placing it in hot water, placing the serving bowl in hot water or gently heating the contents in a double boiler until somewhere between room and body temperature.

It's one thing to decide on a healthy diet plan for your pet. Putting it into effect is another. Food you prepare yourself may be cheaper or more expensive than what you feed already, but menu planning and preparation are sure to take more time, especially as you begin.

Gail Colombo addressed the cost of superior nutrition in the November/December 1994 *Tiger Tribe* (an excellent magazine which is no longer published) and her article offers good suggestions. Among them: Find a meat wholesaler, preferably one who handles organically grown/free-range meat, shop in ethnic neighborhoods such as Chinatown, search for restaurants and butcher shops that give raw meat scraps away, collect bones, plan your own meals with an eye toward your pet's supply of grains and vegetables and learn to identify healthy wild weeds. Sometimes a food co-op can help, and some veterinarians, groomers, trainers and pet supply stores arrange regular deliveries of organically raised meat and bones for their clients.

Now for your time. Like most people who switch from packaged to raw foods, I learned that experience is the best teacher. With practice, you will be organized and efficient. It now takes five minutes to prepare dinner for our dog and cat — not each, but total. Add another minute for cleanup, and I'm done. Shopping isn't time-consuming, either. We buy their foods when we shop for groceries at the supermarket, health food store and local co-op, and their supplements come from health food stores and mail order catalogs. When we made the transition, I seemed to spend half the day planning and preparing our cats' dinners and the other half worrying about whether it was balanced, but now it's easy and automatic.

Cooking and Storage Methods

If you have to choose between a frozen or cooked food, or between a microwaved or boiled food, which is better? Fresh is always at the top of the scale, but when that's not possible, keep this list in mind. From best to worst:

1. Fresh, served raw (most desirable).
2. Frozen and thawed, served raw.
3. Lightly steamed or scalded, not heated through.
4. Fried, baked, boiled or pasteurized.
5. Microwaved, irradiated, pressure-cooked or canned under pressure (least desirable).

Plates and Dishes

Food plates and water bowls should be glass, ceramic or stainless steel, not aluminum, plastic or pottery that might contain lead glaze. The use of plastic food bowls has been associated with the loss of pigmentation on a dog's nose and feline acne, a condition in which eruptions like blackheads form on a cat's chin. Replacing plastic bowls with glass, ceramic or stainless steel has cured these conditions in dogs and cats. Of course, food bowls should be washed after every use and water bowls kept clean.

Food Safety Issues

What About Bones?

Is it safe to feed bones to your dog or cat? Cooked bones are dangerous because they splinter and can cause serious problems. Raw bones, however, are a different story. We're so indoctrinated by the "don't feed bones" rule, we forget that our feline and canine companions spent thousands of years dining on them. Bones provide essential nutrients, hence the importance of bone meal as a pet food ingredient. But there's a world of difference between commercially processed bone meal and the raw bones your dog or cat might gnaw on.

When I switched my cats from cooked food to raw, I had the same misgivings as anyone else, but Anitra Frazier's *Natural Cat*, my first guide, calmly recommended giving cats whole Rock Cornish game hens. I did and they loved them, bones and all. Pepper and Samantha regularly share free-range chickens, and our only problem has been finding poultry shears sufficiently strong to cut them into practical servings.

Holistic veterinarians warn that pets who are not used to eating bones or who are in poor health should start with small quantities. Too much at first may cause either constipation or diarrhea, or the animal may have trouble digesting bones when they are first introduced. However, after adjusting to an improved diet of fresh, raw foods, most dogs and cats are able to digest raw bones without difficulty.

In addition to their nutritional benefits, bones are good for the teeth. As veterinarian Beverly Cappel-King says, "You can always tell a bone-chewing dog; they have the whitest, strongest, cleanest teeth."

Most American holistic pet care experts caution against feeding chicken and lamb bones to dogs because they can splinter, but Ian Billinghurst, an Australian veterinarian, recommends these bones as the foundation of a balanced diet. His book *Give Your Dog a Bone* describes the rapidly deteriorating health of Australia's dogs and cats after the nation adopted commercial pet foods in the mid-1960s. Until then, Australians fed their pets raw bones and table scraps. "Everybody knew how to do it," he says. "It was common sense. As a consequence, most Australian dogs were very healthy."

Billinghurst fed his own dogs commercial food for two years and watched them develop skin problems, runny eyes, scruffy coats, itching skin, hot spots, ear infections, anal sac problems, smelly fur and feces, bad breath, tooth and gum problems, repeated worm infestations, bone and growth disorders and reproductive problems. Previously, his dogs had dined on fresh meat, raw bones and table scraps; they were never wormed or vaccinated, had large litters of robust puppies and stayed healthy with a minimum of effort.

Because Billinghurst was in the habit of asking clients what their animals ate, he was able to document the connection between packaged food and health problems. As soon as he switched his dogs back to their previous diet, their health improved. So did the health of dogs belonging to clients who adopted his feeding plan, about 60 percent of which is raw meaty bones including lamb and raw chicken. The remaining 40 percent is mostly table scraps, including leftover vegetables, gravy, scraps of meat, fruit, small amounts of rice, mashed potatoes or pasta, plus added raw eggs, liver, kidneys, vegetable oils, honey, brewer's yeast, kelp powder, cod liver oil and occasional vitamin supplements.

Lamb, beef, venison, chicken, turkey and other meats are excellent sources of concentrated protein, amino acids, minerals and some vitamins. Pork is not usually recommended as a food for pets. Veterinarian Richard Pitcairn and others suggest cooking wild game and most fish to prevent the spread of parasites.

Using Cooked Foods: A Strategy for Avoiding Leucocytosis

In the 1930s, the French chemist Paul Kouchakoff discovered that as soon as cooked or processed food is tasted, white blood cells rush to the intestines. This phenomenon, called digestive leucocytosis, disrupts the immune system; the body regards cooked food as a pathogen and works hard to destroy it. When Kouchakoff's volunteers ate raw food, their white blood cells remained in place. As Leslie and Susannah Kenton wrote in *Raw Energy*, the implications of leucocytosis are that every time white blood cells flock to the intestines to deal with cooked food, the rest of the body is left undefended. "Continual red alerts, three or more times a day, year in and year out," they observed, "put considerable strain on the immune system." Unlike cooked foods, raw foods leave the white blood cells free for other tasks, thus saving the body considerable effort while strengthening its resistance to disease.

However, if you eat something cooked after eating something raw, leucocytosis doesn't happen. The body responds only to the first bite of food. For that reason, it's sensible to begin every meal with a taste of something raw. If you have to feed your pet something that has been pasteurized, baked, canned, boiled or heated well above body temperature, give him or her a raw food first, such as a carrot or even a piece of grass to nibble on.

Cooked food should always be accompanied by digestive enzyme supplements; see page 99.

Insuring Meat Safety

What about meat safety? No one except the meat industry denies that our meat inspection standards are a scandal. Organically raised beef and poultry are not necessarily problem-free, but reputable brands take pains to provide healthy products. Unfortunately, the organic meat and poultry sold in health food stores is usually frozen and always expensive. Here in New York, Coleman beef and Bell & Evans poultry are the best supermarket brands, and they are often marked down on the last day of sale. Kosher beef and poultry may not be organically raised, but their inspection process insures that no diseased meat goes to market, unlike U.S. Department of Agriculture guidelines that allow inspectors to approve chickens with cancerous tumors. High-speed conveyor belts and a shortage of inspectors make careful examination in most poultry plants the exception rather than the rule.

The phobia Americans share about raw meat is a fear of contamination. Although all the evidence suggests that a healthy animal will thrive on raw meat without any special treatment, we worry about new and lethal strains of *E.coli* in beef or *Salmonella* in eggs and chicken. Supermarket meat, fish and poultry carry warning labels (cook thoroughly or else) and eggs are considered so risky that some lawmakers have tried to ban undercooked eggs in restaurants. That's an extreme measure, but it's prudent to keep dangerous bacteria to a minimum. Many cases of food poisoning have been traced to the careless handling of raw meat and poultry around cutting boards, counters, cupboard doors, refrigerator handles and other kitchen surfaces. Even more are caused by incorrect storage. Don't leave meat, fish or poultry standing at room temperature; refrigerate it and keep it cold until ready to use.

Healthy cats and dogs can eat just about any meat and survive, if not thrive. Their stomachs contain high concentrations of hydrochloric acid and digestive juices and their digestive tracts host an abundance of beneficial bacteria, making it difficult for harmful bacteria to survive. The following disinfecting methods are more for the protection of people than pets, although any animal that's been fed only packaged, processed food probably needs protection, too, until its digestive system recovers.

To disinfect raw meat or eggs in the shell, follow any of the following procedures. The meat should be in large pieces; these procedures are not recommended for ground meat.

1. Soak the meat in a solution of 1/2 teaspoon original formula Clorox bleach per gallon of water for 15 to 20 minutes, then soak in plain water for 10 minutes.

2. Soak the meat in a sink or bowl containing cold water and several drops of 35 percent food-grade hydrogen peroxide. Use enough to create small bubbles in the water but not enough to change the meat's color. Soak for 10 minutes, then rinse in plain water.

3. Soak the meat in a sink or bowl containing cold water and 30 or more drops of liquid grapefruit seed extract; let stand five minutes and drain. Alternatively, add 20 or more drops to a 32-ounce spray bottle of filtered or distilled water, then spray on meat or poultry and rinse in clean water.

Note that any of the above methods can be used to disinfect raw fruits and vegetables. Use a separate soak solution for each type of food. In addition, dilute solutions of bleach, hydrogen peroxide or grapefruit seed extract can be used to disinfect sponges, refrigerator surfaces, countertops, floors and appliance handles.

4. Dip the meat in very hot water. In 1992, the journal *Epidemiology and Infection* reported that meat can be sterilized by placing it for 10 to 20 seconds in water that has been heated to 80° C. (176° F.). Doing so leaves the surface of the meat "virtually sterile." In a large pan, heat water just until active bubbles form at the bottom or check the temperature with a kitchen thermometer; water at sea level reaches a rolling boil at 212° F. Remove from heat. Lift the meat with tongs, immerse it for 10 to 20 seconds and let it drain in the sink.

At about 150° F., hot water from the tap won't disinfect raw meat but it will warm refrigerated meat to body temperature, a recommended step in meal preparation.

Components of a Healthy Diet

The Importance of Fat

Fats, not carbohydrates, are the primary fuel for our furry friends. Dogs and cats should not be fed excessive amounts of fat, such as the thick fat trimmed from a steak, but it's a mistake to try to remove all fat from the diet. A lack of essential fatty acids, which is found in pets fed grain-based commercial weight-loss foods, can seriously disrupt the animal's health. By following Dr. Billinghurst's advice and making meaty bones the foundation of your feeding plan, you can provide most of what your dog or cat needs in the way of fats, protein and minerals with a single food.

Fish is another important source of essential fatty acids, but because pollution is so widespread, try to find fish caught in clean water or raised organically. An immaculate Japanese restaurant, market or sushi bar is a good source of raw fish, for these establishments have strict standards of freshness; other good sources are clean lakes or rivers in which you go fishing yourself, organic fish farms and fish markets that receive prompt shipments of fish from clean waters.

If you prefer to cook fish, try wrapping fish steaks or filets in parchment with a minced clove of garlic, steam it for several minutes and serve with a digestive enzyme after removing the bones. The no-cooked-bones rule applies to fish as well as chicken and other meats.

If you feed raw fish that was caught more than an hour before feeding, scald it in very hot water for a few minutes to soften the flesh before serving. Be sure to feed the heads, which contain the body's richest supply of vitamins. Serve fish often if your breed developed on a fish diet (Portuguese Water Dogs, Newfoundlands, Scandinavian breeds and Arctic sled dogs, for example); otherwise, serve it three to four times a month. Of the canned fish available, the most popular among holistic pet care experts are sardines. The oil from a sardine may be added to other foods for flavor, as may the oil or water from a can of tuna. These additions often help finicky pets adjust to new foods. Because it isn't raw, canned fish should be supplemented with digestive enzymes and raw foods such as pureed greens or finely minced vegetables.

If desired, a pet's diet can be supplemented with essential fatty acid (EFA) or gamma-linolenic acid (GLA) products, such as evening primrose, borage seed, flaxseed, salmon, cod liver and other oils. Avocados are an excellent source of healthy fats, especially when accompanied by unrefined sea salt, which, according to biochemist Jacques de Langre, improves the oil's assimilation.

Rancidity is a serious problem in fats and oils. To avoid it, keep oils refrigerated. Rancid oils destroy biotin and vitamin E, and the fats in meat and meat by-products are sometimes rancid even before they are used in processed pet foods. Dry pet foods stored for long periods are another source of rancid fats. Obviously, an animal eating a well-prepared home diet never encounters rancidity.

Vegetable oils are frequently recommended for both dogs and cats. These oils should be cold-pressed and refrigerated in tightly sealed glass bottles to avoid rancidity. Safflower and corn oil are high in linoleic acid, an important unsaturated fatty acid, but for every vote in favor of safflower oil, there is one against it because of its Omega 3-Omega 6 fatty acid imbalance. Cats don't metabolize unsaturated fats as well as dogs, a reflection of their more restricted carnivorous diet. Dr. Pottenger's cats thrived on cod liver oil, which they received daily. Many holistic veterinarians report good results from feeding cats olive oil or a changing assortment of vegetable and fish oils. For both dogs and cats a variety of supplemental oils such as flaxseed, olive, corn, wheatgerm, salmon, cod liver and other oils fed on a rotating basis should supply whatever the animal needs without creating a nutritional imbalance.

Remember that oils are best accompanied by digestive enzymes for maximum assimilation.

Eggs and Organ Meats

Raw eggs are a health concern because egg whites contain avidin, a protein that interferes with the body's absorption of biotin, a B-complex vitamin. Because cooking neutralizes avidin, many pet nutritionists recommend cooking eggs before serving them to animals. However, foxes, coyotes and wild dogs and cats are fond of raiding bird nests or chicken coops and eating raw eggs, shell and all. In the study that showed avidin's adverse effect on biotin, animals were fed excessive quantities of raw egg white, many times what they would consume in the wild or at home. For these reasons, a growing number of veterinarians and other experts recommend feeding raw egg, although opinion remains divided as to whether the whites should be fed. If your pet has a strong digestive system, you can feed both the whole egg and its shell, which can be pureed in a food processor with other foods; otherwise, feed the yolk by itself.

Some dogs and cats are allergic to eggs. Alfred Plechner described a poodle whose face swelled grotesquely whenever he ate eggs. "Years ago," he wrote, "eggs were used in preparing distemper vaccines for dogs. Eggs were dropped from the formulation, however, after they were found to be causing allergic reactions in many animals."

Dogs and cats raised on a well-balanced raw food diet are less likely to develop food sensitivities or have impaired digestive systems than those fed commercial pet foods; they can usually enjoy fresh raw eggs the way their wild cousins do. As Francis Pottenger proved, eggs from naturally raised free-range chickens are more nutritious, and no doubt less allergenic, than chickens confined to indoor coops.

What about organ meats? Organs are a rich source of nutrients not found in muscle meats and are highly recommended for occasional use. Unless you have access to organically raised meat, liver can be a problem because the liver's task is to remove toxins from the body, and many such toxins remain stored there. The kidneys perform a similar filtering function. Look for the livers and kidneys of organically raised animals, the fresher the better, and other fresh, raw organ meats as available. Always introduce unusual or unfamiliar foods gradually, adding small amounts to your pet's dinner until the new food is accepted.

The herbalist Juliette de Bairacli Levy, still famous in Europe for the Afghan hounds she raised on raw meat and herbs, has written extensively about raw diets for pets. She recommends serving meat in large chunks rather than minced, since animals in the wild don't grind their meat. It's often easier, though, to introduce organ meats or unfamiliar types of meat by grinding them with more familiar fare. If your pet is not used to them, grind organ meats with equal or larger quantities of lamb, beef or chicken, mixing in kelp and other herbs for a nutrient-rich addition to its regular food. This mixture, which freezes well, can be added in small amounts every few days.

On the Use of Grains

Almost all of the veterinarians and nutritionists I interviewed for this book recommend cooked grains for both cats and dogs, noting their impressive nutritional content and pointing out that in the wild these animals consume grains when they eat the digestive organs of prey.

But as Russell Swift, D.V.M., explained in the June 1996 edition of *Natural Pet,* a growing number of veterinarians active in the American Holistic Veterinary Medical Association question the use of grains in commercial and home-prepared pet foods. Their argument is that oats, wheat, rice and barley are really not part of the natural diet of wild dogs and cats because in the true natural setting, grains hardly exist at all. The argument that "dogs and cats eat animals that have grains in their digestive tracts" doesn't hold up to scrutiny, he wrote. Not only are grains not a substantial part of a truly wild animal's diet but dogs and cats do not require the nutrients in complex carbohydrates and the other nutrients in grains are readily available in other dietary ingredients. For example, B vitamins are found in organ meats and trace minerals come from fruits and vegetables. Last, before grains can be digested, they must be cooked or sprouted, then thoroughly chewed. "Carnivores do not chew much," Swift observed, "and they certainly don't cook or grow sprouts."

Why have grains become so "in-grained" in pet feeding? Swift says that to the best of his knowledge, grains were introduced by the pet food industry, where their high carbohydrate content provides cheap calories and helps bind ingredients. Grains give bulk to pet foods, an important consideration in customer satisfaction. A large quantity at a low price makes grain-based foods seem practical and substantial. Thanks to 60 years of advertising and availability, grain-based foods are familiar to all. In fact, notes Swift, "We have become so used to feeding grains to dogs and cats that most of us get nervous when we decide not to use them."

However, grains can generate a host of problems for our animal companions. It is difficult for dogs and cats to produce the quantity of amylase enzyme necessary for carbohydrate digestion and assimilation; the proteins in grains are less digestible than animal proteins; foreign, nonnutritive protein and carbohydrate particles irritate and weaken the immune system, often resulting in allergies and chronic immune problems; and the demand for amylase so stresses the pancreas that Swift and others believe grain consumption is a likely cause of diabetes, pancreatitis and other digestive tract disorders. Add dental calculus problems and you have an impressive list of conditions that may be linked to grain consumption.

Pat McKay, an animal nutritionist and author of the book *Reigning Cats and Dogs,* worked closely with Celeste Yarnall, the author of *Cat Care, Naturally,* when Yarnall established her supremely healthy line of Tonkinese and Oriental shorthair cats. Since their books' publication, both authors have substantially reduced the amount of grain they recommend. "I now feed a small amount of oatmeal or barley flakes for their soluble fiber and gamma-linolenic acid (GLA) to both dogs and cats," Yarnall told me, "about 10 to 15 percent of the total amount by volume for cats and no more than 30 percent for dogs. I prefer vegetables and yams puréed raw in a food processor or thoroughly baked and served with an enzyme supplement."

McKay has completely removed grains from her recipes and uses only raw vegetables, including sweet potatoes, feeding 75 percent raw meat and 25 percent raw vegetables to both dogs and cats.

When feeding grains, here are some steps worth taking. Consider your pet's breed and its history. Breeds developed in Scotland, Ireland and England may have more of an affinity for oats than those developed in other parts of the world. Rye is the common grain of Scandinavian countries. Breeds developed in Asia may tolerate rice well. The most common grain in your breed's country of origin may be easier for the animal to tolerate. According to some authorities, the number-one cause of allergies in dogs is soybeans, followed by wheat and corn. Wheat allergies are common in people, hence the increasing popularity of "alternative" grains such as amaranth, millet, barley, brown rice, teff and quinoa. If you plan to feed grain, experiment with different types.

If your dog or cat has symptoms that might be traced to food allergies or sensitivities, test your pet for specific grains (see food sensitivity testing, page 93). Wheat is by far the most widely used grain in American pet foods, but any grain may cause problems for individual cats and dogs.

Make the grains you use more digestible by soaking raw rolled or flaked grains in raw milk, water or yogurt, or sprout whole grains (see page 108) and, as soon as they sprout, grind or purée them with a digestive enzyme powder containing amylase, the enzyme that digests carbohydrates; let the mixture stand for 20 minutes or longer before feeding. If desired, sprouted grains can be lightly cooked and served with an enzyme supplement.

Dairy Products

Raw milk, especially raw goat's milk, is one of the most widely prescribed foods for puppies, kittens, cats and dogs. Raw cow's milk or sheep's milk is also recommended.

The milk that causes problems for pets is pasteurized, homogenized, condensed, septic-packaged, "long life" or, worst of all, sweetened condensed milk. If it's been heated above body temperature, be suspicious. Also, try to buy organically raised milk, which does not contain the growth hormones, antibiotics or pesticide residues found in most American milk. As Dr. Pottenger showed when he compared the deficient raw milk of the hay-fed dairy cows of Los Angeles with that of foraging cows of Denver in the 1930s, the most nutritious and "alive" milk comes from cows that graze on fresh grass and other vegetation in the open air and sunshine.

Are dairy products good for adult cats and dogs? Here we find a controversy. No adult in the wild has a reliable source of milk, and after weaning, dogs and cats lose their ability to produce lactase, the enzyme that digests lactose or milk sugar. The symptoms of a lactose intolerance include bloating, gas, flatulence, diarrhea and abdominal discomfort.

At the same time, dairy products can be excellent sources of protein and other nutrients. If your dog or cat enjoys dairy products, it is worth experimenting with raw milk products and digestive enzymes. Lactaid, a lactase supplement, digests milk sugar; other enzymes digest the proteins and other nutrients in pasteurized milk. Enzyme supplementation is appropriate whenever using packaged or powdered goat's milk. Nothing compares with milk fresh from the cow or goat, but these substitutes are at least better than milk straight from the supermarket carton.

Yogurt and kefir, which are cultured milk products, contain "friendly" bacteria, combat the overgrowth of pathogens and help restore intestinal balance, which is especially important after an animal takes antibiotics. In addition, yogurt and other milk cultures are associated with reduced rates of cancer, infectious diseases and diarrhea.

Beneficial bacteria are grown in laboratories for use in acidophilus supplements, such as *Lactobacillus acidophilus*, *L. bulgaricus*, *Streptococcus thermophilus* and *Bifidobacteria*. These bacteria have an ancient history, for people have been culturing soured milk foods for centuries. Lactic acid is the common by-product of the fermentation of the milk of cows, goats, sheep, camels and mares. Lactic acid fermentation breaks down fat, sugar and proteins to make milk more digestible.

Cultured milk dishes are always best freshly made, when their taste is superior and their bacteria most lively. As yogurt ages, its *L.acidophilus* competes with *L. bulgaricus,* and the result can be dead acidophilus long before the product's expiration date. For those who want to provide yogurt's health benefits for their companion animals:

1. Buy plain unflavored yogurt labeled with the National Yogurt Association's "live and active cultures" seal, which recognizes yogurts that deliver 10 million or more live bacteria per gram at the expiration date, or check for the words "Contains live cultures."

2. Buy acidophilus powders from your health food store's refrigerator (look for amber glass jars with distant expiration dates) and sprinkle it on your pet's food or give acidophilus supplements after a meal, when the stomach is less acidic. Some acidophilus capsules and tablets are designed to break down later in the digestive process and a few brands claim to survive stomach acid. Check labels. Acidophilus powders can be used as yogurt starters.

3. Use purchased yogurt, acidophilus powder or yogurt starter to make your own. Freshly made yogurt, kefir and other cultured milk dishes contain the maximum number of beneficial bacteria.

Fruits and Nuts

As Juliette de Bairacli Levy wrote, "The dog and even the cat will eat many varieties of fruits and berries with much pleasure," a statement most of us can verify. Some cats crave cucumbers, cantaloupe or watermelon and many dogs enjoy apples. Both the fox in the Bible and de Bairacli Levy's Afghan hounds were famous for their love of grapes, her Irish Wolfhound bitch hunted wild raspberries, spaniels of her acquaintance grazed avidly on currant bushes,Lurcher dogs of gypsies with whom she traveled raided strawberry fields and in the Middle East, jackals were a nuisance in melon fields as they went from fruit to fruit taking bites.

I have spoken with animal nutritionists who claim that fruit is bad for dogs and cats, that it's impossible to digest and causes nothing but problems, but I haven't found this to be so with my pets or other fruit-loving cats or dogs of our acquaintance. Whenever they indulge in apples, mangos, grapes, papayas, blueberries, bananas or other fruit, their stools remain normal although the color sometimes changes, there are no identifiable undigested pieces except for occasional bits of peel, and I assume that the vitamins, minerals and other nutrients in the fruit are digested and absorbed. Fruits are of course a staple food for birds around the world, and occasional fruits supplement the diets of rabbits and other animals.

Nuts are another food pets enjoy. As de Bairacli Levy wrote, "Many dogs will themselves crack open walnuts and hazel nuts and carefully extract the contents, discarding all the bad pieces." Nuts provide natural oils, vitamins and minerals. They can be served whole or chopped, grated or ground and mixed with food.

Vegetables

Carrots, peas, green beans, artichokes, parsnips, squash — there's probably at least one vegetable your dog or cat adores.

When organically grown in fertile soil in abundant sunshine, carrots top the list as one of the best additions you can make to the diet of not just your rabbit but your dog, cat, bird, horse, goat, almost any other pet and yourself as well. Carrot juice alone can sustain life for long periods and, in combination with a balanced diet, finely minced carrot greens, puréed or pressed carrots, freshly made raw carrot juice or the pulp left after making carrot juice in a centrifugal juicer are all significant sources of vitamins, minerals and other healing substances. In fact, whenever you make juice for yourself, save some of the pulp for your dog, cat, bird or rabbit. Dr. Norman Walker, who invented the Norwalk hydraulic juice press, proved that the most nutritious part of fruits and vegetables processed in a centrifugal or macerating juicer is the pulp that most users throw away.

In his book *Live Food Juices,* H.E. Kirschner, M.D., described an 11-year-old Dalmatian diagnosed in 1961 with nephritis, an inflammation of the kidney that caused him to lose bladder control several times daily, and a large intestinal tumor that his veterinarian considered inoperable and probably malignant. One week later, the tumor had grown so rapidly that the dog was expected to die within days. His owner, who had been feeding the dog a canned food recommended by the veterinarian, stopped when the dog grew weak and trembled convulsively for 24 hours. Instead, she gave him carrot juice extracted from a centrifugal juicer, gradually increasing his intake until he was drinking two quarts daily. When the owner reported this in a letter to Dr. Kirschner, the Dalmatian had been drinking carrot juice for a year, during which time his tumor stopped growing, he gained weight, his kidney function returned to normal and he could withhold his urine for eight or nine hours in comfort.

Collard greens, though not as sweet as carrots, may be the most nutritious green vegetable, with exceptionally high levels of vitamin A, vitamin C, calcium and potassium. Like carrots, they contain less well-known compounds with important healing functions. By adding small amounts in your pet's food every day or two, you provide exceptional nutrients and the fresh factors vital to good health.

Collard greens, wheat grass and other grasses are concentrated sources of chlorophyll. Much has been made of chlorophyll's similarity to hemoglobin, for both are blood: chlorophyll is the green lifeblood of plants, hemoglobin the red lifeblood of animals, and their molecular structure is almost identical. The hemoglobin molecule has iron at its center, while the chlorophyll molecule is built around magnesium, but in every other way, these two complex molecules match exactly. No doubt because of this affinity, chlorophyll is easily absorbed by the body, where its healing properties can be dramatic.

Feed your pets a variety of fresh, raw foods, but try to include raw carrots and greens every day.

Parsley, sage, thyme, rosemary, oregano, purslane, cleavers, comfrey, dandelion greens, collard greens, wheat grass, buckwheat grass and other green herbs are appropriate for both dogs and cats, but these animals aren't really designed to digest vegetable fibers. To help your pet benefit from the nutrients in vegetables, an intermediate step is necessary. Either purée, finely grind or grate the vegetables (green herbs, carrots, parsnips), lightly steam them (artichoke, potatoes) and serve them with digestive enzymes or put them through a juicer raw. Some markets and health food stores sell frozen, organically grown carrot juice; many health food stores have juice bars equipped with macerating juicers or hydraulic juice presses which produce juice that keeps for several days without losing nutrients; or you can make your own at home.

Another way to make vegetables more digestible is to slice, grate, chop or purée cucumbers, carrots or other vegetables, layer them with a small amount of unrefined sea salt and press them in a Japanese salad press (see Resources for this chapter in the Appendix) or under a weight, such as a heavy plate. This creates lactic acid fermentation, which improves digestion, increases the absorption of nutrients, feeds the beneficial bacteria that live in your pet's intestines and may reduce the risk of cancer, bowel disease and other illnesses.

Garlic, Onion and the Heinz-body Factor

Because their sulfur compounds and volatile oils are so beneficial to human health, many herbalists and nutritionists assume that garlic, onions, chives, shallots and other pungent members of the lily family are good for all animals, and the more, the better.

Unfortunately, this isn't so. *The American Journal of Veterinary Research* (January 1992) reported that onion-induced oxidation of canine red blood cells has caused severe reactions in some dogs, even those who consumed small portions of the vegetable. If enough onion is ingested, a sensitive dog may develop anemia, weakness, pale mucous membranes and an increased respiratory rate.

More recently, researchers have warned that garlic can be hazardous to cats and to herbivores such as rabbits. There is now a great deal of controversy and confusion over garlic and onions. Can they be toxic? How much is too much?

As herbalist Gregory Tilford explained in the August 1997 issue of *Natural Pet*, Heinz-body anemia is a potentially life-threatening blood disease caused by the excessive and prolonged ingestion of garlic, onions, turnips, kale, rape (canola) and other plants rich in vitamin K. Scientists theorize that chemical compounds in these plants deplete a naturally occurring glucose enzyme, glucose 6-phosphate dehydrogenase or G6PD, whose special function is to protect the cell walls of red blood cells. G6PD depletion causes oxidative damage to red blood cells, leading to the formation of "Heinz bodies," which trigger their rejection from the bloodstream, resulting in dark-colored urine. If this dumping process continues unchecked, the animal can become anemic and eventually die.

Nonetheless, garlic and onions have been fed to animals of all shapes and sizes for centuries. Both of these pungent herbs fight infection, help prevent cancer, expel tapeworms, inhibit protozoan infections such as *Giardia lamblia*, make animals less attractive hosts to all parasites, including fleas, and prevent blood clotting. In parts of France, race horses with clotting disorders are fed garlic to prevent this problem. In short, garlic and onions are powerful medicines.

Most dogs, cats, birds, rabbits and other animals benefit from the occasional addition of garlic and/or onion to their food. It may be that animals fed a raw diet are less likely to suffer from Heinz-body anemia than those fed a monotonous cooked, packaged or processed diet, so the following guidelines may be most appropriate for those making the transition from cooked to raw foods or for those who continue to feed a commercially prepared diet. As Tilford noted, the recorded cases of allium poisoning typically involve onion doses exceeding 0.5 percent of the animals' body weight, so that a healthy dog weighing 60 pounds would have to ingest a 5-ounce onion or several cloves of garlic to begin the Heinz-body process. Red blood cell regenerate quickly in healthy animals, so the overdose would have to be repeated frequently to cause harm.

In general, dogs may tolerate garlic better than cats do, and cats may tolerate onions better than dogs. Some veterinarians recommend that cats never be given garlic, but most agree that small amounts from time to time do far more good than harm. Although any animal can have a sensitivity to any food, it is probably safe to give your dog garlic in the quantities recommended in this book for several days per week, such as five days on and two days off. Smaller amounts of onion or garlic are appropriate for cats on a less frequent schedule, such as two days on and three days off. In either case, going without garlic altogether is appropriate for one week per month.

For birds, rabbits, sheep, cattle, horses and other herbivores, consider feeding garlic once or twice per week. To treat specific illnesses, larger quantities and daily consumption for seven to ten days is probably safe and effective, but prolonged, uninterrupted, high doses may pose a risk. Garlic and onions are not appropriate supplements for infant puppies, kittens and other very young animals because their ability to manufacture red blood cells is still developing; wait until they are three or four months old before feeding these foods on a regular basis.

As with any food or supplement, watch your animal for signs of discomfort or distress. If they occur, decrease the dosage or discontinue the food altogether. Keep in mind that because garlic is a natural blood thinner, it can prevent clotting when it's desirable, such as during surgery. If your animal is about to be spayed, neutered or have any other surgical procedure, discontinue garlic for a week or two prior to the operation.

Chocolate and Carob

Chocolate is toxic to dogs, cats, birds and other small animals, although I know poodles who receive regular handouts and other dogs who swallow occasional candy bars, wrapper and all. Serious problems arise when a dog with a sweet tooth finds itself alone with a Valentine's Day sampler box or a stash of baking chocolate, for overdoses can be fatal. In susceptible animals, chocolate's theobromine triggers epileptic seizures and can damage heart tissue as well as cause internal bleeding in the digestive tract. Gardeners should know that chocolate hull mulch, which is wonderfully fragrant when you first apply it, has killed dogs who swallowed it.

Carob, which dogs enjoy just as much, is a safe alternative. This cocoa-brown seed pod, also known as St. Johns bread, is often used as a substitute for chocolate. Health food stores carry roasted carob, but if you'd like to try raw carob powder, look for Jaffee Brothers in the Resources listed for this chapter in the Appendix. Juliette de Bairacli Levy considers carob an important food for puppies and adult dogs and credits it with preventing hip dysplasia. Even if it doesn't, carob contains protein and is rich in calcium and phosphorus. If you ever find whole carob pods at a health food store or ethnic market, buy them for your dog, teething puppy, bird or rabbit.

Sugar and Honey

Sugar is a frowned-upon ingredient that often appears in commercial pet foods, snack foods and treats. Before putting honey in the same negative category, consider the claims made on its behalf. "I believe I could not successfully rear domestic dogs without this remarkable antiseptic food," wrote Juliette de Bairacli Levy, and her followers around the world agree. Lions, bears and other wild animals are fond of honey. According to de Bairacli Levy, in addition to being a source of energy, honey is a nerve tonic and the only heart stimulant which is not a drug. In addition, it inhibits the growth of harmful bacteria in the digestive tract. She recommends feeding honey to puppies and kittens with their milk and to sick dogs in their water or in balls of honey put in their mouths.

Raw, unpasteurized honey is not recommended for human infants because it may lead to botulism, a result of the infant's immature digestion. Although I have read warnings about giving raw honey to puppies, I haven't found any case of illness resulting from such feeding and wonder if the warnings come from an assumption that all infants — human and canine — are at risk; however, they are entirely different.

Do Pets Require a "Balanced Diet"?

The notion that every meal an animal eats should be completely balanced is a recent invention resulting from the use of packaged foods. If you were restricted to the same food in the same amount every day for the rest of your life, each identical meal would have to be nutritionally balanced because you would have no other source of nutrients. But you don't eat that way, you don't feed your children that way and animals in the wild don't eat that way. It's completely unnatural. What matters is not whether tonight's dinner contains 100 percent of every nutrient your body requires but whether all of the combined foods you eat today or this week provide them.

Monotony is not only boring, it's dangerous. Cats who eat only tuna and dogs who eat only one kind of meat eventually suffer serious health problems. So do pets who eat the same processed food at every meal.

Here in the United States, feathers, beaks, hooves, horns, diseased tissue and cancerous tumors all count as pet food protein, and a pet food label's "guaranteed nutritional analysis" says nothing about the source of whatever it examines. Pet food manufacturers are allowed to use "4-D meats," which are rejected for human consumption because the animals they came from were dead, diseased, dying or disabled on arrival at the slaughterhouse. Animal meal, a primary pet food ingredient, can legally contain ground feathers, nails, claws, cartilage, tendons, bones, blood and fecal waste. In 1983 the Pet Food Institute convinced the U.S. Food and Drug Administration (FDA) to allow changes on pet food labels so that cheese rinds could be called "cheese," corn husks and peanut shells could be called "vegetable fiber," hydrolyzed chicken feathers could be called "poultry protein products," and ground bones could be called "processed animal protein." The Humane Society of the United States and the American Holistic Veterinary Medical Association strongly opposed the changes, which hide important information from the consumer.

The chemical analysis of ingredients on pet food labels is meaningless no matter what their origin because all commercial pet foods are cooked and, as Dr. Pottenger proved 60 years ago, cooked food is deficient by definition. A variety of high-quality meats, bones and other foods served raw or minimally processed in combination with a variety of supplements will supply everything a dog or cat needs for perfect health. The key word here is variety. Why feed your pet under laboratory-controlled conditions when its species evolved on a constantly changing assortment of foods? Yes, cats require more protein than dogs, but neither needs a computer-equipped lab technician for basic menu planning.

Feeding the Adult Dog

The following are guidelines for adult dogs of most breeds. Feed two meals per day and nothing between meals. Depending on your dog's training schedule, the latter instruction may be unrealistic, but the fewer between-meal snacks, the better. If you feed twice a day, concentrate carbohydrates and fruit (including avocado) in the morning meal, then meat and vegetables in the evening. Supplements can be given with either meal. If your dog is exceptionally active, like working retrievers during hunting season, feed as much and as often as necessary.

Quantities depend on many factors: your dog's breed, size, metabolism, exercise and work load, even the weather. Working Alaskan sled dogs need thousands of calories a day, while warm-weather couch potatoes need hardly any. Large dogs need more, small dogs less. Dogs fed a natural diet are guided by an internal appetite control that directs them to eat as much as they need and then stop, so once your dog is used to fresh, raw food, your best guide will be his or her appetite. A general rule of thumb is to feed a daily ration of 2 to 3 percent of the dog's body weight in bones and meat. In a 50-pound dog, this would be about 1 to 1-1/2 pounds of bones and meat. Start with approximately this amount and adjust the quantity as needed.

Suggested Breakfast for a 50-Pound Dog

Serve any two of the following to a dog who spends an hour or more in active outdoor exercise. Increase the quantity and/or selection for more active or larger dogs; decrease for less active or smaller dogs. Serve different foods for breakfast every day to ensure variety. Supply abundant clean, pure water throughout the day.

- 1 or 2 bananas, apples, melon servings or other fruit; *or*
- 1 avocado sprinkled with unrefined sea salt; *or*
- 1/4 to 1/2 cup raw oat flakes or similar raw, whole grain cereal flakes or raw, sprouted wheat or rye, soaked in 1/2 cup raw milk, goat milk, raw fruit or vegetable juice, fresh yogurt or water; *or*
- 1 cup Lactaid-treated cottage cheese, live-culture yogurt or kefir; *or*
- 1/2 cup raw milk cheese and 1 raw egg.

Suggested Dinner for a 50-Pound Dog

• 1 to 1-1/2 lbs raw bones and meat.

• 2 to 4 Tbsp. finely minced fresh wheat grass, dandelion greens, collard greens or other fresh herbs.

• 1/4 cup finely minced or puréed raw vegetables (carrot, parsnip, pepper, cucumber, etc.) or pressed vegetables.

Although some experts prescribe large amounts of bran as roughage, grated or finely cut raw vegetables and raw bones provide all the roughage a dog's digestive tract requires. Grain sensitivities are so widespread, it's worth experimenting with a grain-free diet, or at least substituting other grains for wheat and wheat bran. Constipation should never be a problem on a natural diet, especially if your dog receives sufficient exercise, water and well-planned meals.

Feeding Puppies

Infant Puppies:

When nursing puppies are large enough to drink water from a bowl, keep it supplied with clean, pure water (not tap water) to which you can add a catalyst-altered water extract (see Willard Water concentrate, page 106) and a pinch of unrefined sea salt. Begin supplying warm (barely heated) raw milk, if available, at about four weeks. The preferred milk is raw goat's milk.

If raw milk isn't available, look for pasteurized cow's milk that has not been homogenized (sold in many health food stores and some supermarkets) or buy dried or packaged goat's milk from the health food store. Because these are not raw milks, treat them with Lactaid, use them to make fresh yogurt or kefir and add a digestive enzyme, such as ProZyme, when feeding. Warm the milk, yogurt or kefir to body temperature by placing it in a glass or ceramic cup in a bowl of hot water, or heat it gently on the stove just until warm.

As nursing puppies approach their fifth week, de Bairacli Levy recommends thickening their milk with whole-grain flaked cereals. Her basic recipe for "tree bark gruel" is 2 Tbsp. flaked barley, 1 Tbsp. powdered slippery elm bark, 1 Tbsp. powdered arrowroot and 1 tsp. powdered dill weed. To this you can add 1 to 2 tsp. powdered raw carob (see Resources) or roasted carob powder, which is beneficial for puppies. Mix the combined powders with an equal amount of honey to form a paste. Add a small amount to lukewarm milk to create a thin soup as the puppies' first solid food. Every few days add more of the honey paste to create a thicker gruel until you are mixing about 1 part paste with 3 parts milk.

You may want to give your puppies a colostrum supplement after weaning. Bovine colostrum has become a popular human food supplement because it increases resistance to infection and it may keep puppies at a high level of natural immunity. Adapt label directions to the pups' weight.

Toward the fifth week, begin to add raw meat cut into tiny pieces and sprinkle it with a small amount of an enzyme powder containing bromelain, a proteolytic enzyme derived from pineapple, or any enzyme that digests meat. Apply the powder a few hours before serving and leave the meat at room temperature; warm it to body temperature just before serving.

A first meat meal for an average size puppy is about one teaspoon. Increase the quantity every three days until at eight weeks of age, the average-size breed consumes two tablespoons finely minced meat twice daily. By that time, the puppy should be fully weaned.

Weaning to four months:

Breakfast: Combine raw milk or yogurt with the barley-honey mixture described above, using roughly equal proportions of powder and milk. Lunch: Raw whole grain flakes (oats, wheat, barley, rye or mixed flakes), soaked overnight in yogurt, carrot juice or raw milk. Before serving add 1 finely grated apple, 1/2 tsp. vegetable or fish oil, a pinch of unrefined sea salt and a sprinkle of ProZyme or similar enzyme powder.

Late afternoon: Approximately 4 Tbsp. raw, shredded meat cut into increasingly larger pieces. Beef and other meats can be alternated with fish and chicken.

Dinner: Approximately 4 Tbsp. raw meat with bones or a raw egg plus 1 tsp. cod liver or other oil, a pinch of seaweed or kelp powder, 1/2 tsp. finely minced raw green leaves and any appropriate food-based vitamin/mineral supplements.

Teething puppies need bones to chew on, so keep them supplied with raw bones between meals. A puppy lying in her crate chewing on a bone is doing useful puppy work, nourishing her body, strengthening her teeth and staying out of mischief.

After four months:

Three meals a day, increasing the food supply as needed. After eight months, feed twice daily, at noon and in the evening, feeding cereal with milk in the morning and meat in the evening.

After four months, schedule one day per week for a half-day fast (serve only water and raw but not meaty bones from after lunch until the next morning) and once per month make this a full-day fast (water and raw bones only). Adult dogs can fast on water only one day per week.

Feeding the Adult House Cat

The nutritional needs of cats and dogs are not identical, but the same basic strategies work well for both: the more fresh, raw food you feed and the more variety you offer, the more balanced the result.

Raw bones are essential for good health, and they can be the bones of raw chicken, turkey, game hen, freshly caught fish or other small animals. In addition, occasionally feed your cat the marrow from a beef marrow bone, the kind sold as soup bones.

Raw milk and cultured milk products, such as yogurt or kefir, raw milk cheese, goat's milk, buttermilk or cottage cheese can be fed to cats of all ages, but if they are not used to drinking milk, add Lactaid or a similar milk-digesting enzyme and, if the milk has been pasteurized, add a digestive enzyme such as Prozyme as well. Begin by serving small portions of milk and increase the amount slowly. If desired, add occasional flaked whole grains such as oats or barley to the milk.

Meat and bones, which should make up most of your cat's diet, can be any of the selections listed for dogs. Cut the meat into chunks so your cat can exercise his teeth and jaws, ripping into it. Cats in the wild don't eat ground meat and their domestic cousins are just as well-equipped to deal with chunky pieces or even whole game hens. Of course, if your cat has the dental problems that come with eating commercial pet foods, he may not be able to rip much of anything, so smaller pieces are appropriate. No tabby cat can eat the knuckle bone of a steer, but a healthy cat can bite through all the bones of a raw game hen or small chicken. Invest in the best poultry scissors you can find in order to cut the drumsticks of free-range chicken, which have far denser bones than commercially raised chickens. Try to feed bones every other day or at least twice a week.

Suggested Breakfast for a 10-Pound House Cat

Adjust the following quantities as needed for larger, smaller, younger, older and less or more active cats. Combine ingredients and warm the food slightly before serving.

- 1/2 cup warm raw milk, yogurt or kefir
- 1/8 tsp. borage, evening primrose, fish, vegetable or cod liver oil or an essential fatty acid (EFA) supplement; alternate oils daily
- 1 Tbsp. fresh, raw carrot juice
- 1 pinch unrefined sea salt

  Occasionally for breakfast offer raw watermelon, cantaloupe, cucumber, mango, banana, avocado or other raw fruit. Some cats love raw corn. Encourage your cat to eat a variety of fresh, raw foods, no matter how unlikely this may seem.

  Let your cat determine how much food to supply. Give as much as the animal will eat in 15 to 20 minutes, then remove the food. Supply only water between meals.

Suggested Dinner for a 10-Pound House Cat

- 1/4 lb raw chicken or game hen with bones (include the liver when available) with a pinch of unrefined sea salt and/or a pinch of powdered seaweed (kelp, dulse, etc.)
- 1 tsp. to 1 Tbsp. finely minced fresh wheat grass, collard greens or other greens
- 1 tsp. to 1 Tbsp. finely minced, pureed or pressed raw carrots, peas, beans or other vegetables
- The following are optional ingredients:
  1 minced garlic clove, or capsule equivalent
  Herbal supplements, as appropriate
  Enzyme supplement
  Glandular supplement
  Trace mineral supplement
  Vitamin and/or mineral supplement
  Acidophilus supplement
  As with dogs, the dosages of herbal supplements, vitamins, trace minerals, glandular supplements and other additions depend on conditions being treated and package directions. If the product is designed for human consumption, assume that the human weighs 120 to 150 pounds and adjust the dosage accordingly.

Feeding Kittens

For kittens after three weeks of age, supplement the mother's milk with warm, raw cow's or goat's milk; if raw milk is not available, increase the digestibility of pasteurized milk with Lactaid and other enzyme products, such as Prozyme. De Bairacli Levy encourages kittens as young as two weeks to sip tepid water from a saucer.

After four weeks:

Begin feeding small amounts of tree bark gruel in milk as for puppies (see page 84). Offer four small meals per day, alternating between gruel (honey and tree bark powder) in milk and flaked barley in milk every four hours. One day per week, give smaller amounts less frequently to give the digestion a chance to rest.

After weaning to four months:

Offer the same breakfast, as much as the kitten will eat.

At noon, feed plain milk with any flaked raw grain plus a few drops of vegetable oil (de Bairacli Levy recommends sesame, corn, sunflower or canola oil), plus about 1 tsp. of beaten raw egg, cottage cheese, or buttermilk. On alternating days, add up to 1 tsp. finely ground raw almonds, grated raw carrot or coconut.

At 4:00 p.m., feed raw meat shredded or cut into small pieces with finely minced raw greens. Add up to 1 tsp. raw bran soaked in water for additional fiber.

Four hours later, repeat this dinner with up to 1 tsp. shredded carrot or other vegetable in place of the bran. Add a tiny pinch of unrefined sea salt with the meat.

As the kitten grows, begin feeding small bones, such as those in a chicken breast. Cut the chicken, bones and all, into small pieces. Feed a variety of different meats during the week and alternate oils, greens and puréed vegetables as well. If desired, add occasional food-derived vitamin/mineral supplements, such as Cryofood powder from Standard Process (see Resources), a high quality powdered or liquid brewer's yeast or a multivitamin tablet crushed into a powder. Add a small amount, such as a few drops or a pinch, to one meal every day or every few days.

Feeding Birds

In the wild, birds eat all kinds of things. Parrots, for example, consume seeds, nuts, grains, sprouts, leaves, insects, fruits and occasional mice, small birds and other animals. All birds typically eat a single food if it is plentiful, but when its supply declines, they forage.

Birds kept as pets live on more restricted fare. The basic commercial mix sold for small birds, like finches and canaries, consists of small seeds. Cockatiels eat a mix for small birds with added sunflower seeds. Conures, African greys, Amazons and other large birds are usually fed sunflower seeds, peanuts, red pepper, cracked corn and dried corn. Pelleted food contains these same ingredients shelled and compressed into small morsels. "It looks like gerbil or hamster pellets and is totally nutritious and balanced according to the manufacturers," says Doreen Gluck, "but there are things that birds eat in the wild that we never know about. I think it's important to supplement seed mixes or pelleted food with fresh fruits and vegetables, dried fruit like raisins and all kinds of people food. The only things my birds never eat are chocolate, foods or beverages containing caffeine or anything carbonated. They all eat fresh corn, carrots, apples, grapes, leafy green herbs like dandelion leaves, kelp and a variety of meats. Birds are very sensitive and they have a higher heart rate than other animals, so I don't give them anything that contains chemical preservatives, artificial colors or flavors or anything that might be toxic. I try to feed my birds a well-rounded diet that offers variety, something different every day, not only because it's good for them but because they enjoy change."

According to Fred Bauer, an avicultural nutritionist with 18 years of experience breeding parrots and other birds, "Nutrition-related health problems in captive birds are often traced to the use of synthetic vitamins and isolated minerals. There isn't a pellet on the market that isn't laced with these unnatural substances, and when a bird's diet is changed to supply essential nutrients through whole living foods, persistent health problems often resolve quickly, especially feather plucking and aggressive behavior."

Bauer cautions that the use of disinfectants recommended for use on bird cages and food and water bowls have a long-term deleterious effect because of residue buildup. "Even in very small quantities," he says, "these toxic materials have a profound effect, and it's impossible to rinse away all residual trace of chemical disinfectants or household bleach. Plain soap and water works well, and in the case of a confirmed exposure to serious pathogens, I recommend adding 8 drops of grapefruit seed extract to 2 cups of water as a final rinse or soak."

At the 1994 American Holistic Veterinary Medical Association, veterinarian David McCluggage offered general nutrition guidelines for various birds, emphasizing the importance of organically grown, minimally processed feeds that are free of preservatives and artificial ingredients.

For canaries and finches, which are primarily seed eaters, McCluggage recommends feeding approximately 50 percent mixed small seeds such as rape, niger, poppy and millet. Some species need live animals in their diet, which can be supplied as grubs, meal worms and crickets. Seeds can be sprouted (see page 108) to make them more nutritious and digestible.

Mynah birds can eat a basic seed mix for up 75 percent of the diet, with the remainder including fruits such as apples, raisins, grapes and bananas, plus some meat, such as ground beef.

Bauer, whose China Prairie Psittacine Breeding Facility has tested raw foods and natural supplements on more than 400 parrots of over 50 species, recommends that these birds consume freshly sprouted sunflower seed, yellow corn, oats, brown rice, wheat berries, green peas, garbanzo beans, mung beans, buckwheat, millet, fenugreek, pumpkin seed, sesame seed, quinoa, raddish seed and red clover seed soaked in water containing grapefruit seed extract to prevent the growth of undesirable microorganisms.

McCluggage recommends supplementing all birds with a natural vitamin/mineral product derived from whole foods; his preference is Cryofood from Standard Process, Inc. (see Resources). Bauer supplements his birds' diet with a blend of microalgae, dehydrated barley grass, alfalfa leaf powder, clay, cayenne pepper, garlic, ginger, psyllium, echinacea, pau d'arco, astragalus, ginseng, licorice, kelp, acidophilus and other probiotics and unrefined sea salt. Many birds enjoy whole, fresh cayenne peppers; in some cultures, hot peppers are believed to improve a bird's ability to speak.

Other fresh factors for your bird can include freshly harvested, chopped or shredded comfrey, sage, parsley, chives, carrot tops, beet greens, dandelion greens, dandelion blossoms, calendula blossoms, nasturtiums and other edible flowers, rosemary, cress, chard, spinach, dandelion roots, beets, carrots, fruits and berries. Save the fresh raw seeds from watermelon, papaya, cantaloupe, pumpkin and squash for your feathered friend.

When feeding perishable food, remove leftovers after two to three hours to prevent spoilage. If your bird is used to a single food, he or she may be what McCluggage calls a "seed addict." To help your bird change to a healthier diet, restrict the amount of seed while providing other foods.

Feeding Rabbits

In the wild, rabbits and hares feed mainly on grasses, herbs, tree bark and vegetables. Bugs Bunny is famous for his love of carrots. In addition to fresh air, sunshine, clean water and exercise, your rabbit needs fresh foods for optimum health.

Rabbit books and magazines emphasize the importance of feeding a well-balanced, nutritionally sound diet of pelleted food made of alfalfa hay and other ingredients. They often warn never to give greens such as carrot tops, lettuce or cabbage to rabbits less than six months old because any drastic change in diet can kill them.

That may be true, but not changing from a dried, processed diet can leave your rabbit in the same sad condition as Dr. Pottenger's cats, described at the beginning of this chapter. If your young rabbit has been fed a commercial diet, make the adjustment slowly by adding tiny amounts of greens and carrots, starting with less than 10 percent of the total. In addition, sprinkle an enzyme product like Prozyme on the pelleted food to improve its digestion and assimilation and add a pinch of unrefined sea salt for minute amounts of trace elements.

Older rabbits can make the change more quickly, but with all animals it's a good idea to continue feeding whatever they're used to while slowly changing over to an all-raw diet.

Freshly harvested herbs, grasses, tree prunings, greens, vegetables, edible flowers and occasional seeds and nuts in the shell will keep your rabbit healthy. Grow your own alfalfa, wheat grass, barley grass, buckwheat lettuce and sunflower seedlings in trays as described on page 109; grow carrots, calendula blossoms, sweet peppers and greens such as collards, chard, broccoli de rabe and spinach in your garden; let some carrots and other plants go to seed for your rabbit friend, and offer the seeds from your watermelon, pumpkin and other foods; gather dandelions and other wild herbs away from the air pollution of busy roadways; buy organically grown mixed salad greens at your market or health food store.

If possible, plant a small garden for your rabbit and let her spend some time in it

every day, harvesting whatever suits her fancy. Fresh air and sunshine are just as important to rabbits as other pets, so if you don't have a safe, secure place to let your rabbit run
freely, buy a harness and let her explore at least part of the great outdoors while you hold
the leash.

The Fine Art of Stool Watching

One of the simplest ways to monitor your pet's digestion is to keep careful track of what he or she eats — and to monitor what comes out the
other end.
The most significant difference you will notice as your dog changes from grain-based,
canned or packaged food to more natural fare is that stool size is greatly reduced. Healthy
stools are firm, compact and well-shaped. Depending on the supplements and vegetables you add, they may be colorful — grass green, for example, or carrot orange.

As your dog adjusts to eating raw bones, you will notice mucus-covered stools the
next day as bone residue is eliminated. Remember that too much raw bone too soon can
cause temporary problems in a dog whose digestive tract has been weakened by cooked,
canned or packaged foods. This reaction decreases as the animal's system adjusts and is
unlikely to recur in dogs fed raw bones daily or several times per week.

Obviously, diarrhea is a warning signal. In many cases, diarrhea is a temporary, self-
correcting condition, but diarrhea that doesn't disappear by itself within one day is a
cause for concern. It may be caused by a specific food, which is why food diaries are so
important. Keep track of what your dog eats and, if loose stools always follow a certain
food, eliminate that food and see if the problem disappears. For specific treatments for
diarrhea, see page 370.

The most obvious difference between the stools of dogs and cats fed the natural diet
described here and those fed commercial, grain-based foods is size. With little or no
grain to deal with, dogs fed raw meat produce small, compact stools that are easier to
dispose of.

The fecal matter of other animals deserves attention, too. Dogs are notorious for eating manure, goose droppings, cat litter offerings and even their own stools, a condition
called coprophagia. Although it is usually considered a behavior problem, coprophagia
is probably nutritional. Dogs fed a well-balanced natural diet are less likely to eat their
own feces than dogs on commercial pet foods, and when owners add mineral-rich supplements such as kelp to the food of a dog with this habit, the habit often disappears.

Still, even the best-fed dogs may go out of their way for cow, horse, sheep or goose
manure. Is it disgusting or healthy or what?

Juliette de Bairacli Levy encourages dogs to enjoy these delicacies so long as they
come from vegetarian animals. Manure contains large quantities of active bacteria,

enzymes, minerals and other nutrients. Many holistic veterinarians agree, especially those who keep livestock or grew up on farms. It may not be appetizing to humans, but neither you nor your pet are likely to contract any illness or infection from the animal's habit.

Rabbit owners can inadvertently cause diarrhea in their pets by keeping their cages scrupulously clean. Rabbits produce two types of fecal pellet: pale green droppings that have been through the digestive system once and dark shiny droppings that are the final product. Rabbits must be given access to their first-stage droppings or they develop digestive disorders and vitamin deficiencies.

Allergies in Pets

If your pet has been raised on commercial food, he or she may experience food allergies. Alfred Plechner blames the inferior quality of meat and poultry by-products, brewer's yeast and other pet food ingredients for increasingly common allergic reactions. His "allergic hit list" for dogs includes beef, beef by-products, milk, yeast, corn, corn oil, pork, turkey, eggs, fish, fish oils, wheat and wheat by-products. The list for cats includes beef, beef by-products, tuna, milk, yeast, pork and turkey. In addition, any pet may react to chemical additives, mold, or contaminated drinking water. According to Dr. Plechner, a dog or cat with chronic diarrhea or skin problems, or a cat with urinary tract infections, may be suffering from a food allergy. As an experiment, study the ingredient list of whatever food your dog or cat has been eating, then prepare a high-quality diet based on other foods and supply only clean (filtered, bottled, or distilled) drinking water.

Just as some chemicals provoke allergic reactions in people, they can have a deleterious effect on dogs, cats and other pets. Sodium nitrate, benzoic acid, red dye number 40, blue dye number 2, BHA, BHT, MSG and sodium metabisulfite are commonly used in pet foods as are artificial flavors, sugar, propylene glycol, formalin and ethoxyquin. Pet food manufacturers are defensive about these ingredients, all of which have been approved by the U.S. Food and Drug Administration. As far as the FDA is concerned, no one has proved that any of these ingredients cause health problems in people or pets. At the same time, a growing body of research suggests that artificial colorings have caused cancer, epilepsy and birth defects in laboratory animals, that chemical preservatives have caused liver and kidney disease, birth defects, metabolic stress, behavioral problems, allergic reaction, baldness and brain defects in laboratory animals and that artificial flavors cause nervousness, allergic reactions, and behavior problems in pets.

It would be wonderful if a simple blood or skin test would reveal everything you need to know about your animal's food sensitivities. Unfortunately, blood tests using

RAST and ELISA technologies, as well as skin "patch" testing, are regarded by many veterinarians and researchers as inconclusive or too inaccurate to provide useful guidance. The least expensive and most accurate way to test your pet is at home, using the same type of rotation diet you would use to diagnose food allergies in yourself or your child.

There is much debate in natural nutrition circles about the best "preparation" diet for allergy testing. The point of this project is to give your pet's digestive tract a complete rest from whatever it's been eating in the past, so the best combination is a protein food it has seldom or never eaten (such as lamb, venison or salmon) raw or lightly cooked and a raw or lightly cooked vegetable (carrot, potato, parsnip, etc.). Some veterinarians recommend white rice for this exercise because it is easy for impaired animals to digest. Students of food combining prefer to separate starches from proteins, serving two meals a day, carbohydrates in the morning, and meat at night.

Your pet may find dietary changes stressful at first. It's safe to assume that an animal with severe allergies has been eating cooked, canned, baked or packaged food all its life, so feeding cooked foods at first may help. No matter how you serve it, raw or cooked, this is a very unbalanced diet suitable for short-term use only, but it's an important part of the diagnostic process because it gives the body a chance to eliminate all residues of dinners past. Nothing but hypoallergenic foods and pure water can be fed during the trial — no treats, snacks, vitamins, chew toys or heartworm preventive tablets.

In most cases of food sensitivity, the change is rapid, obvious and dramatic. A scratching pet stops itching, a lifeless coat begins to shine, a tired dog becomes an energetic puppy, a high-strung cat becomes calm and affectionate and symptoms of poor digestion disappear.

After two to three weeks of this rigid, restricted fare, begin testing your pet for sensitivity to a variety of foods. If you haven't already done so, gradually shift from cooked to raw foods, always emphasizing quality and freshness.

There are two ways to approach the "trial" or "challenge" phase of allergy testing. One is to introduce a new food every week and serve it for five to seven days. If the food fails to cause a problem, one can assume it's well tolerated by the dog or cat.

The rotation diet is more complicated, but it tests several foods at once. The basic rule of rotation testing is to wait four days before repeating an ingredient. For example, serve beef on Monday, chicken on Tuesday, lamb on Wednesday, salmon on Thursday, goat milk and goat milk cheese on Friday, fresh tuna or catfish on Saturday and nothing but water on Sunday. Vary the side dishes the same way, starting with boiled potatoes on Monday, rice on Tuesday, sweet potatoes on Wednesday, parsnips on Thursday, etc. These are just examples; create your own plan using foods in any sequence as long as you don't repeat a food until four days have passed.

Every week add a few more ingredients until you are serving a variety of meats, grains, vegetables, fruits and supplements, keeping each category separate. That is, don't serve two types of meat the same day or two kinds of grain. The foods can be served at any time of day, separately or combined. Remember to think in terms of food groups, so you feed chicken and chicken eggs on the same day, not subsequent days. Potatoes are close cousins of eggplants, peppers and tomatoes and should be fed on the same day as these foods or separated from them by at least four days. Keep rotating ingredients so that the next time you try a meat, it's with a different grain, fruit, vegetable and supplement. Always wait four days before repeating any food or its close relatives.

The symptoms of a food sensitivity are not necessarily obvious or immediate. Yes, a dog or cat might suddenly scratch, vomit, break out in hives, have diarrhea, limp, wheeze, shake, drool, or be overcome with fatigue right after eating. But the animal is just as likely to display symptoms a day later. This is why allergy testing requires detective work and careful record keeping. If every time you feed your dog eggs she spends the next morning scratching her fur off, there's a clue. Try avoiding eggs for several weeks. If her reaction is really dramatic, you may want to eliminate them from her diet forever. If you decide to reintroduce eggs at a later time, either to verify your diagnosis (perhaps you overlooked something and eggs were not the real culprit) or to see whether your pet can now tolerate eggs (frequent exposure causes some sensitivities), do so when you can observe her reaction over several days.

The advantage of testing individual foods is to determine specific allergens. Most pet foods, even high-quality foods, contain so many ingredients that an adverse reaction is impossible to trace to its source.

Once you become familiar with your pet's preferences and sensitivities, you can decide on the best long-term feeding plan, one that meets your animal's nutritional requirements, your budget, your schedule and your pet's appetite. You will have become, in the meantime, a zealous reader of labels, an unusually well-informed consumer, a knowledgeable nutritionist and a trained observer of your pet's responses.

Pets as Vegetarians

Food is the social cement that binds us together as families and cultures. It excites our passions. Some of us devote our lives to food—growing it, selling it, studying it, preparing it, teaching people what to eat or how to eat, writing about it and publishing books about it. Everyone talks about food. It's something we deal with every day and there's no escaping it. People argue, debate, discuss and even fight about food. If we worry about our own diets, the feeding of our children and pets is fraught with anxiety and conflicting opinions. In the world of dog people, I rank food as an emotional issue right up there with crates and pinch collars.

Most American dog owners will never feed their pets a raw diet. They believe that canned or packaged food is what dogs are supposed to eat, and people who do weird things like feed their pets raw bones are just asking for trouble.

A smaller group is experimenting with raw diets and telling anyone who will listen about their spectacular results.

An even smaller group is experimenting with vegetarian diets for dogs and cats and they, too, are encouraging others to follow their example.

When I began considering a raw diet for my cats, Pepper and Pumpkin, I had been a strict vegan for years. Vegans are vegetarians who don't use anything that comes from animals, including fish, poultry, eggs, milk and honey. I'd spent most of my adult life balancing a vegetarian diet while fielding the concerned questions of meat-eaters who knew my health must be suffering, so going without meat was not an unfamiliar concept. But the nutritional needs of cats are so different from those of people that the task of creating a balanced, healthy menu for them seemed formidable. In the end, Francis Pottenger's experiments convinced me that raw is always better than cooked and Mother Nature is the best guide.

There are political, religious and philosophical reasons for pursuing a vegetarian diet, but do they apply to our nonvegetarian companion animals? To my knowledge, no spiritual or religious leader has ever suggested that dogs or cats be deprived of meat, for doing so would violate the laws of nature.

Some have argued that dogs can be vegetarians without much trouble but cats, who are true carnivores, cannot. It's true that dogs can survive on vegetarian fare, but do they thrive? The supplements that would make the most difference for vegetarian dogs — bone meal, glandular concentrates, fish oils and whole-food extracts containing liver and other organs — come from animal sources and are therefore inappropriate. It is a dilemma.

In the end, each owner makes a personal choice, and that choice must be respected. I hope that everyone who lives with a dog or cat will let thousands of years of natural selection define their canine and feline menu planning. If that isn't possible, I hope they will do whatever they can within the constraints of their philosophy to provide the nutrition their animals require. When all is said and done, love is probably the most important ingredient in any animal's life. ☙

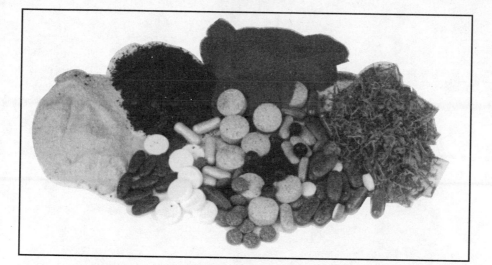

Supplements
for Pets

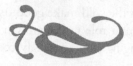

The Importance of Enzymes

FOR THOSE NOT ABLE to provide an all-raw diet for their pets, enzyme supplements are available to replace enzymes killed by the cooking and processing of food. Enzyme supplements (see the Resources for this chapter in the Appendix) have impressive records of safety and health improvement for animals of every description, from dogs, cats and horses to reptiles, birds, fish, primates and humans. The addition of enzymes to processed food improves digestion and assimilation so effectively that the quantity of food may have to be reduced by 15 to 20 percent to prevent unwanted weight gain. Veterinarians who have tested enzyme supplements report improved coats, uniform litters, higher puppy survival rates, fewer problems in pregnancy and increased mobility in older dogs, even improvement in hip dysplasia, all without vitamin or mineral supplementation. Enzymes increase the assimilation of vitamins, minerals and other nutrients in food.

All growing sprouts, grasses and herbs contain enzymes, and health food stores offer an assortment of green powders containing dehydrated barley grass juice, wheat grass juice, chlorella, spirulina and similar plants rich in enzymes. Added to other foods, these concentrated enzyme sources improve digestion and the assimilation of nutrients. Some foods, like raw seeds, contain enzyme inhibitors and are best served in small quantities or soaked and sprouted before serving.

Hormones and Glandular Extracts

In the wild, dogs and cats don't just dine on rib steaks and drumsticks. The first things most foxes, coyotes, wolves, hyenas, feral dogs, lions, tigers and even domestic cats eat are the prey's digestive organs. Then come all the other organs and glands, including the thymus, spleen, brain, eyes, thyroid, pituitary and adrenals. Glands contain hormones, and animals in the wild make good use of these substances.

Hormones play an important role in the growth of new skin and hair; they keep black noses and fur from changing color, intensify coat color and help prevent allergic reactions.

Only a few people feed their dogs and cats glandular supplements, but those who do claim excellent results. Glandulars are not a quick fix; they require months of daily supplementation to make a difference, but they correct imbalances as no other nutrients can.

For best results in glandular supplementation, animal nutritionist Marina Zacharias suggests having a complete blood panel done to test hormone levels and other factors in order to determine which supplements would be most effective. If the animal has no apparent health problems, providing a variety of glandular supplements from organically raised, minimally processed sources on a rotating basis will supply the nutrients otherwise missing in a pet's diet.

Vitamins and Minerals

Many veterinarians believe that supplements are both a waste of money and potentially harmful. Others, such as Wendell Belfield, disagree. Dr. Belfield has found that vitamin and mineral supplements make a dramatic difference in the health of dogs and cats. Of course, his patients all developed their deficiencies eating commercial pet foods. When fresh foods provide all the nutrients an animal needs, supplementation isn't necessary.

In an ideal world, our animals would all be fed as Dr. Pottenger's cats, cows, chickens and guinea pigs were, on fresh, whole, raw foods in fresh air and sunlight. Alas, this is not an ideal world. Unless you provide everything your pet needs from your own bucolic farm or sheep ranch, your dog or cat will probably benefit from occasional supplements, and if your pet has spent a lifetime on commercial pet food, the right vitamins and minerals may save his life.

Because of nutritional studies conducted shortly after World War II, most veterinarians believe that dogs and cats produce all the vitamin C their bodies need. For this reason it is not an ingredient in pet foods. However, when Belfield began using vitamin C on his canine and feline patients, they responded dramatically.

The foundation of this supplement program is an all-purpose multiple vitamin/mineral supplement with added vitamins C and E, depending on the pet's individual needs. According to Belfield, vitamin C prevents a variety of health problems, including degenerative spine disorders, arthritis, skin and coat conditions and ruptured discs. To prevent hip dysplasia, which he considers a subclinical form of scurvy, Belfield recommends feeding puppies between weaning and six months of age 250 mg vitamin C daily for small dogs, 500 mg for medium dogs, 500 to 1,000 mg for large dogs and 750 to 2,500 mg for giant breeds. Increase to these amounts gradually, checking for bowel tolerance, which is the mild diarrhea or loose stool that occurs when the body can no longer absorb vitamin C and begins throwing off the excess; if that occurs, decrease the dosage. Bowel tolerance levels vary from one animal to the next and from one day to the next as the need for vitamin C increases with stress, exposure to infectious diseases, accidents and surgical procedures.

Belfield uses liquid vitamin C for infant kittens, beginning with 20 mg per day at birth and increasing to 65 mg per day at weaning. Weaned kittens receive 250 mg until six months, when they go on the adult dosage of 500 to 750 mg daily. In *The Very Healthy Cat Book* and *How to Have a Healthier Dog*, Belfield devotes long chapters to vitamin C, documenting its ability to improve immunity, treat viral and bacterial infections, detoxify the body, improve collagen, improve the condition of cancer patients and prevent arthritis and joint problems. He also dispels the myth that large quantities of vitamin C can be toxic or cause kidney stones.

For best results, use a natural vitamin C complex that includes bioflavonoids. Adult dogs and cats on a raw diet that includes fresh fruit and vegetables don't need large amounts of supplemental C, but the addition of 500 mg every few days is inexpensive insurance. Whenever the animal is stressed from overwork, breeding, emotional or physical trauma, surgery, an accident or illness, give the vitamin to bowel tolerance.

Vitamin A, a fat-soluble vitamin formed in the body from beta carotene, is essential for night vision, the maintenance of soft mucous tissues and normal growth. Vitamin A deficiencies cause stunted growth, night blindness and other vision disorders. Beta carotene in foods such as carrots and yams converts to vitamin A in the canine body; animal sources such as cod liver or salmon oil are recommended for cats. Many holistic veterinarians recommend giving adult dogs and cats 750 IU of supplemental vitamin A per 10 pounds of body weight daily.

The B-complex vitamins (thiamine, niacin, riboflavin, biotin, folic acid, pantothenic acid and others) are vital to the health of the nervous system, and deficiencies in this group can manifest as symptoms anywhere in the body, most often in the mouth, eyes and reproductive organs. These are among the most fragile and heat-sensitive vitamins. Like vitamin C, they are water-soluble and are not stored in the body. Liver and other organ meats, fish, poultry, brewer's yeast, eggs, beans, peas, dark green leafy vegetables, whole grains and dairy products are rich sources of B-complex vitamins. The individual B-vitamin dosages often recommended for adult dogs per 20 pounds of body weight are 0.5 mg B1, 0.5 mg B2, 15 mg B3, 0.75 mg B6, 6 mcg B12, 3 mg pantothenic acid, 33 mcg folic acid, 12 mcg biotin and 20 mcg inositol. For adult cats the average recommendations are 0.4 mg B1, 0.4 mg B2, 7.5 mg B3, 0.4 mg B6, 1.5 mcg B12, 1.5 mg pantothenic acid, 16.5 mcg folic acid, 6 mcg biotin and 11 mcg inositol. However, the raw diet described here is so rich in B-complex vitamins that little supplementation is necessary. Once or twice a week you may want to give your pet a supplement derived from whole-food sources for humans, such as Standard Process Cataplex B, and adjust the dosage for your pet's weight.

Vitamin D is called the sunshine vitamin because exposure to sunlight manufactures it in the body. Vitamin D, which is also supplied by fatty fish, is necessary for healthy bones. Veterinarians recommend up to 100 IU per 20 pounds of body weight, but half an hour in the sun can produce that much and more. Because vitamin D is fat-soluble, the body stores what it can't use and excessive amounts can be toxic.

Vitamin E is essential during every phase of life, including gestation. Animals with high vitamin E levels tend to have stronger, healthier litters and easier birthings than those with low levels. Vitamin E speeds the healing of wounds and burns, improves the assimilation and distribution of nutrients throughout the body, keeps the heart healthy, invigorates older animals, slows the symptoms of aging, protects cats against steatitis, a painful disease of fatty tissue resulting from diets high in the unsaturated fats of fish oils, improves the skin and coats of all animals and boosts resistance to disease. Food sources of vitamin E include vegetable oils, nuts, dark green, leafy vegetables, organ meats, seafood, eggs and avocados. Recommended supplementation: 100 IU per 20 pounds of body weight daily.

Vitamin K regulates blood clotting and other clotting factors; it is also essential for kidney function and bone metabolism. Food sources include beef liver, cheese, oats, cabbage, turnip greens and other dark green, leafy vegetables. Healthy animals on a natural diet receive ample amounts of this vitamin.

Vitamins A, C and E and the mineral selenium are antioxidants; that is, they protect fatty acids in cells from damaging oxidation. Belfield has described several chronic cases that responded to antioxidant therapy after conventional treatments, such as antibiotics, failed. These included ear infections, the gum disease gingivitis, miliary dermatitis, colitis, heart disease (valvular insufficiency) and cancer.

The amino acid taurine is essential to all mammals, especially cats. It is interesting that the taurine content of a typical mouse (2.4 mg per gram) is more than 10 times that of most foods your indoor pet is likely to encounter, including beef (.2 mg), beef liver (.1 mg), chicken (.2 mg), eggs (.1 mg) and milk (.05 mg). Clams are high in taurine (1 mg per gram). There is no significant vegetable source of this amino acid. All mammals create taurine, but cats seem to use it faster than they can replenish it, hence their need for taurine-rich foods. Even though dogs haven't suffered the dramatic symptoms of taurine deficiency documented in cats, remember that cats weren't known to need taurine until recently.

Natural vs. Synthetic

In any discussion of supplements, it's necessary to examine the differences between natural vitamins and amino acids such as taurine from food and their synthetic counterparts made from chemicals. Nobel Prizes have been won for vitamin synthesis; the scientific community regards synthetics as identical to natural vitamins, and the low cost of synthetic supplements makes them affordable to all.

But are synthetic and natural vitamins really the same? Their molecular structures may match, but they are mirror images of one another. Living bodies can tell the difference, and the difference can be debilitating. In the 1930s, Barnett Sure at the University of Arkansas conducted several experiments on the links between nutrition and fertility. In one, he divided identical laboratory rats into four groups, all of which were fed a natural diet that supplied B-complex vitamins. In addition, each group was given pure crystalline thiamin hydrochloride (synthetic vitamin B1) manufactured by Merck, either 10, 100, 200 or 400 mcg daily.

The fertility and lactation of the 10 mcg group remained normal for two generations. When the dose was increased to 200 mcg, lactation efficiency dropped from 95 to 41 percent and one female became sterile. The second group, which started the experiment on 100 mcg daily, was fine for one generation; then in the second generation, two females were sterile. When this group's dose was increased to 400 mg, all of its third generation's offspring died at birth. In the third group, which began the experiment on 200 mcg daily, sterility appeared in the first generation, and when the third generation's dosage was increased to 600 mcg daily, four of its six females were sterile or their offspring died within days of birth. The fourth group, which began on 400 mcg daily, suffered a pronounced failure of lactation in its third generation, and when mothers were given 800 mcg daily, their infant mortality rose to 88 percent. The more synthetic vitamin B1 these animals ingested, the worse their reproductive health.

Natural vitamin C is derived from citrus fruits, ascerola cherries, amla berries, rose hips, red and green peppers and other fruits and vegetables. Be sure to check labels for sources as some vitamin C supplements are labeled "natural and organic" because they are synthesized from corn sugar (glucose), which technically fits that definition but is not the same as a natural vitamin C complex from whole food.

Synthetic and natural vitamins interact differently with minerals in the body. For example, many nutritionally oriented physicians, such as Bruce West, M.D., warn their patients not to take ascorbic acid because it depletes copper levels. Natural vitamin C does not. When beta carotene failed to protect heavy smokers from heart attacks, headlines condemned vitamin therapies without mentioning that the supplement tested was synthetic, not natural. Hundreds of studies have shown that people who eat foods rich in beta carotene have lower heart attack and cancer rates than those who don't.

In response to the increasing demand for natural or food-based vitamins, more manufacturers are supplying them; see the Resources for this chapter.

Minerals

Minerals are another concern because, since the late 1800s, America's farm soils have been stripped of their minerals and trace elements. The result is such a severe mineral depletion that the mineral levels of our industrially grown staple crops are insufficient to provide and maintain good health. The most widely used chemical fertilizers contain only two or three minerals, not the 72 trace elements found in nature.

Mineral deficiencies interfere with vitamin absorption, digestion and the health of every body system, from the brain's electrical circuitry to the healthy operation of the heart, circulatory system, reproductive organs, skeleton, skin, lungs and everything else. A lifetime of health problems can be prevented by feeding puppies, kittens and other young animals the minerals their growing bodies require.

Seaweeds such as kelp and dulse provide dozens of minerals, including iodine. Brazil nuts are rich in selenium. Blackstrap molasses and wheat germ contain substantial magnesium. Organ meats provide substantial iron and potassium. Bones offer calcium, magnesium, phosphorus and other minerals in perfect balance; bone marrow is rich in copper and iron. The advantage to food-derived minerals is that they are easy to assimilate and in proportions that living bodies utilize well. Ian Billinghurst based his dog diet on bones because they provide a puppy's most complete and balanced supply of minerals, preventing hip dysplasia, growth defects, wobbler syndrome, dropped hocks, spayed feet and bone cysts. "We have been breeding Great Danes and Rottweilers for years," he explains. "The bone problems our dogs had been experiencing disappeared the moment we began to raise our puppies on a bone-based diet." Billinghurst cautions breeders and owners that the larger the breed, the more important it is not to use calcium supplements because these supplements have been shown to disrupt the balance of minerals needed by the body and exacerbate bone and growth problems.

Whenever it's necessary to provide a mineral supplement, consider using a liquid or powder that contains most or all of the elements found in nature rather than a product that contains only one, two or five minerals. Mineral supplements derived from plant material, ocean water or salt lakes are easily absorbed, well tolerated and in natural balance.

In fact, one of the most important supplements for any dog, cat, horse, cow, llama, goat, rabbit, bird, tropical fish, reptile or other pet may be salt — not any salt, but unrefined, unprocessed sea salt, which contains only 80 to 83 percent sodium chloride, with the remaining 17 to 20 percent consisting of moisture and 84 trace elements in the proportions needed by all of the earth's animals, human and canine included.

Recommended uses: Sprinkle a small amount of unrefined sea salt on fatty foods to improve digestion and assimilation. Add a pinch to each bowl of drinking water and to every meal, using more for large animals and tiny amounts for small pets.

Do not use refined table salt, kosher salt or sea salt that has been boiled or heated during processing. If the salt is bright white or has the familiar taste of table salt, it won't contribute to your pet's good health. Look for naturally dried sea salt that is slightly gray in color with a taste that's very different from that of table salt.

Other Supplements

Apple Cider Vinegar

Many herbalists recommend vinegar for pets, especially because it can be poured over garlic and other herbs to make medicinal tinctures. Even without those herbs, cider vinegar is an important ingredient in your pet's diet. Use any raw, unpasteurized, unheated, organic vinegar; apple cider vinegar is the most common, but rice and wine vinegars are also available. Do not use a vinegar that is uniformly clear and clean looking, such as cider vinegar sold in supermarkets for pickle making or most of the rice and wine vinegars sold in markets and health food stores. These are "dead" vinegars with none of the enzymes and other live factors that make raw, unpasteurized vinegar so valuable.

Long a folk remedy, cider vinegar has been shown to improve the health of dairy cows, horses, dogs and other animals. It reduces common infections, aids whelping, improves stamina, prevents muscle fatigue after exercise, increases resistance to disease and protects against food poisoning. Cider vinegar is rich in the vitamins, minerals and trace elements found in apples, especially potassium; it normalizes acid levels in the stomach, improves digestion and the assimilation of nutrients, reduces intestinal gas and fecal odors, helps cure constipation, alleviates some of the symptoms of arthritis and helps prevent bladder stones and urinary tract infections.

Add cider vinegar directly to food or drinking water, starting with small amounts and building up to 1/2 to 1teaspoon per 15 pounds of body weight for dogs and cats (1 teaspoon per day for the average cat, 1 tablespoon for a 50-pound dog or 2 tablespoons for a 90-pound dog). Dip carrot greens in cider vinegar for your rabbit or bird or sprinkle it on other foods that they like. By gradually adding small doses to your pet's food over time, you can help even the most finicky eater to accept this valuable food.

See page 126 for making herbal tinctures with raw vinegar; see page 187 for using cider vinegar externally as a flea and tick repellent.

Willard Water (Catalyst Altered Water)

Willard Water, also called catalyst altered water, is a concentrate sold in some health food stores. John Willard, Ph.D., a professor of chemistry, developed this substance while working in oil fields, and after much experimentation he patented two forms of the concentrate. Willard Water is sold as a clear or dark concentrate for mixing with "good" water, good being defined as uncontaminated spring water, distilled water or filtered tap water. The treated water, which reduces stress and improves digestion and the assimilation of nutrients in humans and animals, was the subject of a 1980 *60 Minutes* television program and two subsequent books.

I was interested in Willard Water's ability to destroy chlorine and to act as a preservative and disinfectant, so in 1991, the year he died, I corresponded with Dr. Willard. In a letter dated April 16, he wrote, "In answer to your question, I will give you some information that is not public knowledge. Put one-third of an ounce (10 c.c.) of clear Willard Water extract into one gallon of good water (use distilled or deionized water if you're not sure). Put the dilute solution in a mist sprayer and spray it on hair, wounds, food, raw meat, etc., to disinfect. It reacts with the air to become a powerful oxidizing agent and preservative. I have cleaned up two hospitals with very hazardous contamination. For all other purposes, the dilution of one ounce clear concentrate per gallon of water (or two ounces of the dark concentrate) is best. For raw milk or fresh juice, add one ounce of either clear or dark Willard Water per gallon, or one and one-half teaspoons per quart. Milk tastes richer and keeps fresh longer."

I always add a pinch of unrefined sea salt and a splash of Willard Water concentrate to our drinking water. Willard Water has been used and tested on animals for decades, and the result is a long list of documented improvements with no adverse side effects. The most frequently reported claims from farmers, veterinarians, breeders, trainers, handlers and pet owners are improved digestion, calmness, improved coat luster and eye sparkle, improved gait, resistance to stress-related illness and increased immunity. Willard Water seems to improve the body's assimilation of vitamins, minerals and other nutrients.

A Note on Yeast

Brewer's yeast has become a controversial pet supplement in recent years because of the low-quality yeast used in many products. Veterinarian Alfred Plechner considers it a dangerous allergen and Juliette de Bairacli Levy has denounced it for decades. Brewer's yeast was originally a waste product of beer brewing and the brewer's yeast sold to pet food manufacturers was literally and figuratively the dregs of the process. A yeast residue might have been used and reused until it had no life left, at which time it was discarded and sold as an animal feed.

Allergic reactions are common among animals fed a low-quality brewer's yeast. A high percentage of dogs with skin allergies have been shown to be yeast-sensitive. Another claim is that dogs cannot digest brewer's yeast.

At the same time, nutritional yeast and brewer's yeast are the foundation of many popular supplements, including those developed or endorsed by Richard Pitcairn, Anitra Frazier, Robert Goldstein and others. Whenever researchers announce that brewer's yeast does not repel fleas, readers of health magazines write letters of protest, claiming the opposite.

The primary yeast cultivated by supplement manufacturers is *Saccharomyces cerevisiae*. Its nutritional content depends on the growth medium used to produce it, and its label name depends on the maker. For example, one manufacturer grows *S. cerevisiae* on hops and labels the product brewer's yeast; the same company grows *S. cerevisiae* on molasses and calls it nutritional yeast; a second company grows *S. cerevisiae* on sugar beets and calls it brewer's yeast. Some pet supplement makers claim that all brewer's yeast has a parasite-repelling high sulfur content and bitter taste unless the yeast has been debittered to make it more palatable. However, neither of the brewer's yeasts described here is debittered and both have a low sulfur content and sweet taste, while the nutritional yeast grown on molasses has a high sulfur content and bitter taste. If you hope that yeast will help your pet deter fleas, compare the sulfur content of different brands.

Yeast has been shown to help animals resist infection. In a poultry study, *Saccharomyces boulardii,* the strain used to grow torulla yeast, was added to the feed of half the chickens being tested; then all of the chickens were orally inoculated with *Salmonella* bacteria. Only five percent of those fed the yeast developed salmonella colonies in their intestines, compared to 70 percent of the control group. Some owners feed their birds and other pets brewer's yeast, a close cousin of torulla yeast, to help prevent the growth of undesirable bacteria.

Whatever its growth medium, premium quality brewer's or nutritional yeast was never used in beer brewing and is not a waste product. It is a rich source of B-vitamins, amino acids, selenium, chromium, potassium, phosphorus, magnesium, copper, manganese, iron, zinc and other trace elements.

As nutritious as it is, even the highest quality brewer's yeast can disrupt the life of an animal who is sensitive to yeast. If your dog or cat displays any allergic response to brewer's yeast, read labels carefully and avoid products that contain yeast of any type. After several weeks, if you would like to reintroduce yeast, try a high quality yeast (see Resources for this chapter in the Appendix) in small doses at widely spaced intervals and observe your pet's reaction.

Growing Wheat Grass and Other Green Sprouts

Nothing brings fresh factors to your pet's food like growing grasses and other sprouts. Some veterinarians are suspicious of these foods because they may harbor mold or bacterial contamination, but those problems are easy to prevent.

During summer months or warm weather, grow wheat grass outdoors in direct sunlight; in freezing weather, grow it indoors under full-spectrum lights. Small seeds can be sprouted in the kitchen year round.

The following method can be used for growing the grasses of wheat, rye, oat, kamut, spelt, barley, buckwheat, sunflower seeds and other grains. Barley grass is especially recommended because of its B-vitamin content, but grow a variety, alternating grains from one week or month to the next. Start with organically raised seeds; you don't want to use a seed or grain that might have been treated with pesticides or fungicides. For convenience, use raw, hulled sunflower seeds; that spares you from having to pull empty shell husks from the sprouts.

Depending on the amount of grass you want to grow, use plastic planting trays, plastic restaurant trays, lined cardboard boxes or any similar container that's between one and two inches deep and has no drainage holes or, for smaller sprout gardens, use flower pots. Fill trays with an inch of potting soil or garden compost; fill pots to the top. Have on hand a wide-mouth quart canning jar with plastic mesh sprouting lid (available at most health food stores) or a piece of cheesecloth tied in place with a rubber band. Sprouting requires warm temperatures, preferably 70 to 80 degrees Fahrenheit.

Soak a small amount (1/4 cup or so) of seeds in a quart of water to which you have added 5 or 6 drops of grapefruit seed extract. Soak wheat, buckwheat, oats, barley, sunflower seeds and other large grains 10 to 12 hours or overnight. Eight hours is recommended for medium seeds and about five hours for small seeds. For increased mineral content, add a pinch of powdered or liquid kelp, a splash of Willard Water concentrate or several drops of liquid trace minerals. Adding an ounce of 3-percent hydrogen peroxide is another technique for increasing germination.

After soaking and with sprout lid or cheesecloth in place, drain the seeds well, then lay the jar on its side. Leave it undisturbed in a warm place away from direct sunlight for one or two days.

As soon as they sprout, grains and seeds can be used as food. For dogs and cats, mix sprouted grains with a digestive enzyme containing amylase and let stand for half an hour or longer to more accurately duplicate the predigested grain found in the digestive tract of prey animals. For birds and rabbits, feed directly.

To grow wheat, rye, oat, barley, kamut or spelt grass, buckwheat lettuce or sunflower seedlings, plant the sprouting seeds. Water the planting tray's soil until moist but not wet. Spread the seeds in a thin layer, covering the surface. Cover the tray or flower pot with an inverted tray or with a wet paper towel covered with plastic to keep light out and moisture in. After two days, remove the cover, water the sprouting greens and place them outside in indirect light; on the second day move them into direct sunlight. Indoors, place trays under full-spectrum plant lights. Water daily until the grass is about six inches high, which takes about a week. If mold forms on the soil's surface from overwatering, spray the grass with 3-percent hydrogen peroxide or with 1 part liquid grapefruit seed extract diluted in 2 to 3 parts water.

Harvest grass by cutting it with scissors or a knife just above the soil surface. It will keep well in the refrigerator for about a week in zip lock bags that you press the air out of or wrapped in layers of damp newspaper or paper towels.

After harvesting your grass, recycle the soil mat by placing it in your compost bin and start over.

If you have a wheat grass juicer (forget about centrifugal juicers; you need a hydraulic press, screw press or macerating juicer for this task), add a small amount of wheat grass juice to the animal's food or water. Green juices are like concentrated vitamin/mineral/chlorophyll supplements. Freeze juice in ice cube trays, transfer the frozen cubes to heavy plastic bags for freezer storage and thaw the cubes as needed.

Every day, offer freshly cut grass to your pet, mincing it finely for dogs and cats. Buckwheat lettuce, which is a rich source of rutin as well as chlorophyll, makes a colorful addition to your own salads as well as your pet's dinner. Its red stems and green leaves are ready to harvest after seven days. Sunflower seedlings are thick and succulent at about the same time.

To grow sprouts without soil, use sprouting jars or tightly woven untreated bamboo or natural fiber baskets in small to medium sizes. Soak the seeds as directed and drain. If using glass jars, set the jar on its side, plastic sprout lid or cheesecloth top in place. If using a sprouting tray system, follow the manufacturer's directions. If using a bamboo basket, rinse it well, empty the seeds into the basket, rinse again, drain well and place the basket in a large plastic bag left partly open. This creates a greenhouse that allows air to circulate but prevents the seed from drying out. Your use of grapefruit seed extract in the soaking water should prevent mold, but if it occurs, rinse the seeds vigorously under a strong spray, drain them well, then spray or soak the sprouts with 3-percent hydrogen peroxide or diluted grapefruit seed extract.

If your sprouting area is dark, move the growing sprouts into indirect sunlight on the third or fourth day.

If growing a crop that produces empty hulls, such as alfalfa, radish, red clover or mung beans, wait until the hulls begin to separate and fall off, then submerge the sprouts in a sink of cool water and agitate them. Empty hulls will separate from the sprouts and either sink to the bottom or float to the surface. If using bamboo baskets, simply submerge and agitate the basket (the sprouts will cling by their roots) and let it drain; if using jars, lift the sprouts into a strainer, then replace in the jar.

To sprout dried beans or lentils for improved digestibility, soak lentils for four hours or beans overnight, then drain well and leave them undisturbed for one or two days or until sprouts are visible. This procedure reduces cooking time dramatically. We humans, with our longer digestive tracts, have a hard enough time digesting beans. Poor dogs and cats! For both of us, Beano, an enzyme supplement, makes beans and bean products easier to digest. Liquid Beano is sold as a pet product under the name Curtail.

Diatomaceous Earth

Diatomaceous earth is a powder made from fossilized, microscopic one-celled plants called diatoms. Deposits of diatoms, which are ground to create diatomaceous earth, cover large areas around the world. Two types of diatomaceous earth are sold in the U.S., one used in swimming pool filters, the other an untreated "food grade" powder sold to gardeners as a slug and snail deterrent. A growing number of pet owners are adding the second type to their animals' dinners.

When diatoms were tested as a grain protectant, feeding tests were conducted on laboratory animals to determine toxicity. Researchers noticed that the animals fed diatoms were in better health than those fed a normal diet and, in subsequent tests, young diatom-fed animals gained weight faster than control animals and had fewer problems with intestinal parasites. Diatoms remove existing worms and prevent reinfestation by scouring the intestines, irritating and damaging the parasites' soft bodies. When added to a cat's food, diatomaceous earth helps prevent hair balls.

While diatomaceous earth is considered a safe addition to livestock grain and other dry foods, keep in mind recent warnings of lung damage caused by inhaling this powder. Diatomaceous earth works because of its sharp edges, which cut soft tissue. This is how it kills flea larvae, garden slugs and other soft-bodied animals. Diatomaceous earth should be handled carefully and gently stirred into wet food or combined with dry food, such as seeds for birds, and sprayed with just enough water to reduce dust. The recommended amount is 1/2 teaspoon per 10 pounds of body weight.

Dr. Goldstein's Health Cocktails

In the 1970s, when Robert Goldstein, D.V.M., and his wife, Susan, began to study alternative medicine, they traveled to the Bahamas to work with Dr. Lawrence Burton, creator of Immuno-Augmentive Therapy, the cancer treatment the Goldsteins now use at their veterinary clinic. Many of the island's human cancer patients were weak from chemotherapy, radiation therapy and other allopathic treatments received in the United States. To improve their immune systems, many of them drank a concentrated blend of nutrients nicknamed Radiation Cocktail.

Its concentrated nutrients can help nearly any ailing pet. Goldstein recommends it for most debilitating, degenerative or chronic diseases or conditions, including cancer, liver or kidney disease, colitis, inflammatory bowel disease, degenerative conditions of the pancreas such as pancreatic insufficiency, feline leukemia, feline AIDS, infectious peritonitis, arthritis, skin problems, lupus and Lyme disease.

Using only fresh, organically raised ingredients (substitute organic egg yolks for the calves' liver if organic liver is not available), combine the following in a blender.

Health Cocktail No. 1 (Radiation Cocktail)

1/4 cup distilled or filtered water
1/2 cup raw organic calves liver or
2 raw organic egg yolks
1 Tbsp. powdered dulse or kelp
1 Tbsp. nutritional yeast
1 tsp. organic apple cider vinegar
1/2 tsp. ground rosemary
400 I.U. vitamin E (open capsule and add)

Add fresh juices just before feeding:
1/2 cup freshly extracted organic carrot juice
1 Tbsp. freshly extracted parsley juice
1 Tbsp. aloe vera juice

If your pet is allergic or sensitive to yeast or eggs, omit those ingredients. Cats and small to medium-size dogs can take 2 to 5 tablespoons per day, while large and giant breeds can take just over 1/2 cup. Divide the recipe in half to make a smaller portion; for best results, blend everything but the fresh juices and refrigerate this base, adding freshly made juice at the last minute. This is especially important if you use a centrifugal juicer. Juices made with a macerating juicer or hydraulic press retain most of their nutrients when refrigerated.

Health Cocktail No. 2

Goldstein recommends a simpler version of the above recipe for all pets on a weekly basis:

1/4 cup distilled or filtered pure water

1/2 cup freshly extracted organic carrot juice

1/2 cup freshly extracted celery juice

1 Tbsp. aloe vera juice

1 Tbsp. powdered wheat grass or barley grass, or
   use freshly extracted wheat grass juice

1 Tbsp. nutritional yeast

400 IU vitamin E

Use the same dosages as above and divide the recipe as needed. Or, as Goldstein suggests, give some to your pet and drink the rest yourself.

The suggested schedules for Dr. Goldstein's recipes are for dogs and cats in ill health or making the transition from cooked to raw foods. A dog or cat on an all-raw diet can be fed carrot, apple, celery, wheat grass and other juices daily. Wheat grass and other grass juices should be fed in smaller quantities (a teaspoon rather than a tablespoon, for example) because they are so concentrated. Fruits and vegetables can be juiced together.

Skin-Saver Cocktail

Rich in zinc, beta carotene and vitamin B6, this health cocktail has detoxification and anti-inflammatory benefits for the pet with skin problems. Juice the following ingredients:

   3 sprigs parsley

   1 cucumber

   1 medium apple

   1 small beet

   4 carrots

   1/4 cup peas

   1/4 inch ginger root

Dosage for dogs and small cats: 2 tablespoons three times daily; for dogs up to 50 pounds: 5 tablespoons daily.

Juices can be fed straight, diluted in drinking water or added to meals. ☙

Chapter

4

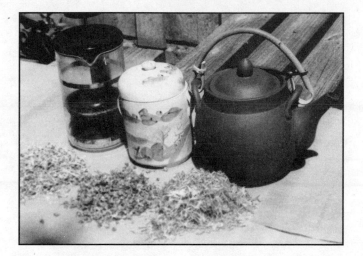

Herbs
for Pets

IN OUR AGE OF MODERN MEDICINE, when illnesses are treated in high-tech hospitals with laser surgery and powerful prescription drugs, it is easy to forget that until the 20th century, plants were the medicines that kept people and their companion animals well. In fact, most of the prescription drugs in use today were derived and synthesized from plants, and outside of Canada and the United States, plants remain the world's primary healing agents.

The surgical techniques and pharmaceutical drugs that define Western medicine work well in acute or crisis conditions, but they are far less successful in the treatment of chronic illnesses. This is because Western medicine as practiced by physicians and veterinarians is allopathic, which means that its focus is the alleviation of physical symptoms, not finding and treating the cause. Chronic conditions like arthritis, skin and coat problems, gingivitis, ear infections, asthma and allergies may improve temporarily when their symptoms are masked, but they usually recur and, over time, grow worse. For this reason, conventional or orthodox medicine considers these conditions irreversible and incurable. In addition, drugs and surgery carry hidden costs in adverse side effects that range from negligible to fatal.

The advantage of natural remedies is that they often work as well as or better than conventional treatments, have fewer side effects and address the cause of a condition, resulting in its improvement or cure. It is because of allopathic medicine's limitations that so many Americans have begun to explore more natural approaches to health and healing. This is not to say that natural therapies are successful in treating every condition in every person or pet, but they offer a first line of defense in the prevention of problems and, when an illness is well-established, they can help speed healing.

By far, the world's most widely used natural therapy is herbal medicine. Every culture on every continent has experimented with local plants and developed a tradition of diagnosis and use, a repertoire based on experience and observation.

My teacher, Rosemary Gladstar, offers sensible advice to those who are new to these old traditions. "In order for herbs to be effective," she says, "they must be used with consistency. This is probably the most difficult aspect of herbalism for people in the 20th century. In our age of quick fixes and instant medicine, the old art of brewing and using herbal tea seems antiquated and time-consuming." On the contrary, she explains, it's really easy and practical.

What are the advantages of brewing teas for pets? Although herbs can be given directly in food or capsules, teas provide an herb's medicinal benefits in a form that's easy to assimilate even when the animal's digestion is impaired. Herbal teas can be added to food or drinking water, given directly or applied externally.

Some herbal blends are famous, such as Essiac, a 20th-century tea used as a support therapy for people and pets with serious diseases, such as cancer. Some simples, or single-herb teas, have been used for centuries, such as chamomile and peppermint. Other medicinal teas are less well known to American consumers, although they were probably familiar to our great-grandparents and to their grandparents.

This chapter reviews some of the ways in which we can use the plants around us to prevent and treat common problems in household pets.

Whole Herbs and Standardized Extracts
A Conversation with James Green

In 1969, a Canadian Indian medicine woman introduced James Green to the healing power of plants and his life changed. Green became an herbal practitioner, medicine maker and educator; he is now director of the California School of Herbal Studies and the owner of Simplers Botanical Company, which makes herbal products. His books, *The Male Herbal* and *The Herbal Medicine Maker's Handbook,* are popular references, and he teaches workshops throughout the U.S. and Canada.

Through the end of the 19th century, herbs were popular medicines here in America. When did they fall from favor, and why?

GREEN: After World War II, the pharmaceutical industry chose to make a full switch from plant medicines to mineral medicines because they are easier to control. You don't have to deal with insects, availability problems or variations in the plants' constituents due to growing conditions, and you can make clear liquids or white powders that can be chemically standardized. Medical doctors adopted these products and used them as their official medicines and one by one, slowly but surely, plants were eliminated from the U.S. pharmacopoeias, the official medicine texts.

At the same time, even though physicians stopped using whole plant products, plants were examined for active ingredients that could be synthesized and patented. Unfortunately, when you pull one ingredient out and throw the rest away, you lose the plant's synergy. If you use the whole plant, which has a variety of nutritional components, you experience a gentle process that produces a variety of beneficial effects with minimal side effects.

How did medicinal herbs make their comeback?

GREEN: Well, in other countries they never went away, but here in the U.S., the tradition was pretty much extinct by the 1950s. Then in the '60s, a bunch of renegades like myself realized you can take whole plants home with you and make medicines out of them that are very safe and that really work. We experimented, tried things out, taught what we'd learned, studied with whatever healers we could find and encouraged everyone to do the same. The marketplace began to introduce people to an effective alternative to prescription drugs, and whole-plant herbalism became popular again.

Unfortunately, we've come full circle and now the emphasis is back on the one magical active ingredient in a plant that makes it work. For years, the European marketplace has emphasized standardized products in which an herb is treated with solvents or other extraction methods to create a consistent product with the same percentage or amount of its active constituent in every capsule. Now American herb companies are adopting the European model.

Altering the natural chemistry of a plant means creating something different and unfamiliar, especially when the resulting product may contain the residue of toxic solvents used to isolate and extract an "active ingredient."

My main objection to standardization is that it places the emphasis on science. When we embrace standardization because it's scientific, we accept the notion that science will make things better, and in doing so we disempower ourselves. Herbalism thrives in the home. Plants are accessible to all of us, they're whole and perfect the way they are. You can go out and identify a plant, harvest it and make your own medicine for yourself, your family and your pets. You have all the personal power you need to make the finest medicines available. In fact, your result can be a medicine that's superior to anything technology can offer. The beauty of herbalism is that you can do it yourself; in fact, it's already done.

I hope that your readers will consider involving themselves more deeply in their own wellness process and that of their pets by growing their own plants, identifying and collecting them in the wild or finding sources of whole, unprocessed, organically grown or wildcrafted herbs and making their own tinctures, blending their own teas, preparing their own salves and using these highly effective, healing materials to keep themselves and their animals healthy.

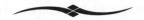

How to Judge an Herb's Quality

The best dried herbs are fragrant, flavorful, colorful and pungent. They don't look like shredded hay or smell like cardboard. These plants are dried at low temperature with lively air circulation and stored away from heat, light and humidity, the enemies of all dried herbs. The best herbs for medicinal use are grown organically or wildcrafted from pollution-free sources, then handled with care at every step of their drying and storage. By their look, smell and taste you can recognize these plants — the peppermint is obviously peppermint and the chamomile is obviously chamomile.

Here are some simple rules to keep in mind as you evaluate dried herbs. The larger the piece, the longer it lasts. Powdered herbs begin to lose their flavor as soon as they are ground. The more a leaf is exposed to heat, light, the open air and humidity, the faster it loses its healing properties as well as its taste.

This information will help you answer a commonly asked question: "How long can a dried herb be kept before it loses its effectiveness?" The answer is, "It depends." While most herbs should probably be replaced after a year, the most sensible rule is to look, smell, touch and taste. Roots and bark hold their fragrance, color and taste longer than delicate leaves and flowers, yet even blossoms and leaves can retain their herbal identity for much longer periods if properly stored.

Harvesting Your Garden's Herbs

If you are able to grow your own herbs, you have a real advantage for you can control their quality every step of the way. Home-harvested herbs, with their bright color and intense flavor, are usually superior to anything you can buy. In the middle of winter, nothing from the store will match your garden's lemon balm or sage.

Herbs should be planted in fertile soil and watered until well-established, but for best flavor and medicinal benefits, don't overfertilize or overwater during the growing season. Obviously, you will want to keep your herb plants far from pesticide sprays.

Try to pick culinary, medicinal and tea herbs on a clear morning after the dew has evaporated. To dry herbs successfully, you need an absence of sunlight, plenty of circulating air, low humidity and an undisturbed location. Although it's promoted as a fast and easy way to dry herbs, don't put medicinal plants in the microwave. If your attic or sheltered area outdoors is not appropriate because of high humidity, you can arrange the herbs on wire racks placed on trays in a barely heated oven. Small quantities can be dried in the refrigerator; just leave them in an open, empty jar until they're brittle. Many herbalists use food dehydrators. In hot, humid New York summers I drape herbs over a wooden laundry rack in the basement in front of the dehumidifier with a fan blowing, and they're brittle by morning.

Store dried herbs in glass jars, plastic bags or cellophane away from heat and direct light. Amber glass jars are the preferred storage containers, but use whatever does the job. Paper bags are not recommended for obvious reasons: they can't protect against humidity, and some herbs, like valerian root, contain delicate essential oils that paper absorbs. Plastic-lined paper bags, which are used by some herbal tea companies, work well. Because kitchens are usually warm and humid, they're not the best place to keep your harvest. The cooler the room, the better. Transfer small quantities to the kitchen as needed.

If you decide to cut, chop, sift, grind or powder your dried herbs to reduce their size, prevent deterioration by storing them at once in tightly sealed glass jars in a cool, dry, dark place or in your freezer. Don't leave any dried herbs, especially crushed or powdered herbs, exposed to heat, light or humidity.

A Note on Wildcrafting

Wildcrafting, the harvesting of herbs in their natural habitat, has always been recommended by herbalists. However, because of urban growth, destructive logging practices and overharvesting, America's medicinal plants are disappearing from the countryside.

Rosemary Gladstar and other leading herbalists now recommend that medicinal herbs be cultivated instead of wildcrafted wherever possible. Common lawn weeds like dandelion and plantain will always be abundant, but echinacea, goldenseal, ginseng and many other popular plants have become scarce in the wild. Consider growing medicinal plants in your garden, fields or woods, and purchase herbal products from companies that grow their own medicinal plants.

> **If you gather plants in the wild, please follow these guidelines.**
>
> 1. Identify the plant carefully before harvesting. Study herb guides so you know what part of the plant to use (leaves, blossoms, roots) and when to harvest it.
>
> 2. Learn what plants are endangered in your area and do not gather threatened or endangered plants. Instead, plant their seeds or seedlings, which you can obtain from herb farms or catalogs, in the wild or on your own property.
>
> 3. Harvest only from abundant stands of healthy medicinal herbs growing far away from busy highways, farms that use chemical sprays or polluted water.
>
> 4. Leave plenty of healthy, mature seed-producing plants so the herbs can reproduce. Unless the plant is abundant throughout your area, harvest no more than 10 percent of a native plant or 30 percent of a naturalized plant in any area. Do not harvest the same area repeatedly.

For information on what you can do to lessen the impact of wildcrafting on endangered plants, contact United Plant Savers; see the Resources for this chapter in the Appendix.

Herbal Preparations

There are many ways to take herbs: in teas, capsules, tablets, syrups, lozenges and tinctures, not to mention all their external applications in compresses, poultices and washes.

For best results, use herbs that were grown organically or wildcrafted (gathered in the wild, far from chemical exposure and automobile exhaust), then dried at low temperature to maintain their flavor, color, essential oils and other properties. See Resources in the Appendix for herbal tea companies that specialize in high-quality medicinal herbs.

If you are new to herbal medicine, remember that the recipes given here and in herbal reference books are flexible and forgiving. If you can't obtain an ingredient, find an appropriate substitute. Quantities are flexible, too. As you gain experience, you will be able to develop your own recipes. As you do so, be sure to refer to two or three different herbal references for information about each plant so that you have a clear understanding of its benefits, potential side effects and special requirements.

Simples and Blends

A simple is a single herb. Your cat has been a nervous wreck since the puppy arrived, so you put valerian in his food to help him relax, or the pup bruises her shoulder and you apply arnica. Whole schools of herbal healing have developed around simples, in which a single herb treats a condition until it improves.

Blends are combinations of herbs. You want to unwind after a hectic day, so you mix chamomile, skullcap and peppermint for tea. A blend can combine two herbs or dozens. Chinese medicine uses teas and tinctures that contain 10, 20 or 30 different herbs, and long ingredient lists are not unusual in European and American herbal handbooks.

There are no hard and fast rules in herb blending, but for beginners it makes sense to work with simples until you feel comfortable with individual plants, then begin combining two or three herbs together. If you work with only a few plants at a time, it will be easier to identify any plant that generates an allergic reaction or that is unusually effective. Keep a notebook, for individual reactions vary.

A specific is any herb known for its effectiveness in the treatment of a condition, such as crampbark for muscle spasms or milk thistle seed for liver disease. Specifics can be used alone, in which case they are simples, or combined with other herbs, in which case they act as the blend's active ingredient.

A catalyst, stimulant or activator herb is often used in herbal blends to increase circulation and digestion. The world's most widely used stimulant is caffeine, which is an ingredient in many over-the-counter medications because it helps them act faster. Some stimulant herbs are used alone, but most make up a small portion of an herbal recipe. Lobelia and ginger are examples of catalyst herbs added in small doses to many teas and tinctures. Cayenne pepper is a more powerful catalyst, but its hot taste makes therapeutic doses difficult to take by mouth. Small amounts of cayenne can be added to food and some animals — notably dogs and birds — often seem to relish it. Cayenne can be given in capsules for its own beneficial effects or to enhance the performance of other herbs or supplements taken at the same time. In fact, by giving cayenne at the same time, it is often possible to reduce the dosage of a therapeutic herb without reducing its effectiveness.

How to Brew an Herbal Tea

To brew loose tea, which is usually recommended, you will need some kind of strainer. Loosely woven bamboo strainers are attractive, but they let so many particles through that they work best with teas made of whole leaves; for smaller pieces, such as cut and sifted herbs, line the bamboo strainer with a piece of cheesecloth or cotton muslin. My favorite strainer is made of fine stainless steel mesh.

Paper coffee filters can be used, but finely chopped or ground herbs may clog the filter long before the tea is strained. Stainless steel "tea balls" are widely sold, but if you decide to use one, be sure to fill it less than half full. Dried herbs swell in water, and a ball that's full will not allow water to circulate for optimum brewing.

If you are making a medicinal tea, most herbalists recommend using loose tea that floats in the pot for best results. Tea bags are convenient, but they contain only a teaspoon of herb, so you will need quite a few. In addition, they alter the flow of liquid around and through the herbs.

Use only the best quality cookware and teapots. Avoid anything chipped, rusty or cracked. If you use a wire mesh strainer, be sure it is made of stainless steel. Brew your tea in clean ceramic tea pots or glass jars. Obviously, you will want to avoid using ceramic ware that might contain lead pigment.

The coffee maker called a French press, sold in kitchen supply stores, makes loose tea brewing especially convenient. Most people associate the French press with coffee, but it's a great way to brew tea as well. Press the perforated disc down to strain the brew, and the result is a clear beverage with superior flavor.

Although it's common to make beverage teas by the cup, that's an impractical way to make medicinal teas. Most herbalists make all their teas, medicinal and beverage, in large quantities, at least a quart at a time and often by the gallon. For pet use, a pint or quart jar is convenient and easily fits in the refrigerator for storage.

Parts and Other Units of Measure

Herbal tea recipes are usually given in parts rather than tablespoons, cups or other familiar units of volume. When a recipe calls for 1 part peppermint and 2 parts lavender, your parts can be anything: a teaspoon, a tablespoon, an ounce (measured by volume, not weight), a cup or a bucket. The herbal ingredients should be of similar size, usually cut and sifted, crushed by hand or powdered just before blending. Once the tea is blended, you will use it like any other herb tea, measuring a teaspoon of the mix to make a cup of beverage tea or a tablespoon per cup for medicinal tea.

Infusions or Tisanes

The simplest teas are infusions, also known as tisanes (pronounced tee-SAHN in French). An infusion or tisane is made from fresh or dried herbs and hot water. Chamomile, peppermint and most other leaves and blossoms lend themselves to this method although a few leaves, like those of uva ursi, an herb used in the treatment of urinary tract and bladder infections, do not release their medicinal constituents unless simmered the way roots and barks are. Only a few delicate roots are brewed as infusions; one is the relaxing herb valerian, which contains fragile essential oils that would evaporate if the tea were boiled. Infusions extract mucilage, volatile oils, some vitamins and other nutrients. Water quality is always a concern. For best results, use distilled, filtered or bottled spring water, not chlorinated tap water. The water should be heated to just below the boiling point.

Proportions of herbs to water for most beverage teas:
- 1 teaspoon dried herb per cup of water
- 1 to 2 tablespoons fresh herb per cup of water
- 4 to 6 teaspoons dried herb per quart of water
- 1/4 to 1/2 cup fresh herb per quart of water

These are guidelines, not hard and fast rules. For example, use less of an herb that is dense and heavy, more of an herb that is light and fluffy, less of an herb that is fragrant and in excellent condition and more of an herb that is old and tired. Everything depends on the quality of the herb and the tea's purpose.

European recipes measure herbs by weight, which makes measurements more exact, but in the U.S., recipes almost always measure quantity by volume. To follow a European herb tea recipe, invest in a kitchen scale that measures metric units (grams and kilograms).

There is more than one way to brew an infusion. Here are four.

1. Place the herbs in a preheated ceramic teapot, glass jar, French press or ceramic cup. Pour the right amount of boiling water over the herbs, cover tightly (if using a cup that doesn't have a lid, cover it with a saucer) and let the tea steep 10 to 15 minutes or until cool; serve at room temperature. Add to your pet's food or water, use as a rinse after shampooing or apply externally as needed.

2. To make a stronger infusion, place the herbs in a pan with the proper amount of cold water. Cover and heat the water over low or medium heat until it just reaches the boiling point. Before it can come to a boil, remove the pan from the stove and let it stand without removing the cover for another 10 minutes, or until cool.

3. Solar infusions are fun to make, and some believe that the rays of the sun make this type of tea more therapeutic. On a hot sunny day, fill a clear glass gallon jar with cold water and one cup of loosely packed dried herbs (use less if the material is dense rather than fluffy) or 3 to 4 cups loosely packed fresh herbs. Place the jar in direct sun and leave it there for six hours or longer. See cold infusions, below, for an effective way to position the herbs in the jar.

4. Some recipes call for a cold infusion. To brew this type of tea, soak fresh or dried herbs in a measured amount of cold water for 10 hours or overnight, stirring occasionally, then strain and gently heat until warm. Cold infusions can be made with leaves, flowers, roots, seeds and bark. Be sure to cut, chop, shred or grind any hard or tough plant material before soaking. The most efficient way to brew a cold infusion is

to place your dried herbs in a roomy muslin or cheesecloth bag, dampen the bag as you fill a quart jar with cold water, then tie the bag so it's suspended at the top of the jar. Be sure the bag is large enough to allow the herbs inside to drift and move. Close the lid and let it stand overnight. A natural current will move from the bottom of the jar to the top and back, releasing the tea's constituents.

Decoctions

A decoction is a simmered or boiled tea. Roots and seeds are brewed by this method, though some roots with volatile oils require the more gentle infusion procedure, and some leaves must be simmered instead of steeped. Always check individual descriptions in herbal reference books.

To make a decoction, use a stainless steel, glass or enameled pan with a tight-fitting cover. Roots, whether fresh or dried, should be cut into small pieces. Use the same basic proportions of tea and water as for infusions.

1. Stir the herbs into cold water, cover the pan, bring it to a boil, then reduce the heat and simmer for 15 to 20 minutes. Be sure the pan's lid fits well to prevent steam from escaping. Remove the pan from heat and let the tea steep an additional 5 to 10 minutes; strain and serve. If you have to take the lid off for any reason, put it back quickly; high temperatures and an open pan allow volatile oils to escape.

2. Alternatively, bring the water to a boil by itself, then add the herbs, lower the heat and simmer for 15 to 20 minutes. Remove from heat, let stand an additional 5 to 10 minutes; strain and serve. Unlike leaves and blossoms, roots and seeds can be reused, usually three to four times. As flavor and color decrease with use, you can extend the brewing time or replenish herbs by adding small amounts of new material.

Combination Infusion/Decoctions

Some herbal blends combine leaves that need infusing and roots that require decoction or flowers that should be infused and seeds or bark that should be decocted. To make a combination tea, start with the roots, bark or seeds and brew a decoction using the full amount of water required for the combined tea; then remove from heat, lift the lid, add the leaves and flowers, replace the lid and let the tea stand another 10 to 15 minutes. If the tea is a premixed blend containing some herbs that should be defused and some that should be decocted, take half the recommended amount of herbs and brew a decoction; then add the other half and let it steep.

Medicinal Teas

A medicinal tea is made by increasing the proportion of herbs to water, increasing the brewing time or both. Use up to twice as much plant material as for a beverage tea; again, the quantity depends on the quality of the herb, so you may need less.

To brew a medicinal infusion, place the herbs in a pan of cold water. Cover with a tight-fitting lid and heat just to the boiling point. Do not allow it to reach a rolling boil. Remove from heat and let stand, covered, for an hour or longer or overnight.

To brew a medicinal decoction, place the herbs in water, cover, heat to boiling, then turn the heat down to a slow simmer and simmer gently for 15 to 20 minutes. Let stand for an hour, several hours or overnight before straining.

Alternatively, use a 1-pint or 1-quart canning jar to make a medicinal infusion the way the Chinese use ceramic ginseng cookers. This method is appropriate for all plant material (leaves, blossoms, stems, roots, bark and seeds) for it extracts the plants' constituents at a controlled temperature and prevents evaporation while brewing close to the boiling point for as long as desired.

Place cold or room-temperature distilled, filtered or pure spring water with the measured herbs in your canning jar, leaving about an inch of empty space at the top. Screw the lid on and place the jar upright on a wire rack. It is important to elevate the jar slightly from the bottom of the pan so the jar doesn't rattle or break; ceramic ginseng cookers have tiny feet for this purpose.

Fill the kettle with enough water to cover most or all of the canning jar. Put the kettle's lid on, bring the water to a boil, then turn the heat down and let the water simmer gently for one or more hours. You can also use a crock pot or slow cooker for this purpose. Place the tea jar on its roasting rack, fill the crock pot with boiling water and leave it on low heat with the lid on while the tea brews. For jars too tall for the crock pot's lid, use aluminum foil to fashion a lid to prevent evaporation.

For teas made of fragile plant material, such as most leaves or blossoms, the tea will be fully infused within an hour. For teas made of woody stems, bark and most roots and seeds, let the tea simmer as long as two or three hours or even longer. Using a jar lifter or wearing insulated rubber gloves (a pair of cotton gloves inside household rubber gloves works well), remove the jar to check the tea's color, which will usually darken as the tea brews.

Let the tea cool, then strain and use. Store leftover tea in the refrigerator.

Units of Measure by Volume

1 tablespoon (Tbsp.)	= 3 teaspoons (tsp.)			
1 fluid ounce (oz.)	= 2 Tbsp.	= 6 tsp.		
4 oz. =	1/2 cup =	8 Tbsp.		
1 cup =	8 oz. =	16 Tbsp.		
1 pint =	2 cups =	16 oz.		
1 quart	= 2 pints	= 4 cups	= 32 oz.	
1 gallon	= 4 quarts	= 8 pints	= 16 cups	= 128 oz.

Tinctures

Tinctures are liquid extracts, usually made with alcohol or vegetable glycerine. Alcohol is the most widely used tincture solvent because it extracts more constituents and preserves them longer than anything else. Unfortunately, alcohol has its own side effects, especially in children and small animals. While a large dog may safely take an alcohol tincture, cats, kittens, puppies, birds, rabbits and other small creatures should have minimal exposure to alcohol. Health food stores and herb companies offer tinctures from which the alcohol has been removed, or you can buy tinctures called glycerites, which are made with vegetable glycerine. If only alcohol tinctures are available, place the recommended amount in a cup and pour a small amount of boiling water over it, causing much of the alcohol to evaporate. Tinctures can also be diluted in food, water or juice and given in small doses during the day, which reduces alcohol exposure.

Another approach is to make your own tinctures using fresh or dried herbs and a combination of alcohol and glycerine. This combined solvent will extract all of the plant's medicinal constituents while reducing alcohol levels; by making a double-strength tincture, you can divide the recommended dosage in half, further reducing alcohol exposure. So many commercial tinctures are of questionable quality that your homemade tincture will be superior to many popular brands.

The preferred alcohol for most tincture-making is 80-proof vodka, which is a standard proof throughout the U.S. Eighty-proof vodka is 40 percent alcohol (proof is the alcohol percentage multiplied by two) and 60 percent water.

To reduce a tincture's alcohol content without losing its benefits, mix 80-proof alcohol with an equal or lesser amount of vegetable glycerine. To eliminate alcohol altogether, substitute vegetable glycerine, apple cider vinegar or a blend of cider vinegar and glycerine, but keep in mind that the result will not be as concentrated as an alcohol tincture; it may not contain some of the plant's key constituents, and its shelf life will be shorter.

To make a tincture, fill a glass jar 1/4 to 1/3 full with fresh or dried herbs that you have cut or shredded into small pieces. The herbs should be loose, not tightly packed. Cover the herbs with the solvent of your choice. At least an inch of liquid should cover the top; allow several inches for dried herbs, which will expand as they rehydrate. Seal the jar and place it in a warm location. Every day or two, turn it upside down and shake it gently. Add more liquid if necessary so the herbs float freely. Some recipes call for 1 part plant matter to 6 or more parts alcohol, but using less alcohol and/or more plant material results in a more concentrated, medicinal tincture. Let the tincture stand for a month or longer before filtering. Some herbalists recommend straining and bottling tinctures at the full moon. A popular six-week cycle begins tincturing at the new moon and ends at the second following full moon. There is no specific deadline but longer is often better; a tincture left for six weeks or two months will be far more potent than one left for just two weeks. Strain the tincture through cheesecloth or muslin, pressing out as much liquid as possible before discarding the spent plant material.

For a more concentrated tincture, pour your filtered tincture into a jar containing new plant material and repeat the process. Small quantities of this "double-strength" tincture will have a powerful medicinal effect at reduced dosages. Compared to some popular brands of tincture, yours will be "quadruple-strength" or even more concentrated, a significant advantage for children, pets and those who wish to use as little alcohol as possible.

Alcohol tinctures have an indefinite shelf life. Stored in amber glass jars away from heat and light, they last for decades.

Capsules

Capsules are convenient if you're giving a dog or cat something that tastes really awful or if you simply find them more convenient than measuring powders or making teas. Herbal capsules are widely sold and, if you need a special blend of herbs in capsules, some of the mail order herb companies listed in the Resources for this chapter in the Appendix blend and encapsulate custom orders for a nominal fee. Or you can put your own herbs into capsules. For best results, leave dried herbs whole or in large pieces until needed to preserve their essential oils and medicinal properties. Herbs should be stored away from heat and light in well-sealed glass containers for maximum shelf life. When ready to use, grind them in a blender, spice grinder or coffee grinder until powdered. To reduce exposure to herb dust, which can irritate nasal passages, wear a pollen mask. Two-part gelatin capsules, including vegetable gelatin capsules for vegetarians, are sold in health food stores and herb catalogs in sizes ranging from 0 (smallest) to 00 and 000 (largest). Many herb companies sell mechanical capping devices that hold several capsules in place for faster and easier filling.

Poultices

A poultice is a wet herbal pack applied directly to an inflamed, irritated, swollen, infected or injured part of the body. Poultices are made of fresh mashed herbs or the residue left after brewing tea. They are usually applied cool rather than hot. Use whatever will hold the poultice in place for as long as possible: bandages, plastic wrap, cheesecloth, muslin, etc. A layer of plastic over the poultice helps prevent fabric stains. If the affected area is difficult to treat this way, either because of its location or the animal's reaction, place the plant material on folded gauze and hold it in place by hand for as long as the animal will lie still.

Comfrey poultices are an excellent first aid measure in the treatment of cuts, burns, abrasions and other injuries, for comfrey contains allantoin, a cell growth stimulant that speeds healing. Practically everyone who works with herbs and dogs, cats, birds or rabbits has a comfrey story, and most involve its direct application. A widely published warning about comfrey is that it should not be applied to puncture wounds or infected cuts because its rapid healing action may cause the wound to close, trapping infection beneath it. I have asked many herbalists if they have experienced this problem because I have used comfrey this way several times with good results, such as when my husband's hand was badly swollen from a spider bite or when a cat scratch on my hand became infected.

Recently my dog had a bump on her nose that looked like a tiny mushroom and felt warmer than the skin around it. The tiny scab on top suggested a scratch. I applied diluted tea tree oil twice a day and nothing happened. Ignoring it for a few days didn't change anything, either. Finally I applied a dark green comfrey salve and the bump disappeared without a trace that same afternoon.

To guard against infection, clean the wound first with topical disinfectants such as tea tree oil, grapefruit seed extract, lavender essential oil or echinacea tea or tincture before applying the comfrey and give echinacea or grapefruit seed extract internally in therapeutic doses for several days. Another technique is to alternate comfrey and other herb poultices before the wound closes.

Any plant can be used as a poultice, but green plants seem to have a special affinity for infections and toxins. Wheat grass is a good example. A friend treated an infected dog bite on his leg by putting fresh wheat grass through a juicer, recombining juice and pulp and holding it in place with bandages. He did this only once and the bite healed quickly without leaving a scar.

Compresses and Fomentations

A compress is the application of cold herbal tea on a saturated towel or thick cloth. Use medicinal-strength infusions or decoctions for this purpose. To treat a fever, brew a strong peppermint tea, which has a cooling effect. To cool it quickly, pour it into a cold metal bowl (store it in the freezer while brewing the tea) and add ice cubes. The ice will melt and dilute the tea, so use as much as 2 or 3 tablespoons of dried peppermint or a large handful of fresh for each cup of boiling water. Soak the cloth and wring it just until it stops dripping. The compress should be wet enough to stay cold for several minutes. Apply it to the animal's head, legs, feet or abdomen and hold it in place. The circulating blood is close to the skin in these extremities, making them important cooling points. When the compress warms to body temperature, soak it again, adding ice as needed to keep the tea cold. Repeat until the treatment has lasted 15 to 20 minutes. Dry the skin and fur gently.

Cold compresses can be applied to any bruise or injury to help reduce swelling.

To make a fomentation, which is a hot compress, brew a medicinal strength tea and pour it into a bowl. Wearing rubber gloves to protect your hands from the heat, saturate a washcloth or other absorbent fabric with the hot tea. Let it cool slightly by exposing the fabric to the air until it's no longer hot enough to scald or burn but still very warm.

Tea is also good toner and to be used. Fold the fabric to an appropriate shape and size, then apply it to the affected area and hold it in place. Fomentations are sometimes recommended to soothe and help clear impacted anal glands.

Washes and Rinses

These preparations are just what they sound like. Any beverage or medicinal-strength tea can be used to flush a cut or rinse debris from a wound or abrasion. Teas can be used as a final rinse after shampooing or even in place of soap.

When our red tabby kitten began to scratch the furniture instead of his scratching post, I filled a small squirt gun with water. As Pumpkin clawed industriously, I spritzed his back to discourage his inappropriate behavior. To my surprise, Pumpkin turned, delighted, and begged for a shower. Every week from then on, I brewed a strong chamomile tea, which is recommended for blonds and redheads, filled a hydraulic sprayer, spread towels on my lap and soaked him to the skin while he purred and kneaded. A thorough towel drying and an hour in the sun returned his sweet-smelling coat to its fluffy, dander-free glory.

Oil Infusions

To make an oil infusion, such as an oil for treating ear infections or in preparation for salve-making, you can use the stove, an oven, the sun or an electric cooker. Although any carrier oil can be used, olive oil is the standard medicinal infusion oil.

Fresh chopped garlic and fresh or dried mullein blossoms are traditional ingredients in ear oils for dogs, cats and humans, especially children. Use either or any combination of both. Cover the plant material with olive oil and heat it gently in the top of a double boiler above simmering water or in a closed glass jar set on a rack in a pan of simmering water for one to two hours or longer. If using dry herbs, additional oil may be needed as the plant matter absorbs it. Use enough oil to cover the herbs well but not so much that your result is weak and ineffective. Start with 2 cups oil to 1 cup dried herbs and adjust the proportions as desired. Fresh herbs, which should be allowed to wilt before using, will absorb less liquid, so simply cover them with oil.

To make a solar infusion, let fresh plant material wilt slightly to reduce its water content, then loosely pack a clean glass jar with fresh herbs (or fill a jar half way with loosely packed dried herbs), then fill it to the top with oil, clean the top of the jar so that no oil or plant material interferes with a tight seal, put the lid on tight and leave the jar in the hot sun for several weeks or months. My favorite oil for salve-making is a blend of fresh St. John's wort blossoms, calendula blossoms and chopped, wilted comfrey that stays outdoors from July through October. The unusually potent healing properties of this oil, which the St. John's wort colors a deep red, may be due to its prolonged photosynthesis or to some magical effect of continual sunlight and moonlight.

Another way to infuse herbs in oil is to use the oven. Pour olive oil over fresh or dried herbs in a stainless steel pan, cover with foil and bake at low heat (200º to 250º F) for two or more hours, or at a higher temperature for a shorter time. Check the pan from time to time to prevent scorching or burning. The oil is "done" when it takes on the color and fragrance of the herbs. Electric turkey roasters, slow cookers (crock pots) and other heat sources also work well.

When ready to use, strain the oil through cheesecloth and add a few drops of tea tree oil or grapefruit seed extract as a disinfecting preservative. Pour into a clean glass jar, label with ingredients and date of preparation and store away from heat and light. Stored correctly, oils can last for years, though most herbalists prefer to make them annually for maximum freshness. Note that these oils are for external use only. Discard any oil that becomes rancid.

Herbal Salves

To turn an herbal oil into an herbal salve, just add beeswax. One of the best all-purpose salves you can make begins with fresh or dried comfrey, calendula blossoms and St. John's wort blossoms. Either infuse oils separately or pour olive oil over the combined plants (equal proportions are nice, but they work well in any combination) and heat until the oil absorbs the color and fragrance of the plants. The more comfrey you use, the darker green the oil will be; the more calendula, the more yellow; and the more St. John's wort blossoms you use, the deeper red.

Basic Salve Recipe

   1 cup infused oil
   1/2 tsp. tea tree oil
   1/4 tsp. grapefruit seed extract
   Several drops essential oil (lavender or other)
   1 oz. beeswax
Combine ingredients in a double boiler or over very low heat until the beeswax has melted. Test the salve by placing a spoonful in the refrigerator. As soon as it hardens, check to be sure the salve is soft but not runny. If it's too soft, add more beeswax; if too hard, add more oil. Pour into clean baby food jars or other containers. Herbal supply catalogs sell small tins for salve.

This antiseptic, analgesic, soothing salve speeds the healing of cuts, burns and other wounds. Cats tend to dislike the fragrance of tea tree and lavender, and many dogs are attracted to the olive oil in salve and lick it off as fast as you put it on, which may present a logistical problem. None of the ingredients are harmful if swallowed; in fact, this type of salve can be used on the sore nipples of a nursing mother without harming her puppies or kittens. Even if the salve stays in place for only a short time, it will speed the healing of most skin conditions.

An Herbal Glossary

Here are brief definitions of terms you are likely to find in herbal reference books and field guides.

Abortifacient. Induces the premature expulsion (abortion) of the fetus. Same meaning as ecbolic. *Example:* Pennyroyal.

Adaptogen. Gradually corrects imbalances, such as by raising or lowering blood pressure, reducing or increasing pulse rate or correcting blood sugar levels. *Examples:* Ginseng, Siberian ginseng, fo-ti, schizandra, ashwagandha, astragalus.

Alterative. Gradually restores normal body functions. Also known as blood purifier. *Examples:* Burdock root, dandelion leaf and root, echinacea, red clover, goldenseal, Oregon grape root, nettles, yellow dock root.

Analgesic. Relieves pain; also called anodyne. Used internally or externally, depending on the herb. *Examples:* Skullcap, lobelia, chamomile, crampbark, valerian, catnip, cloves, passionflower.

Antacid. Neutralizes acid in the stomach and intestinal tract. Most also contain demulcent properties to soothe, protect and heal the stomach lining. *Examples:* Irish moss, fennel seed, slippery elm, dandelion leaf and root, most seaweeds.

Anthelmintic. Destroys and expels worms and parasites from the intestines. Same as vermifuge. *Examples:* Aloe, chaparral, cloves, wormwood, garlic, pomegranate (white rind), rue, black walnut hull.

Antiabortive. Counteracts abortive tendencies. *Examples:* Crampbark, lobelia, red raspberry, witch hazel.

Antibilious. Combats nausea, abdominal discomfort, headache, constipation and gas caused by excessive secretion of bile. *Example:* Barberry, dandelion, goldenseal, vervain, mugwort.

Antibiotic. Inhibits the growth of germs, bacteria and harmful microbes; also called antimicrobial, antizymotic. *Examples:* Clove, chaparral, echinacea, eucalyptus, garlic, goldenseal, grapefruit seed extract, myrrh, tea tree, thyme.

Anticatarrhal. Helps eliminate and prevent excessive respiratory mucus. *Examples:* Cayenne, sage, goldenseal, mullein, yerba santa, ginger, echinacea, garlic, yarrow.

Antiemetic. Prevents or alleviates nausea and vomiting. *Examples:* Black horehound, cayenne, cloves, dill, fennel, ginger, lavender, lemon balm, meadowsweet, peach leaves.

Antilithic. Aids in preventing the formation of stones in the kidneys and bladder. *For urinary stones:* Gravelroot, marshmallow root, cleavers, cornsilk, parsley root, dandelion root, buchu, stone root. *For gallbladder stones:* Oregon grape root.

Antiphlogistic. Counteracts inflammation or swelling. *Examples:* Arnica, chamomile.

Antiseptic. Helps prevent the growth of bacteria and resist pathogenic microorganisms. *Examples:* Goldenseal, calendula, chaparral, myrrh, sage, garlic; essential oils of tea tree, eucalyptus, pine, clove, juniper berries, thyme; grapefruit seed extract.

Antispasmodic. Prevents or eases cramps in the body and muscle spasms. *Examples:* Crampbark, black cohosh, skullcap, wild lettuce, blue cohosh, lobelia, lady's slipper, valerian, wild yam.

Aromatic. Herb with a pleasant fragrant scent and pungent taste. *Examples:* Angelica, aniseed, balm, basil, caraway, cardamom, celery, chamomile, cinnamon, cloves, coriander, dill, fennel, hyssop, ginger, meadowsweet, pennyroyal, peppermint, rosemary, valerian, wood betony.

Astringent. Constricts tissue, reducing discharge and secretions. Most astringents contain tannins. *Examples:* Bayberry bark, witch hazel bark, wild oak bark, prince's pine, uva ursi, oak gall, cranesbill.

Bitter. Herb having a bitter taste and serving as a stimulant tonic to the gastrointestinal mucous membranes. *Examples:* Centaury, goldenseal, gentian, horehound, wormwood.

Carminative. Contains volatile oils that help prevent intestinal gas from forming and assist in expelling it. *Examples:* Angelica, anise, caraway, cardamom, calamus, ginger, dill, cayenne, chamomile, peppermint.

Cathartic. Causes evacuation of the bowels. A cathartic may be either mild (laxative) or vigorous (purgative). See those definitions.

Cholagogue. Stimulates the flow of bile from the liver into the intestines. *Examples:* Balmony, barberry, black root, fringe tree, wahoo, wild yam.

Demulcent. Has mucilaginous properties that are soothing and protective internally to irritated and inflamed surfaces and tissues. Important in formulas. *Examples:* Licorice, chickweed, chia, aloe vera, mullein, slippery elm, Irish moss, psyllium, flaxseed, fenugreek, oatmeal.

Deodorant. Eliminates foul odors. *Examples:* Blackberry, echinacea, wheatgrass, numerous essential oils.

Diuretic. Promotes the production and secretion of urine. Used to treat water retention, cystitis, overweight, edema and types of skin infection. *Examples:* Parsley, cleavers, buchu, dandelion, nettles, cornsilk, horsetail, yarrow.

Emetic. Induces vomiting and causes the evacuation of stomach contents. *Examples:* Ipecacuanha, lobelia in large quantities.

Emmenagogue. Often used to describe tonic herbs for the female system, helps promote menstruation in humans. *Examples:* Black cohosh, angelica, rue, blue cohosh, pennyroyal. Emmenagogue herbs should be avoided during animal breeding and pregnancy.

Emollient. Used externally to soften, soothe and protect skin surfaces. Similar to demulcents, which are used internally. *Examples:* Flaxseed, slippery elm, comfrey, chickweed.

Expectorant. Helps expel excess mucus from the system. *Examples:* Eucalyptus, elecampane, lobelia, coltsfoot, yerba santa, grindelea.

Febrifuge. Reduces body temperature and fever; same as antipyretic or refrigerant. *Examples:* Angelica, cayenne, elder flower, lobelia, peppermint, Peruvian bark *(Cinchona succiruba)*.

Galactagogue. Increases the secretion of mother's milk. *Examples:* Fennel, aniseseed, raspberry, fenugreek, blessed thistle.

Hemostatic. Generally internally astringent, arrests hemorrhaging or internal bleeding. *Examples:* Cayenne, shepherd's purse, goldenseal, yarrow, cranesbill, wild oak bark.

Hemetic. Rich in iron and manganese, augments and enriches the red corpuscles of the blood. *Example:* Yellow dock root.

Hepatic. Promotes the wellbeing of the liver and increases the secretion of bile. *Examples:* Dandelion, Oregon grape root, goldenseal, wild yam, yellow dock.

Hypnotic. A powerful nervine relaxant and sedative that induces sleep. *Examples:* Hops, Jamaican dogwood, passionflower, valerian, mistletoe, skullcap.

Laxative. Promotes bowel movement. Laxatives are not as drastic as purgatives. *Examples:* Cascara sagrada, flaxseed, senna, rhubarb root.

Lithotriptic: See antilithic.

Local anaesthetic. Produces loss of sensation where applied locally. *Examples:* Caraway oil, coca, oil of cloves, echinacea.

Mucilaginous. Has a soothing effect on inflamed mucous membranes. *Examples:* Comfrey, fenugreek, flaxseed, Iceland moss, Irish moss, mallow, marshmallow, quince seed, slippery elm.

Nervine: Calms and soothes the nerves and reduces tension and anxiety, a healing tonic for the nerves. *Examples:* Catnip, passionflower, oatstraw, valerian, chamomile, lady's slipper, peppermint.

Parisiticide See anthelmintic.

Peristaltic. Stimulates and increases peristalsis or muscular contraction, as in the bowels. *Example:* Bitter rind of aloe vera.

Pectoral. Healing to complaints of the broncho-pulmonary area, having a strengthening effect on the respiratory system. *Examples:* Coltsfoot, elecampane, licorice, comfrey, mullein.

Purgative. Promotes vigorous evacuation of the bowels. Usually used to relieve severe constipation or to help rid the body of toxins. *Example:* Castor oil.

Rubefacient. Draws inflammation and congestion from deeper areas, increases circulation and promotes warmth. *Examples:* Cayenne, horseradish, ginger, clove, mustard.

Sedative. Lowers the functional activity of an organ or part of the body, thereby tending to calm, moderate or tranquilize. *Examples:* Black cohosh, passionflower, chamomile, valerian, lady's slipper, skullcap.

Sialagogue. Promotes the secretion and flow of saliva and aids digestion. *Examples:* Echinacea, black pepper, ginger, cayenne, gentian.

Soporific. Helps produce sleep. *Examples:* Skullcap, valerian, passionflower.

Stimulant. Increases functional activity and energy in the body. *Examples:* Cayenne, peppermint, sarsaparilla, rosemary, prickly ash, horseradish, ginger, ginseng, sage, astragalus, mustard.

Styptic. Arrests hemorrhage and bleeding. *Examples:* Yarrow, cayenne, shepherd's purse, essential oil of lavender, clean cobwebs.

Tonic. Restores and strengthens the entire system, producing and restoring normal tone. Most tonics have general effects on the whole body and specific effects on different organs. *Examples:* Ginseng, dong quai, nettle, dandelion, raspberry leaf.

Vulnerary. Used in treating fresh cuts and wounds, usually as a poultice; a healing substance that promotes cell growth and repair. *Examples:* Aloe vera, goldenseal, comfrey, chickweed, plantain, St. John's wort, calendula.

Dosages

Most of the herbs recommended in this book are safe to administer to pets in teas, tinctures, capsules, tablets or simply mixed into food several times daily for several days or even weeks at a time. Many commercially prepared tinctures are weaker and less concentrated than those you can make at home, either because the proportion of alcohol to herbs is higher, creating a more dilute solution; the commercially produced tinctures are made quickly, allowing insufficient time for complete extraction; or the quality of the raw materials is inferior.

Because concentration and quality vary among tinctures, just as the pets and people who take them vary in size, weight and physical condition, it is impossible to specify a single dosage for best results. If you don't notice improvement after using a tincture as directed, your pet may need more. In general, if you purchase a tincture that is clear in color and has no distinctive herbal taste or smell, it is less likely to be effective than one made of the same herb that has a strong taste, smell and color.

If you purchase herbs in capsules, try to buy them from a retailer whose stock rotates quickly or who powders herbs for capsules as needed. Powdered herbs lose their potency when exposed to heat, light or humidity.

As you become familiar with herbs, experiment with small doses of single herbs in tea, tinctures or capsules before giving therapeutic doses.

Suggested Dose for the First-time Use of Any Herb

Animal's Weight	Tincture	Size 00 Capsule	Tea
5 to 10 lbs	2 drops	1/2 cap	1 tsp.
10 to 20 lbs	4 drops	1 cap	2 tsp.
20 to 30 lbs	6 drops	1 cap	1 Tbsp.
30 to 50 lbs	6-10 drops	2 caps	4 tsp.
50 to 70 lbs	10-14 drops	2 caps	5 tsp.
70 to 90 lbs	14-18 drops	3 caps	2 Tbsp.
90 to 110 lbs	18-22 drops	4 caps	3 Tbsp.

All preparations should be given 3 times daily.

If your pet displays any adverse reaction to an herb or herbal preparation, such as diarrhea, rapid pulse, dizziness, vomiting, itching, rash, loss of appetite or any other unusual symptom that seems to result from using the herb, substitute something else. Adverse reactions to the herbs recommended here are unusual, but just as people have allergic reactions to different foods and herbs, so can their companion animals.

For most of the herbs recommended here, the dosages above are conservative and cautious; they are smaller than the therapeutic doses you would use to treat an acute condition but are appropriate first doses to gauge an animal's response.

Depending on the condition (chronic or acute, mild or serious) and the nature of the herb, larger or smaller doses may be appropriate. Herbal preparations used on a regular basis as nutritional supplements or preventives are often given in courses. A typical course of treatment is five days on and two days off, which is the schedule de Bairacli Levy recommends. In the treatment of chronic conditions, therapeutic herbs can be given according to this schedule, or herbs with a similar action can replace each other at regular intervals. For example, to treat a long-standing arthritic condition, an herbalist might use one anti-inflammatory herb for three to five weeks following the five-days-on, two-days-off schedule, then switch to another anti-inflammatory for the next three to five weeks. If an herb is given every day of the week and every week of the year, the body may become accustomed to it and fail to respond as efficiently as it would otherwise. For the same reason, herbs used to treat acute conditions, such as echinacea for bacterial or viral infections, should not be given in therapeutic doses every day as a preventive; they should be saved until needed.

On the Safety of Herbs

To say that herbs are controversial is to make an understatement. Warnings about their potential toxicity abound. Is the user really in danger?

In a few cases, yes. Foxglove, the source of digitalis, is a poisonous plant, as is belladonna. No one should ever make a tea from either, but there have been cases of mistaken identity, such as when a novice herbalist mistook foxglove for comfrey with fatal results, or more recently, when the FDA documented the contamination of a commercial supply of plantain by foxglove.

Laxative herbs, such as cascara sagrada, should be used in small doses and for a limited time to avoid diarrhea and bowel irritation; powerful stimulant herbs, like ma huang (ephedra) should not be used by people with high blood pressure and are seldom if ever recommended for pets. The same is true for herbs that contain caffeine, such as green tea, guarana and kola nut.

Some common herbs cause skin irritation and must be handled with care. One woman who read that rue is a natural insect repellent rubbed fresh rue on her skin and broke out in a terrible rash. Rue is an insect-repellent when used as a companion plant in the garden, but it has never been recommended for use on the skin. Another insect-repelling plant is tansy, which, although less irritating than rue, affects some people adversely. A longhaired dog or cat might not be affected, but anyone stroking her fur can be. Even aloe vera, one of the most widely known medicinal herbs, can be irritating: it has a harsh laxative effect when taken internally unless the gel is removed from its leaves with care so that none of the plant's cathartic ingredients come with it.

Still, according to experts on the subject, most warnings about toxic herbs stem not from experience but from theory and the way in which herbs are researched, regulated and reported. According to Mark Blumenthal, executive director of the American Botanical Council and publisher of the journal *HerbalGram,* toxicologists determine the relative safety of a drug by weighing its benefits against anticipated risks. This is why chemotherapy and radiation therapy, which often cause hair loss, severe vomiting, weight loss, immune disturbances, brittle bones and other side effects, are considered appropriate for the treatment of terminal cancer. The widely used pain relievers aspirin and ibuprofin cause between 10,000 and 20,000 human deaths per year, a statistic that receives little publicity. In contrast, herbs used medicinally are so rarely toxic that a former president of the American Association of Poison Control Centers says the association considers the category too insignificant to track in its computer banks.

Because herbs cannot be patented, there is no economic incentive for their testing in the United States, and little meaningful research is conducted here. But in Europe, Japan, China and other countries, herbal remedies are widely used and tested. Most herbs in common use have a long history of safety.

Some confusion in the U.S. stems from the Food and Drug Administration's "GRAS" or "Generally Recognized as Safe" list, which contains about 200 herbs commonly used as extracts, flavorings, oils and seasonings. An additional 200 herbs in common use do not appear on the list, such as slippery elm bark, burdock root, arrowroot, catnip, coltsfoot, echinacea, flaxseed, goldenseal root, gotu kola, hibiscus flowers, horsetail, uva ursi, stinging nettle, saw palmetto berry, skullcap, senna, tormentilla, blue vervain and yellow dock root. Such herbs are not unsafe; they are simply unlisted.

Burdock root is a common Japanese vegetable called gobo, sold in thousands of grocery stores and sushi bars and used in many herbal formulas. In one instance, a batch of burdock was contaminated with belladonna root, which contains the poisonous compound atropine. It happened only once, but some medical authorities still refer to burdock as toxic because of its presumed atropine levels. Burdock root contains no atropine and is as safe to eat as potatoes. In fact, potatoes, which belong to the belladonna or nightshade family, are more dangerous because green potato skins, sprouting eyes and all above-ground parts of the potato plant are toxic. Burdock root is an important herb for pets, as it helps cleanse the blood and supports the immune system.

Chamomile is often blamed for allergic reactions, especially in people who have ragweed allergies. In one case, a man with a severe ragweed allergy went into anaphylactic shock while drinking chamomile tea. In the past hundred years, only five cases of chamomile allergy have been reported in the medical literature, and some research suggests that chamomile actually helps alleviate allergic reactions such as hay fever. Chamomile is an exceptionally safe herb for pets, and it has important digestive, anti-inflammatory and relaxing benefits for all animals, including people.

Sassafras contains safrole, a substance that the FDA tested in large quantities on rats in the 1950s. When the rats developed liver cancer, a compound in sassafras was blamed. The same compound, safrole, is found in nutmeg, black pepper and mace, but these seasonings were never implicated. Because safrole is not soluble in water, someone drinking sassafras tea can ingest very little of it and no case of liver damage from sassafras tea has ever been reported. The southeastern U.S., where most sassafras tea is consumed, has a lower liver cancer rate than other parts of the country. Sassafras is used in some worming blends for dogs and cats, and their recommended doses and schedule are unlikely to cause problems in pets.

The Herb Research Foundation is one of the organizations gathering scientific data pertaining to herb safety from around the world. If you have questions about the safety of any herb or if you'd like information about an herb's uses, contact the HRF (see Resources for this chapter in the Appendix).

Common sense and education are your best guides to herb use. Don't use an herb without learning about it first. Mislabeled herbs are rare, and a company that grows its own herbs and tests what it buys helps insure product safety. The safest herbs may be those you grow yourself using organic methods, plants you harvest from areas that are free of pesticides and far from highways and automobile exhaust and dried herbs purchased from reputable sources, labeled organically grown or wildcrafted. Unfortunately, nearly all herbs imported into the United States are fumigated on arrival, a consideration for anyone using herbs medicinally. No discussion of herb safety would be complete without a mention of this concern.

Herbs for Dogs and Cats
A Conversation with Deb Soule

Every herbalist's dream is to live and work surrounded by plants. Deb Soule realized that dream in 1985 when she founded Avena Botanicals Herbal Apothecary on the coast of Maine. Now housed on a 24-acre farm half a mile from its organic gardens and teaching center, Avena is an active business with eight dedicated partners and a catalog listing hundreds of extracts, infused oils, salves, essential oils, teas and a special line: Herbs for Animals. Over 60 percent of the ingredients come from Avena's own gardens, nearby woods, fields and the seashore. Soule is the author of *The Roots of Healing: A Woman's Book of Herbs,* published by Citadel Press.

What is the most effective thing people can do to improve the lives of their companion animals?

SOULE: I can answer that question in one word: food. No herb or supplement can bring perfect health to a poorly fed dog or cat. Once you have the right diet in place, I like to add herbs like nettle, alfalfa, rosemary, calendula flowers and the seaweeds kelp and dulse. These plants are rich in vitamins and trace minerals, so they help with a healthy coat of fur and proper pigmentation. The mucous membranes in the body benefit and so do all the organs, bones and teeth. This formula's high mineral content reduces a dog's interest in eating stools. We recently added spirulina to the formula because of its minerals and chlorophyll and because it's cleansing to the kidneys and liver.

I use a lot of garlic, too, because I think it's really good for animals. I make a garlic vinegar and put a little in their food every day. You can do this at home by filling a pint jar with chopped up garlic and then covering the garlic with an organic brown rice or apple cider vinegar, something that's raw and hasn't been heated or distilled like white vinegar. Let it stand a few weeks and you have a strong vinegar tincture with all kinds of healing properties. You can give a teaspoon a day to a large dog, half a teaspoon to a medium size dog, down to an eighth of a teaspoon for a cat or very small dog.

I don't have a regular schedule for garlic, but I feed it most of the time. It's probably a good idea to give animals a break so they don't eat the same herbs in the same quantities every day. A few days on, a few days off–that usually works well.

What are some of the common conditions in dogs and cats that are easy to treat with herbs?

SOULE: One is flea allergies and the itching, scratching and coat problems that come with them. To help the animal feel better, I like to make a tea using equal amounts of fresh or dried red clover, nettle, calendula, rosemary and yarrow, which are some of my favorites, brewed as a strong infusion that steeps for eight hours or so. If the herbs are fresh, I use a lot, like a handful for each cup. If they're dried, it's one or two tablespoons per cup of water. Then I apply the cool tea to the affected area with a cloth or just pour it on directly as a rinse, repeating the application every few hours. This tea is so cooling and healing that it reduces the inflammation right away.

To get rid of fleas, we have a flea soap that I've been making for 12 years. It's a liquid castor oil soap with essential oil of pine as the main ingredient. We add calendula and rosemary extracts to keep the skin and fur clean and soft, but the pine in what smothers and kills the fleas. You don't even have to leave it on for five minutes; just lather it up, rinse it off and the fleas fall off dead.

We used to use eucalyptus, but that was a problem for animals taking homeopathic remedies at the same time because eucalyptus is a well-known antidote; it interferes with homeopathy. I found that pine oil doesn't have this side effect, so that's why we changed the formula. When homeopathy isn't a factor, eucalyptus works very well. You can take any liquid soap or shampoo and add several drops of essential oil just before you put it on the cat or dog. I like to use a natural castor oil or olive oil castile soap because these are simple soaps that clean well and don't contain harsh detergents or chemicals.

What about ear mites?

SOULE: Garlic, rosemary and rue infused in olive oil work well together at killing ear mites. Our other ear oil contains mullein in addition to other herbs, and it clears up ear infections and excess ear wax in people and animals.

Do you combine homeopathy with herbs?

SOULE: I do because they're so compatible. The homeopathy usually works immediately and the herbs stimulate healing in a different way. Take puncture wounds. It might be a porcupine quill, the bite of a sharp tooth or the wound caused by a thorn or splinter. Homeopathic Ledum is an excellent treatment for all puncture wounds, so that's the first thing to give. Then chop, pulverize or puree some fresh plantain, a weed that grows in lawns all over America, and apply it to the wound because this will pull any infection out. At the same time, I usually give the animal a glycerite of goldenseal and echinacea internally. This combination stimulates rapid healing with no complications.

What are the most common health problems in dogs and cats?

SOULE: Arthritis is probably the most common chronic condition in dogs, just like people. In fact, my mother has arthritis, and she has been getting relief from glucosamine sulfate, which is the same supplement holistic vets often recommend for arthritic dogs and horses. That, in combination with alfalfa, would be my first choice, but the real culprit is diet. I think it's impossible to cure any chronic condition in an animal who isn't eating fresh raw foods.

Another common condition is urinary tract infections in cats. For that I like to give a cleavers or cornsilk tea because they're soothing kidney tonics and mild diuretics, so they keep the fluids moving. Often I'll add a little echinacea or goldenseal glycerite because they're infection fighters, and uva ursi, which is a specific for this condition. The dosage schedule I use for a glycerite or tincture is one drop per five pounds of body weight. If it's acute, I give it once every two or three hours until the infection clears; if it's a long-term problem, I'll give it three times a day for five days, then take two days off and continue on that schedule, five days on and two off, for as long as necessary.

For incontinence in older cats, one of the best herbs to use is couch grass. You can make couch grass tea for dogs or cats or just put it in their food if they'll eat it. Couch grass is one of the ingredients in our daily tonic for animals, which is a tincture. The other ingredients are garlic, kelp, nettle, milk thistle seed, meadowsweet and hops. This is an all-purpose tonic for dogs and cats. We focus on herbs that help prevent worms and infections, provide trace minerals, protect the liver, strengthen the kidneys, improve digestion and in general have a tonic effect on the body.

What should America's pet lovers know about using herbs?

SOULE: The information the public receives about herbal medicine is often trendy and superficial. Because our culture is so accustomed to the methods of allopathic medicine, it is easy to look at herbs as simple replacements for pharmaceutical drugs but this is a mistake. Herbs aren't a quick fix the way drugs often are; they go deeper, to the source of a health problem, and they are usually gentler and slower acting. Learn how to work with herbs not only to help repair problems your dog, cat, bird or other animal may have but to prevent problems altogether. Don't be afraid to experiment. When you use whole plant ingredients like blossoms, leaves and roots, whether fresh or dried, in teas or powders or tinctures, you're using versatile materials that don't have to be measured like prescription drugs. These are forgiving, living substances; they're food for the mind, soul and body. Plants deserve our care and appreciation. I hope pet lovers everywhere will want to study them and that their animals will enjoy the benefits.

A Pet's Apothecary: Herbs for Animals

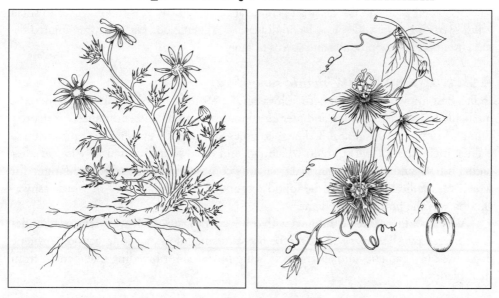

Remember that there are hundreds of medicinal herbs from around the world used for every type of condition imaginable. Here are just a few of the roots, barks, leaves and blossoms that are useful for pets. Representing Chinese, European, North and South American and African traditions, they demonstrate the wide variety in Mother Nature's pharmacy.

Aloe vera *(Aloe vera)*

The same succulent that offers relief from sunburn, insect bites and skin irritation has practical uses in pet care. The juice or gel, which is sold as a beverage, can be added to food to aid the treatment of arthritis and digestive problems; use up to 1 tablespoon per 20 pounds of body weight. Externally, the leaf's inner gel can be applied to hot spots, skin conditions, burns and wounds. The bitter inner rind of aloe vera is a powerful laxative; if giving fresh aloe vera in food, use only the gel.

Arnica *(Arnica montana)*

Arnica is a small alpine plant with yellow blossoms. The flower heads, made into tea, tincture or massage oil, are anti-inflammatory and relieve the pain of bruises, sprains, rheumatism and inflammation. The plant is not recommended for internal use. In *Medicinal Plants of the Pacific West*, Michael Moore noted that the primary uses for arnica have remained unchanged for centuries. The tincture, oil, salve, tea, or bruised fresh plant is used externally for bruises, hyperextensions, arthritis, bursitis, and myalgia. "Arnica works by stimulating and dilating blood vessels," he wrote, "particularly the specialized capillaries that control whether blood is piped into the small peripheral capillary beds or is shunted over to small veins, bypassing more widespread blood dispersal." When blood circulates into injured tissues, it removes waste products and speeds healing.

Ashwagandha *(Withania somnifera)*

India's best known adaptogen herb, ashwagandha root has long been used in Ayurvedic medicine to facilitate learning and memory, increase stamina and endurance, lift depression and improve overall health. There is some experimental evidence to support these claims, including a 1994 study in which rats and mice swam substantially longer after taking ashwagandha. In human trials, patients complaining of lethargy and fatigue for which no medical cause could be found responded to a tonic blend in which ashwagandha was the primary ingredient.

Ashwagandha is often combined with other adaptogens, such as ginseng, schisandra or licorice. Like all adaptogens, it can be taken in small doses for long periods. Athletic dogs, tired or apathetic animals and pets being prepared for breeding may benefit from such blends.

Astragalus *(Astragalus membranaceous)*

One of the most popular Chinese herbs, astragalus root is revered as a powerful immune system strengthener. Traditionally used to treat anxiety and fatigue, astragalus has general tonic properties; that is, it heals, repairs and supports the entire body, increasing stamina and building resistance to disease and infection. Its diuretic properties make it a specific for the kidneys and urinary tract; it is also recommended for conditions relating to the spleen, lungs and blood. In lab tests, astragalus has been shown to kill viruses, destroy cancer cells and induce interferon production.

Astragalus root can be brewed as a decoction or used in capsules or tinctures. It is an excellent herb to give after exposure to infectious diseases, during training for athletic events, in times of stress or overwork or whenever an animal develops symptoms of a respiratory or infectious illness.

No dangerous side effects have been reported, but some human users have experienced mild diarrhea or abdominal bloating. Reducing the dosage eliminates these symptoms.

Black Walnut Hull *(Juglans nigra)*

Black walnut hull powders and tinctures are popular anthelmintics: they help expel worms and other parasites from the body. In addition, this astringent herb is an effective treatment for diarrhea. Walnut hulls are green when they fall from the tree in fall and turn black within a week. The green hulls of black walnut are prized for their superior benefits, making "green" black walnut hull tincture the preference of many herbalists.

"Every day in the summer I put black walnut capsules in my dogs' food," says Beverly Cappel-King. "I take it myself and nothing bites me, either. It works great for mosquitoes. Black walnut tincture keeps the bugs away, too. A farmer in Italy once told me, 'Look at a black walnut tree. You'll never see any insects on it. Even moss doesn't grow on it. It's so nasty that nothing grows on it.' He said that what he and other farmers did was shave the hull of green, immature black walnut hulls and throw it in the food of all their animals. His horses and cows don't get bots, those insect larvae that live in the skin and come out through the spine, leaving holes in the animal's back. The sheep and goats don't get lice. The black walnut makes them taste terrible so the insects won't bite them."

Boswellia *(Boswellia serratta)*

A large, branching tree native to India that produces a gummy resin with a long history of medicinal use in that country, boswellia is a potent anti-inflammatory herb that effectively shrinks inflamed tissue by improving circulation and increasing synovial fluid viscosity. It is approved in India for use against osteoarthritis, rheumatoid arthritis, soft-tissue rheumatism, low back pain and fibromyalgia (fibrositis).

In the U.S., much of boswellia's favorable publicity comes from veterinarians and pet owners, for it is used with much success on dogs, cats and horses. Mark Heimann, D.V.M., of Bay City, N.Y., put two of his most difficult canine arthritis patients on boswellia with excellent results; Gary L. Schmid, D.V.M., of Ellensburg, Wash., has tested boswellia in dogs and horses for over three years and reports that dogs with spinal arthritis and hip dysplasia respond favorably. Ronald Blackwell, D.V.M., and Gary Kaufman, D.V.M., veterinarians in Kentucky and Arizona, have treated horses with chronic arthritis and injuries such as stifle problems, sore backs, bowed tendons and bone spurs, all with good results. Boswellia capsules and powders are sold for human and animal use; boswellia creams help relieve pain and inflammation externally. Note that boswellia does not appear to reverse or cure arthritis, for when pet owners run out of the herb, their animals regress quickly.

Bupleurum *(Bupleurum spp.)* **or Bei Chau Hu**

A Chinese herb, bupleurum has a long history of use in a variety of conditions, including liver disease and allergies. Its anti-inflammatory effects make it an effective treatment for arthritis and related illnesses, though it is better known for its sedative, relaxing properties, its reduction of sugar cravings and its use in the treatment of premenstrual symptoms and migraine headaches in humans. In animals, bupleurum can be used in the treatment of arthritis, liver disorders, skin and coat problems and stress. Bupleurum strengthens the immune system and, because of its antibacterial and antiviral properties, can be taken to ward off upper respiratory infections.

Burdock Root *(Arctium lappa)*

Burdock is a biennial weed that grows throughout the northern U.S. and Europe, where its round, prickly seeds make its name obvious. In Japan burdock is not a weed, it's a cultivated vegetable as widely used as our potato. Gobo, the Japanese name for burdock root, can be found in Oriental markets and sushi bars everywhere.

Burdock root is a blood cleanser and blood builder as well as a kidney tonic. It has a nurturing, repairing quality, helping to build up the system and increase immunity. In addition, it has been used in the treatment of arthritis, and skin and coat conditions often improve with its regular use. In France it is given to diabetics, and tests have shown that the fresh root lowers blood sugar levels in laboratory animals. Burdock is an ingredient in Essiac tea, which is often recommended for animals with cancer and other serious illnesses.

According to John Lust in *The Herb Book,* burdock can be used for stomach ailments and to neutralize and eliminate poisons in the system.

Calendula *(Calendula officinalis)*

The cheerful orange and yellow blossoms of calendula, also known as pot marigold, are easy to grow and can be used fresh or dried in food, teas, oil infusions, salves and tinctures. Dried calendula flowers can be added to pets' food whole or powdered. Internally, the herb is a blood cleanser with an affinity for the digestive organs. The Austrian herbalist Maria Treben used the tea for gastrointestinal disorders, stomach cramps, ulcers, inflammation of the large intestine, blood or bacteria in the urine, fluid retention, viral infections, infectious hepatitis, liver disorders and worms. Externally, it disinfects wounds, helps heal the skin and treats sores, burns and fungal infections.

Calendula blossoms are often combined with comfrey and St. John's wort in healing salves and oils.

Chamomile *(Matricaria chamomilla, Anthemia nobilis)*

Also spelled camomile, chamomile is one of the most widely used herbs in the world. Even those who know little about its medicinal properties enjoy its fresh apple fragrance and relaxing influence. Chamomile is a nervine, carminative, tonic, sedative, emmenagogue, antispasmodic, aromatic, stimulant and anthelmintic herb. In short, it soothes mind and body, helps prevent infection, heals wounds, relieves indigestion and ulcers, relaxes the nerves, alleviates inflammation and skin irritations, prevents insomnia and relieves both headaches and muscle cramps. Chamomile is so safe that it is recommended for newborn babies.

Only the blossoms are used in chamomile tea, which makes it interesting to do this fragrant work. If you grow your own, try planting both the tall annual German chamomile *(Matricaria chamomilla)* and the prostrate perennial Roman or English chamomile *(Anthemia nobilis)* to see which you prefer. Both can be used for tea and are said to have similar properties, but the sweet apple fragrance that is the plant's signature is stronger and more pleasant in the taller-growing annual.

Research shows that chamomile tea can calm nervousness, relieve pain, promote deep sleep and lift the spirits. Fresh or dried flowers can be fed directly or brewed as an infusion or tinctured. The liquid preparations are appropriate additions to food or water.

Chamomile tea strained through a paper coffee filter makes a soothing wash for the eyes and is well-known as a hair rinse. Unless your pet's coat is extremely light in color, try a final rinse of chamomile tea after shampooing; even dark-coated pets smell wonderful and are dander-free after a thorough soaking. A strong infusion of chamomile tea may temporarily darken white fur, so test a sample before applying.

Comfrey *(Symphytum officinale)*

Every part of the comfrey plant is medicinal: its leaves, roots, stalks and flowers. A demulcent, astringent, nutritive, tonic, mucilaginous herb, comfrey has a soothing and healing effect on every organ it contacts. The most significant plant source of the cell-growth stimulator allantoin, comfrey dramatically speeds the healing of wounds and even broken bones. In fact, some herbalists have fed comfrey to dogs after surgical pins were placed in their broken bones following traffic accidents, and the bones healed so quickly that they forced the pins out, requiring additional surgery. (Comfrey's common name is "knit bone.") Among its hundreds of therapeutic applications are digestive disorders, urinary tract infections, diarrhea, hernias, hemorrhoids and ulcers.

Comfrey has been removed from many pet supplements because of the negative press it has received in recent years. The herb contains a class of compounds that, when isolated and fed in large doses, can cause liver damage and cancer in rats. In hundreds of years of use, no cases of human problems with comfrey ever appeared, but in 1984 a woman who had been taking comfrey-pepsin tablets developed liver toxicity and, since then, three additional cases of human liver disease have been documented in people who took the herb.

The potentially harmful ingredients in comfrey are its pyrrolizidine alkaloids (PAs). Because these alkaloids are less concentrated in the comfrey commonly grown in America than in other varieties and because of the plant's long history of safe use, many herbalists and pet owners continue to use it on a regular basis, feeding chopped, fresh comfrey, dried comfrey in capsules or comfrey tinctures to their animals. Skin and coat conditions often respond quickly. A cockatoo arrived at her new home with only the feathers on her head, for she had plucked all the others, but within a few days of eating foods supplemented with fresh chopped comfrey, the bird's skin irritations subsided and she soon grew a beautiful coat of white feathers. Similar reports regarding dogs, cats, rabbits and other pets are common.

At the same time, veterinarian Beverly Cappel-King cautions that she has seen dogs who began vomiting after taking several comfrey capsules daily for three to five weeks. When she tested the blood of these dogs, Cappel-King found elevated liver counts. She therefore recommends giving comfrey in food with caution, if at all. PA-free comfrey tinctures are available for those who wish to take advantage of the plant's exceptional properties without the risk of liver disease (see Resources), and small quantities of fresh or dried comfrey are unlikely to cause problems. Comfrey products can be contaminated by incorrectly identified plants, so a product's source is critical.

In addition to its internal uses, comfrey is one of the most effective healing plants for topical application; see page 127.

Dandelion *(Taraxacum officinale)*

The familiar dandelion, from woody root to toothy leaf, is one of nature's most medicinal plants. Dandelion is a tonic herb for the digestive tract, a blood cleanser and a diuretic. Add its fresh leaves to food for improved liver function. Michael Tierra notes that serious cases of hepatitis in humans have been cured with the use of dandelion tea in combination with dietary restrictions in as little as one week; a similar protocol has helped dogs with the disease. Dandelion is also effective in the treatment of arthritis.

The entire plant is medicinal: leaves, stems, blossoms and roots. Any of these can be fed fresh to birds, rabbits, dogs and cats. Chop, mince or puree the plant before adding to food as necessary. To brew dandelion tea, make an infusion of the leaves and flowers; make a decoction of the root.

Dandelion is a tonic herb that can be given daily in just about any quantity for months or even years. It's nontoxic unless gathered near busy highways or other sources of air pollution or chemical weed killers applied by gardeners and lawn services.

Devil's Claw Root *(Harpagophytum procumbens)*

Devil's claw has become, especially in Europe, a primary treatment for arthritis and rheumatism. Native to South Africa, devil's claw was tested in African and German hospitals and clinics after World War II. In 1958, the first published report of this research described its effectiveness in reducing inflammation and swelling in experimentally induced arthritis.

After the plant's active component, harpagoside, was identified, it was tested in rigorous pharmacological screening trials that validated its anti-inflammatory properties. Whole root preparations were found to be superior to pure harpagoside, and both were determined to be safe. Early review papers on devil's claw called it a good stimulant of the lymph system and a detoxifying herb for the whole system. Recent studies have shown it to be well suited for various types of arthritis, rheumatism and lower back pain and as effective as commonly prescribed drugs in reducing inflammation and improving range of motion. Not all arthritis patients benefit from devil's claw, but enough do to make it one of the most popular treatments for joint pain in humans, dogs and horses.

Echinacea *(Echinacea purpurea, E. angustifolia)*

One of America's best-selling herbs, the purple coneflower *(E. purpurea)* and its close cousin *(E. Angustifolia)* are often recommended for the treatment of colds and flu in humans and upper respiratory infections in animals, but it effectively fights bacterial and viral infections throughout the body by stimulating immune responses. Echinacea can be given to a pet who has suffered a puncture wound, cut, burn or abrasion for this purpose.

Many assume that because echinacea is so effective at fighting disease, therapeutic doses given daily will keep a person or animal in perfect health. There is controversy among herbalists regarding this strategy, with a growing number now recommending that people and pets take only tiny amounts or none at all until exposed to an infectious disease, suffering an injury likely to result in infection or developing the symptoms of an acute illness, such as upper-respiratory congestion, vomiting, fever or diarrhea. Echinacea is most effective when taken in large doses in capsules or tincture for short periods every two or three hours for one to three days.

For best results, use a tincture made from the fresh rather than dried plant; look for a dark color, sharp fragrance and pungent taste. The entire echinacea plant is medicinal, from dramatic blossom to leaf, stem, seed and root.

Feverfew *(Tanacetum parthenium)* or Wild Feverfew

A bitter-tasting green plant that blossoms with daisy-like white petals around a yellow center, feverfew remained an obscure herb until its ability to prevent migraine headaches put it back into nurseries, seed catalogs, home gardens and health food stores around the world.

Not only does feverfew prevent migraine headaches in most users, it often relieves arthritis, psoriasis, premenstrual and menopausal symptoms, insomnia and stress.

Horse and dog owners who feed their animals herbs and other supplements for arthritis report that they know the product is working because as soon as they run out of it, their animals begin limping again. This reveals that while the supplements relieve pain and increase mobility, they don't reverse or cure the condition. Because so many arthritis patients report that feverfew's positive effects continue for days, weeks or even months after they stop taking the herb, it appears to do more than alleviate symptoms. There is no mention of feverfew for arthritis in pets in the herbal literature, but its lack of adverse side effects makes feverfew safe for experimentation. When a friend's middle-aged mixed breed lost much of his mobility to arthritis, she gave him a capsule a day. Within a week, and with no change of diet, the dog showed improvement; after two weeks, he was jumping on furniture, running up stairs and moving the way he used to. A possible beneficial side effect is that feverfew's bitter taste may make animals less appealing to mosquitoes and other biting insects.

Fo-Ti *(Polygonum multiflorum)* or Ho Shou Wu

Fo-ti, a member of the buckwheat family, has an important place in Chinese medicine, where it is considered an important herb for longevity. The plant can grow for over a hundred years and is said to improve with age. Its root is a liver tonic and diuretic; it strengthens the kidneys, liver and blood and plays an important role in the treatment of deficiency diseases, hypoglycemia and diabetes in pets as well as people. In addition, fo-ti is an adaptogen that helps correct imbalances in all systems. Like other adaptogen herbs, such as ginseng, fo-ti can help balance the hormones of spayed and neutered pets, increase the stamina and endurance of canine athletes and improve resistance to disease in all animals. Throughout China it is believed to prevent premature aging. The root can be powdered and added to food or brewed as a decoction by itself or in combination with other herbs.

Ginkgo *(Ginkgo biloba)*

The elegant ginkgo tree is a familiar sight in America, where it has been a popular landscaping tree for more than two centuries. Because it is so resistant to disease and pollution, the ginkgo thrives in cities. Its distinctive fan-shaped leaves, extreme hardiness, pleasing form and spectacular show of autumn gold make it an enduring favorite of landscape gardeners everywhere. Young ginkgo trees grow an average of two feet per year and mature trees can reach heights of a hundred feet. Some ginkgo trees are over a thousand years old.

Today's ginkgo research focuses on the plant's ability to increase the flow of blood through aging vessels, especially in the brain. This explains its effectiveness in the treatment and prevention of problems as varied as asthma, hearing loss, stroke, heart attack, dementia, depression, tinnitus (ringing in the ears), fatigue, vision problems such as macular degeneration, high blood pressure, kidney problems, allergies, brain function impairment, memory loss, dizziness, impotence and poor circulation. The hundreds of papers that have been published in scientific and medical journals around the world reporting on laboratory tests and clinical trials examining ginkgo preparations have made it one of the most popular herbs in veterinary medicine.

Because it interferes with blood clotting, ginkgo should not be given to animals with clotting disorders. Some human users, after taking extremely large amounts of gingko extracts, have reported restlessness, irritability, diarrhea, vomiting and nausea. Gingko is considered nontoxic in normal doses.

Most experts agree that ginkgo preparations have to be taken consistently for two to four months before significant results are noticed. Gingko leaves are often mixed with gotu kola (another memory-enhancing herb) in memory tonic tea blends and tinctures. Rosemary Gladstar mixes two parts ginkgo leaf with one part each of gotu kola, lemon balm and peppermint to make a tea for increased memory, emotional stability and energy. This blend is helpful to dogs who are learning a new sport or competing in obedience trials — and to their handlers as well.

Ginkgo preparations are a special boon for older pets. For animals in the show ring or participating in activities that require focus and concentration, ginkgo and its herbal partners offer numerous benefits.

Ginger *(Zingiber officinale)*

The knobby rhizome of this familiar spice is enjoyed around the world in main dishes, desserts, cookies and gingerbread. It's also among the mostly widely used tea ingredients, both for its aromatic flavor and for its warm, stimulating, carminative influence. Long prescribed in China for colds, flu, coughs, respiratory problems and kidney disease, ginger was recently discovered in the West as a treatment for nausea. Both motion sickness and morning sickness respond to large doses of powdered ginger in capsules taken on an empty stomach.

Because ginger so quickly improves circulation and digestion, it is an important catalyst or stimulant herb in medicinal tea blends. It is safe and well-tolerated by people and pets of all ages. Try adding dried ginger root to decoction blends and fresh, grated root to infusions. To help pets that suffer from motion sickness, give 1 capsule per 25 pounds of body weight half an hour before leaving home and see whether that is effective. If not, increase the dosage next time.

Ginger is a specific for improved digestion. Add small amounts to your pet's food as a digestive tonic and in larger amounts, as needed, to help prevent flatulence.

Ginseng *(Panax ginseng, P. quinquefolius)*

Ginseng, an unassuming leafy plant that's both hard to grow and expensive, is the world's most researched medicinal herb. Since the 17th century it has been the subject of over a thousand books and papers, but the result of this international investigation has done little to reduce the controversy surrounding ginseng.

There are eight ginseng species, but only three are widely used: *Panax ginseng,* also called Korean ginseng, *Panax quinquefolius* or American ginseng and *Eleutherococcus senticosus* or Siberian ginseng. Research shows their effects are similar, though experts disagree on their potency. All of the ginseng species are "adaptogens" or regulating herbs that help balance the system. For example, an adaptogen herb will help lower high blood pressure in one person while it helps raise low blood pressure in another. Adaptogen herbs boost the immune system, improve stamina and endurance and reduce stress. Some owners and trainers use it to help an animal train and compete; others feed it to stud dogs and claim it improves their performance. Although ginseng is said to have a special affinity for the male system, it is appropriate for both sexes.

As reported in the February-April 1996 *Journal of the American Holistic Veterinary Medical Association,* a recent study suggests that *Panax ginseng* may prove especially effective in the restoration of normal adrenal function and in the prevention of adrenal atrophy in patients treated with corticosteroids. This is a significant finding for holistic veterinarians because so many of America's pets have been treated with steroid drugs or have impaired adrenal function as a result of poor nutrition, stress and other factors.

Ginseng can be powdered, brewed as a tea or made into a tincture for use with animals. For tea, ginseng should be simmered for 10 to 15 minutes in a covered pan, or as described on page 125 simmered in a glass jar or ginseng cooker. Store leftover tea and root in the refrigerator; the root can be used once or twice more, although the resulting tea will be weaker. You can combine an old piece with a new one to maintain the brew's strength without wasting ginseng. Ginseng roots are white (dried) or red (steamed and dried). The red root is more expensive and is said to be more effective. Tea from white root turns brown as it brews, while tea made from red root remains clear. The more bitter the taste, the stronger the brew. According to one saying, ginseng's medicinal value lasts as long as the root does, no matter what its taste. After its final brewing, the root can be added to your pet's food.

It is difficult to say exactly how much ginseng to give because preparations vary as much as the people and animals taking them. In general, the smaller the animal, the smaller the dose. The typical recommendation for a 150-pound human is 5 to 10 grams (1/4 to 1/2 ounce) of high quality root daily. If you brew between 1 and 2 cups of tea with this amount of root, give 1/2 cup daily to a 75-pound animal, 1/4 cup to a 35-pound animal, 1/8 cup to an animal weighing 20 pounds and 1 tablespoon to one weighing 10 pounds. If you prefer to add powdered ginseng to food, divide the human dosage as above.

Ginseng can be taken daily for prolonged periods; in fact, it often takes weeks or months to show results.

Grapefruit Seed Extract or Citrus Seed Extract

In the 1970s an immunologist, Dr. Jacob Harich, searched for a natural alternative to antibiotics, a nontoxic substance that would help the human body resist bacteria, viruses, parasites and fungi. He found it in the seeds and connecting tissue of grapefruit.

Holistic physicians and veterinarians experimenting with grapefruit seed extract, which is safe for internal use, have found it effective in treating staphylococcus, streptococcus, salmonella, *amoeba histolytica* and other parasites, viruses, *Candida albicans,* herpes, sore throats, ear infections, gum disease, fungus infections, traveler's diarrhea and drug-resistant bacteria.

According to Allan Sachs, a nutritionist and chiropractor, "Many prestigious universities and independent laboratories have tested grapefruit seed extract against more than 30 fungi, 20 bacteria and a host of viruses and protozoa. In almost all of these cultures grapefruit seed extract exhibited significant antimicrobial activity at low concentration."

Unlike tea tree oil, with which it shares many properties, grapefruit seed extract can be taken internally in therapeutic quantities with no adverse side effects. The liquid extract has a bitter, unpleasant taste, but manufacturers offer a debittered powder in capsules. Both are convenient for hikers and campers who travel with their dogs. Nearly every lake in North America carries *Giardia lamblia,* a microscopic parasite that causes intestinal disease, and unfamiliar bacteria can cause traveler's diarrhea in dogs as well as people.

Because grapefruit seed extract is so new on the holistic health scene, it doesn't enjoy the decades of medical research and journal reports that document the growth of the tea tree oil industry. Holistic veterinarians are just beginning to use grapefruit seed extract as a natural antibiotic, immune system booster, candida treatment and parasite preventive. Some theorize that its antimicrobial activity enhances the action of herbs such as goldenseal and echinacea, which can be used to prevent or cure respiratory diseases, viral infections and other contagious illnesses. For example, blends of grapefruit seed and echinacea clear *Chlamydia* infections in cockatiels and other birds, mastitis and uterine infections in dogs and farm animals, infections in infant puppies and kittens and a host of other conditions. The extract has been used in combination with astragalus, barberry, white oak bark, witch hazel, calendula, slippery elm bark, pao d'arco bark, artemesia, milk thistle seed, dandelion, plantain and other herbs to augment their healing activity.

Grapefruit seed extract is also called grapefruit extract or citrus seed extract. It is often confused with grapeseed oil or extract; however, that is an entirely different product. Liquid grapefruit seed extract is very concentrated even in the dilute formulas sold for home use and should be used carefully. It can be diluted with an equal amount of water or herbal tea and applied to ringworm, pustules or abscesses; be careful to avoid the eyes and mucous membranes when applying this concentration. Dilute in 5 to 6 parts water or tea and spray on or apply directly to hot spots, burns, infected cuts, sores, puncture wounds, rashes or infected ears. A few drops added to liquid soap or shampoo helps control flaking.

Nutri-Biotic liquid extract is 33 percent grapefruit seed extract; ProSeed is 40 percent extract. These and similar liquid products can be diluted in 3 to 4 parts water to create a disinfecting spray of about 10 percent extract for use in kennels, training schools, catteries, veterinary clinics and grooming salons to prevent the spread of kennel cough, upper respiratory infections and other contagious diseases.

A capsule of powdered, debittered extract can be opened and the powdered extract sprinkled on food or mixed with water. One capsule is equivalent to approximately 10 to 15 drops of liquid extract and can be used for the same purposes. Pet owners and veterinarians have reported to Dr. Sachs that using 1 capsule (100 or 125 mg) per 10 pounds of body weight up to a maximum of about 8 capsules per day for very large dogs has successfully treated or helped prevent conditions such as diarrhea and bacterial, fungal or viral infections. Many conditions clear up within a day or two but some require longer treatment. Because powerful infection fighters are most effective in short-term rather than long-term use, Sachs recommends therapeutic doses for several days to a few weeks; then substitute another natural healer, such as echinacea.

Hops *(Humulus lupulus)*

The fruit or catkin of this flowering vine, best known as a beer ingredient and sleeping aid, is also a diuretic, stimulant, anthelmintic, alterative and astringent herb that promotes digestion by increasing the flow of bile. More commonly sold as a tincture than as a tea, hops help lower blood sugar and has an anti-diabetic effect. Because of its profound effects on the endocrine system, fresh hops and tinctures made from fresh hops can be used to treat hormonal imbalances. Dried hops do not have this effect.

The National Animal Poison Control Center at the University of Illinois in Urbana has recorded eight fatal cases of hops toxicity; the victims were seven Greyhounds and a Labrador Retriever mix whose ingestion of spent hops from home beer-brewing kits resulted in malignant hyperthermia, an uncontrollable fever rising as fast as two degrees F every five minutes. Warnings soon appeared in dog magazines, veterinary journals and herbal publications about the potential dangers of hops to dogs, especially Greyhounds.

There is a world of difference between a bucketful of hops residue from beer making and the small amounts used in herbal teas, powders and tinctures. More important, no further cases of hops toxicity have been reported since 1995.

Herbalists everywhere agree that a massive overdose of any herb can cause problems. Hops residues should be stored where foraging dogs can't reach them, and any that do should be given an emetic (see Chapter 12) and treated by a veterinarian. But there is no reason to stop using blends that contain this important nervine or to assume that fresh or dried hops is inherently dangerous to dogs or other pets.

Horsetail *(Equisetum arvense)*

Long a folk treatment for mending bones and connective tissue, horsetail's healing properties have been proven in clinical research. This herb stimulates the metabolic processes that repair bones and connective tissue, and its effectiveness may result from its ability to replace lost silicon in the body. Silicon levels decline with age, possibly due to a drop in hormone levels.

Horsetail tea is known for its beneficial effects on the kidneys, bladder and urinary system, the heart and circulation and joint and bone conditions such as rheumatism, gout and arthritis. Its special affinity for the hair and nails in humans suggests similar activity in the fur, feathers and claws of animals. Taking horsetail internally improves the skin, coat and nails from the inside; applying it externally as soaks or rinses speeds results. Any itching rash, inflammation of the nailbed, festering wound or abscess can be treated with the topical application of horsetail.

Kelp and Other Seaweeds *(Laminaria longicruris and other species)*

Best known for their abundant minerals and trace elements, kelp and other sea vegetables have a nourishing and tonic effect on all of the body's systems. Juliette de Bairacli Levy was the first in the West to recommend kelp as a nutritional supplement for animals, which she did in the 1930s. Her suggestion was greeted with scorn from the veterinary world, but opinions have changed and it is now widely used.

In addition to correcting mineral deficiencies, kelp and other seaweeds contain alginates that soothe and cleanse the digestive tract while preventing the absorption of toxic metals including mercury, cadmium, cesium, plutonium, strontium and other radioactive isotopes. Seaweeds improve glandular function, promote rapid hair growth and correct pigmentation, making black fur and noses truly black. They are important for healthy reproduction and protect against heart and kidney disease.

Any sea vegetable can be added to your pet's food. Most health food stores offer a variety of North American and Japanese seaweeds, such as nori, also known as laver; kelp, also called kombu; wakame, hijiki and arame, which are brown; and dulse, which is red and contains the highest iron concentration of any food source. Agar-agar, known as kanten in Japan, is used as a jelling or thickening agent, and Corsican seaweed is sold as an anthelmintic or vermifuge (worming herb). Agar-agar and Corsican seaweed come with special instructions; the other sea vegetables listed here can be powdered and added to your pet's food. Add a small pinch for small animals, a large one for large animals.

Licorice *(Glycyrrhiza glabra, G. uralensis)*

Licorice root, familiar to generations of candy lovers, is more than a sweet taste. This versatile herb is a specific for the respiratory system, digestion and adrenal glands. If your pet has a cough, bronchial congestion, asthma, acute gastritis or suffers from stress and exhaustion, licorice root may be just what the holistic doctor ordered.

Chinese licorice, *G. uralensis,* is the most commonly used herb in Oriental medicine. It is said to benefit all of the systems and organs, slow and prolong the effects of strong tonic prescriptions, antidote mushroom poisoning and soothe peptic ulcers.

In large quantities, licorice causes fluid retention and raises blood pressure; it is not recommended for use during pregnancy or for those with heart conditions, cautions that apply to pets as well as people. In moderate doses for short periods, licorice stimulates the adrenal cortex, prolongs the action of adrenal hormones, balances the metabolism, aids recovery from overtraining or stress and helps compensate for the lack of estrogen and testosterone in spayed and neutered animals.

See page 434 for a licorice root course of treatment and its effects on hormone production.

Microalgae (Chlorella, Spirulina, Blue-Green Algae)

Billions of years ago, algae covered the oceans. The first photosynthesizing organisms on our planet, they are believed to have made the earth hospitable to future life by converting carbon dioxide to oxygen, thus creating our atmosphere. Spirulina, chlorella and blue-green algae are among the world's most widespread herbs, and in recent years they have become among the most popular. Nearly every line of pet supplements has at least two or three products containing microalgae.

Not every strain of algae is edible, but the species sold as food supplements are nontoxic and rich in chlorophyll, amino acids, vitamins, minerals and protein.

Spirulina, named for its cell's spiral shape, is the only microalgae visible to the naked eye. First studied by scientists in the 1940s, spirulina was found to contain 65 to 70 percent protein, the eight essential amino acids, abundant vitamin B12 and other nutrients.

Chlorella, another ancient single-celled algae, derives its name from its high chlorophyll content. Chlorophyll repairs cells, increases hemoglobin in the blood and speeds cell growth. In addition to being sold by itself, chlorella appears in many pet products that combine "green" ingredients, such as the other microalgae, wheat or barley grass juice, alfalfa and green vegetables. Processing that breaks chlorella's cell wall is said to improve assimilation.

Blue-green algae, the popular name for a strain of *Aphanizaomenon,* grows on lakes and ponds. Like spirulina and chlorella, blue-green algae contains chlorophyll, vitamins, minerals, protein, amino acids and other nutrients.

Are there significant differences between spirulina, chlorella and blue-green algae? Or between wild harvested and cultivated strains? According to researchers not affiliated with manufacturers, there is little to be gained from comparing their individual merits. Nearly all descriptions of one type's superiority or another's inferiority come from manufacturers' promotional literature. Research conducted in Japan, Mexico, the United States and other countries indicates that similar results can be expected from all three.

While spirulina and chlorella have long safety records, the blue-green algae harvested from Oregon's Klamath Lake is newer and less widely used. Occasional reports of dogs dying after drinking algae-contaminated water from Klamath Lake have appeared in dog magazines, and in November 1996, *Vegetarian Times* reported that *Microcystis,* a toxic algae that can cause fatal liver damage, had been discovered in Klamath Lake. Owners considering the use of this supplement should look for updated safety reports from the manufacturers and from pet-related newsletters and magazines. As with any herbal supplement, consider using any algae product in courses, such as five days on and two days off for four to six weeks, then switch to a different microalgae.

Milk Thistle Seed *(Carduus marianus)*

Milk thistle seed preparations are best-sellers in health food stores because they are such effective liver stimulants, tonics and healers. This is one herb that truly reverses liver damage in both pets and people. Because of its importance in the treatment of mushroom poisoning, hepatitis, cirrhosis, drug damage and the damage caused by environmental toxins, milk thistle has been scientifically researched in Europe for over 45 years. In addition to improving the liver, milk thistle seed can be used for gall bladder problems.

Any pet that has been fed a commercial diet or exposed to chemical pesticides such as garden sprays or flea and tick repellents will benefit from this herb, especially during and after the transition to a natural diet. Brew the seeds as an infusion, grind them and add them to food or give milk thistle seed capsules or tinctures.

The Medicinal Mints

They grow around the world and their family, identified by the plants' square stems, is enormous. Not all its members are sweet (the bitter horehound is a mint), nor are all recommended for internal use, but familiar culinary mints double as the world's most widely used medicinal plants.

Because they release a pleasing fragrance when bruised, peppermint and spearmint were popular strewing herbs. Even today, mint is an instant air freshener: just crush a piece and wave it in the air, simmer it on the stove or steep 1 cup coarsely chopped peppermint or spearmint in a gallon of water, strain into a spray bottle and spritz wherever you want a fresh, cool scent.

Peppermint *(Mentha piperita),* with its concentrated menthol, is one of the best digestive aids known. It encourages bile production and promotes liver and gallbladder functions, helps prevent fermentation, gently disinfects the stomach when there is abnormal decomposition and relieves spasms and flatulence.

Spearmint *(Mentha spicata or M. aquatica)* is just as familiar, thanks to the popularity of spearmint chewing gums, breath mints, toothpastes and mouthwashes. Like its cousin peppermint, spearmint is a powerful digestive aid that helps prevent flatulence. Traditionally used to reduce fevers, spearmint is a mild diuretic that helps alleviate fluid retention.

Peppermint, spearmint and the other culinary mints (curly mint, apple mint, etc.) are nontoxic and well tolerated, though the distilled oils of these plants may be too concentrated for use with very young animals. The tea, usually an infusion but occasionally a simmered decoction, is well tolerated by pets and people of all ages.

Lemon balm *(Melissa officinalis)* is another member of the mint family. Also simply called balm, this pleasant herb with a strong lemon mint fragrance has a long history of medicinal use dating back to the ancient Greeks and Arabs. Lemon balm tea, made from fresh or dried leaves, helps relieve insomnia, anxiety, nausea and fever. Applied externally, the crushed leaves help reduce the itch and swelling of insect bites.

Catnip *(Nepeta cataria)* is America's best-selling herb for pets because everyone who lives with a cat is likely to have at least one catnip-filled toy. Pampered kitties are given fancy packages of organically grown catnip. Kittens usually become interested in catnip at around seven months or when they reach sexual maturity. Some describe it as a feline aphrodisiac. Not all cats are affected, but those who are usually exhibit dramatic behavior changes, rolling on the floor, leaping in the air and eventually lying down in a glazed-eyed stupor. For best results, most experts recommend sprinkling catnip for recreational purposes occasionally, not every day. It can be added to any animal's food as a digestive aid or to relieve nervous stress. In the garden, catnip grown from seed is unlikely to attract attention, but after you transplant catnip or whenever you break off fresh leaves, neighborhood cats may dismantle, uproot and otherwise enjoy your plant.

All of the mints are said to repel ants, other insects and some rodents.

Note: The strong aroma of mint can antidote homeopathy, so most homeopaths suggest that mint products be avoided during treatment.

Also, the frequent use of any mint for improved digestion may weaken its effects. For best results, add mint to your pet's food every few days rather than at every meal, or save mint for use when symptoms of indigestion are obvious.

Mullein *(Verbascum thapsus)*

Mullein is practically synonymous with the respiratory system. A demulcent herb with anti-inflammatory properties, it is is also an expectorant, antispasmodic, soothing nervine and astringent. Its dried leaves and flowers tone the respiratory system's mucous membranes, reducing inflammation and alleviating congestion. Dr. John Christopher, an American herbal physician, called it "the only herb known to man that has remarkable narcotic properties without being poisonous or harmful." He considered mullein a great painkiller and soporific (sleeping aid) that also soothes and strengthens the intestines and kidneys. Fresh or dried mullein can be added to any pet's food on a regular basis as a tonic for the nervous, respiratory and digestive systems.

Mullein's yellow blossoms are the active ingredient in herbal ear oils, which fight infection and reduce ear wax.

Nettle *(Urtica dioica)*

Stinging nettle is a perennial plant found all over the world, usually growing in gardens and along roadsides and fences. Nettle gets its sting from bristly hairs that act like tiny hypodermic needles, injecting an irritating substance when touched. Most people develop tiny blisters and an itching rash from live nettle (wear heavy gloves whenever handling this plant), but its sting is destroyed by boiling water. Despite frequently published reports to the contrary, very young fresh nettle and dried nettle of all ages hold their sting and can irritate your pet's mouth; don't add fresh or dried nettle to food without pureeing or powdering it first. Include sprigs of fresh nettle while juicing carrots or other foods for your pet. Nettle contains protein and impressive amounts of calcium, phosphorus, iron, magnesium and potassium, plus beta carotene and vitamins A, B-complex, C and D.

Nettle is an expectorant, alterative and antispasmodic with a long history of medicinal application, especially in Europe, where it was traditionally used for tuberculosis and is today used to treat arthritis, eczema, anemia, gout, excessive menstruation and kidney problems. It is an appropriate herb for animals with respiratory problems, skin and coat disorders, arthritis and conditions involving the kidneys or urinary tract.

Nettle's most researched application, however, has nothing to do with these ailments. It is nettle's effectiveness in treating respiratory allergies that has made it a best selling herb. A double-blind study showed significant hay fever relief from capsules containing freeze-dried nettle, and herbalists involved in the treatment of asthma report good results treating that ailment as well. Nettle doesn't work for everyone who has allergies or asthma, but for those it helps, improvement is evident within a week of beginning treatment. Pet owners with allergy problems may find relief from nettle tea, capsules or tinctures, and this is an appropriate herb for any animal suffering from the same conditions. Nettle adds nutritional support to any blend or formula and it is often combined with mullein, especially in the treatment of asthma.

Nettle infusions have many uses, especially in the care of human hair and the skin and coats of animals. A strong nettle tea will temporarily darken a light coat, but on dark-furred animals, it's a conditioning final rinse that helps reduce dander and flaking skin. Massage well into the coat and skin and let dry.

Oatstraw *(Avena sativa)*

Oatstraw or oatgrass, the stems and leaves of the familiar oat, is best known as a nervine that soothes, calms and relaxes. Oatstraw tea, made by infusion or decoction, is said to be effective for kidney and chest ailments.

Both the straw and seeds are a nutritive tonic for the nervous and reproductive systems in people, farm animals and pets. Their tea, usually an infusion, helps relieve nervous exhaustion, irritability, stress and anxiety. Oatstraw is often combined with other nervines, such as chamomile.

Red Clover Blossoms *(Trifolium pratense)*

The common red clover has a long history of magical as well as medicinal uses. We no longer use it to protect against witchcraft and evil spirits, but red clover remains a highly regarded alterative, sedative and antispasmodic. It appears in many preparations for sore throats, colds, coughs, skin diseases, nerves, cramps, spasms and chronic diseases. It is a blood-cleansing herb and potent aid to detoxification. Like chamomile, it is highly recommended for children and pets.

Red clover is easy to identify and harvest. Use any infusion method for making tea or add fresh or dried blossoms to food. For skin conditions, brew a large amount of strong tea and use as a wash.

Schisandra *(Schizandra chinensis)*

Schisandra berries are astringent, demulcent, a kidney tonic, a diarrhea therapy and a specific for the respiratory system. One of the most highly regarded Chinese herbs, schisandra is an adaptogen; like ginseng and other herbs in this category, it gradually corrects imbalances and brings the body's systems into equilibrium.

Schisandra is popular among human athletes as an endurance tonic and it benefits animal athletes as well. Race horses and polo horses tested by scientists increased their stamina and quickly recovered from exertion while taking the herb. Schisandra is appropriate for working dogs and for any animal being treated for respiratory or urinary disorders.

According to Western researchers, schisandra contains antioxidants and helps protect the liver. It has no adverse side effects and, like other adaptogen and tonic herbs, can be taken for long periods. Schisandra works well with other herbs and is an ingredient in many tonic blends.

Slippery Elm Bark *(Ulmus fulva)*

The inner bark of the slippery elm tree is a demulcent, emollient, nutritive, diuretic, slightly astringent and tonic source of mucilaginous, water-soluble fiber. Mixed with milk, water or juice, it helps nourish the body while relieving stomach complaints. This is an ideal food for infant puppies and for any pet recovering from an illness. A small amount of powdered bark in water forms a thick jelly, similar to psyllium husk powder. Slippery elm bark is an ingredient in Juliette de Bairacli Levy's tree bark gruel and in Essiac tea.

Valerian Root *(Valeriana officinalis)*

There is no mistaking the woody root of this tall, swaying, white-flowered plant. Its pungent, earthy fragrance fills the room with an odor that stops people in their tracks and reminds some of old sweat socks. And there is no escaping it: despite frequently published claims that only dried valerian has a strong smell, freshly dug roots have it, too, and if you grow valerian in your garden (it is often sold under the name garden heliotrope), you can sometimes smell it even as it grows.

Despite its scent, valerian is one of the most popular medicinal herbs for pets and people because it is a highly effective nervine, an herb that calms and soothes the nerves, reducing tension and anxiety. In addition, it is recommended for any pet suffering from muscle pain, stress, intestinal cramps, nervousness, restlessness, muscle spasms or bronchial spasms. Valerian is probably best known as a soporific — that is, as an aid to sleep. Boarding kennels, veterinary clinics and breeders use valerian to soothe visiting dogs and cats.

Despite its nighttime applications, valerian does not interfere with coordination or thinking; in fact, some studies have shown that it improves concentration, focus and coordination in factory workers. This makes it ideal for dogs on their way to obedience class or competing in the show ring. Their owners could probably use it, too.

Brewing valerian tea means giving your house an aromatherapy treatment that may or may not be to your liking. If it is, remember that valerian is a fragile root that should not be simmered or boiled; brew an infusion instead. Animals don't mind its fragrance, and cats sometimes crave it. Whenever an animal is stressed, upset or overly excited, valerian can help. Add strongly brewed valerian tea or tincture to food or drinking water; add fresh or powdered root to food.

Although most users respond well to valerian, an estimated seven percent of the human population has a different reaction: for them valerian is a stimulant, not a sedative. This reaction has not been documented in dogs, cats, birds or rabbits but an occasional pet may have this unusual reaction. When giving valerian for the first time, start with a small dose. Within 20 to 30 minutes, the animal should feel more relaxed. If instead he or she appears more agitated or uncomfortable, leave valerian and try other calming herbs such as passionflower, chamomile or skullcap.

To preserve its medicinal properties, valerian root should be stored away from heat and light and in glass jars. Valerian's essential oils are absorbed over time by paper, cardboard and other porous materials.

Wormwood *(Artemisia absinthium)*

An important bitter herb, wormwood lives up to its name by helping rid the body of intestinal parasites. In addition, its antiseptic, antispasmodic, carminative and stimulant properties make it a tonic for the stomach and digestive tract. The essential oil of wormwood is toxic and addictive, which is how Absinthe, the notorious liqueur, ruined some of Europe's best minds a century ago. Wormwood tea and powdered wormwood capsules are considered safe in small quantities even for prolonged use; in more concentrated doses, such as in the treatment of intestinal worms, it can be taken for several days.

See page 403 for wormwood's antiparasite applications.

Yucca (*Yucca baccata* and other species)

Native to the American Southwest, yucca has a variety of uses. Its attractive leaves and dramatic white blossoms make it a popular landscaping plant, its stems and foliage produce a coarse fiber with industrial uses, its fruit is cooked when green and eaten raw when purple and its roots can be used as a detergent for cleaning hair and washing clothes. In addition to all that, it's medicinal.

Yucca's saponin content makes it a friend to arthritics, for it reduces stress and swelling in the joints. In human studies, over 60 percent of patients tested with yucca supplements experienced diminished pain, swelling and stiffness; in addition, their blood pressure and cholesterol levels dropped and intestinal toxicity improved as well. Yucca has no known side effects and in recent years it has become a popular ingredient in arthritis blends for pets.

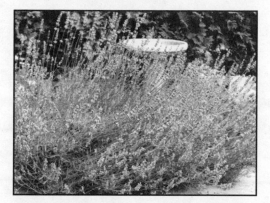

Chapter 5

Aroma–therapy:
More Than Just a Pretty Smell

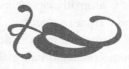

AROMATHERAPY IS THE USE OF FRAGRANCE to enhance the health of mind and body. It is the volatile essential oils in plants that give them aroma, and the extraction of their essential oils, usually by steam distillation, concentrates and preserves their substance. Essential oils are not fats, but they combine easily with vegetable oils, fats and waxes. Alcohol dissolves them partially. They do not dissolve in water.

Essential oils are prescribed to help balance and restore good health, improve circulation, repel insects, kill worms and other parasites, reduce pain, enhance skin and hair, disinfect and speed the healing of wounds, treat burns, prevent infection, clear respiratory congestion, boost the immune system, elevate moods, relieve stress, improve energy levels, prevent insomnia and alleviate anxiety. It is difficult to imagine a health problem in people or their pets that cannot be improved directly or indirectly by the use of aromatherapy.

Most Americans consider aromatherapy a branch of the perfume business. But in France, a nation we associate with perfumes, the professional practice of aromatherapy does not emphasize fragrance at all. Rather, aromatherapy is the realm of medical doctors, who prescribe essential oils internally to treat infections of the urinary tract, reproductive organs, respiratory system and other parts of the body. Essential oils are used internally in Germany as well.

In Great Britain, where essential oils are applied externally, aromatherapy is used in hospitals to prepare patients for medical procedures, speed their recovery and replace sedatives. Julia Lawless, a British aromatherapist, notes in her *Encyclopedia of Essential Oils* that the London-based International Federation of Aromatherapists advises against taking essential oils internally because of their high concentration and the potential toxicity of a small number of essences. This cautious approach is usually followed in the United States, but some American aromatherapists are experimenting with the oral use of essential oils, using French and German guidelines. Those recommendations are mentioned here where appropriate. To make informed decisions about the internal use of essential oils for yourself and your companion animals, study the recommended references listed for this chapter in the Appendix. Remember that some oils that are safe for external application are toxic when ingested. Some that are usually safe for internal and external use should be avoided during breeding or pregnancy. Only a few unusually gentle and well-tolerated oils should be used on or around puppies, kittens, birds, rabbits and other small animals.

How Essential Oils Are Made

Essential oils are a natural product. Their fragrance varies according to the species or variety of plant used, its growing conditions and other factors. For example, a bottle labeled rose oil might contain cabbage rose *(Rosa centifolia)* from Morocco, Tunisia, Italy or France or damask rose *(Rosa damascena)* from Bulgaria or Turkey.

Because of their cost, essential oils are often adulterated with other oils before reaching the consumer. To test the purity of an essential oil, place a drop on blotter paper and let it dry. If the drop disappears without a trace, it was not diluted with a vegetable or mineral oil; if a greasy residue remains, it was.

Although synthetic oils are available, true essential oils are distilled or extracted from fresh herbs or flowers, and there is a difference. No synthetic oil has ever matched the complex oils made by Mother Nature. Even our inadequate human noses can detect the difference. More important, our bodies' response to a synthetic fragrance differs from our reaction to the real thing.

Essential oils are expensive for good reason: their production requires substantial quantities of fresh plant material. It takes 340 pounds of angelica, 50 pounds of eucalyptus, 120 to 160 pounds of lavender or 1,000 pounds of neroli (bitter orange) blossoms to produce a single pound of oil. Fortunately, a little goes a long way, so the cost per use is greatly reduced. Some aromatherapy catalogs offer sample sizes, making experimentation more affordable.

Price alone is not a guarantee of quality, but if one brand costs substantially less than another, it may contain synthetic ingredients or it may have been blended with a less expensive oil from an entirely different plant. See the Resources for this chapter in the Appendix for recommended suppliers and make every effort to locate pure, unadulterated essential oils before using aromatherapy for your pet's ailments. Responsible retailers, such as Jean Argus, whose Jean's Greens Herbal Tea Works carries a selection of essential oils, rely on wholesale sources that test the oils they import for purity and accurate identification. Unfortunately, incorrect identification and adulteration are the most serious and widespread problems in this rapidly expanding worldwide market.

When sampling an essential oil, don't just smell an open bottle. As Argus explains, "The scent of an essential oil is so concentrated that opening the bottle releases only part of the fragrance. I've watched people smell a high-quality lavender oil from the bottle and announce that they don't like it or it doesn't smell right. In order to really test an essential oil, you have to use it. In the open air or applied to the skin or in a blend with other oils, essential oils are transformed."

Using Essential Oils

One need not work with distilled or extracted essential oils to employ the principles of aromatherapy, for any fragrant herb can have a pleasant, healthful effect. Medieval strewing herbs were fragrant flowers, stems and leaves placed where they would be stepped on, releasing pleasant odors. In colonial days, sweet spices in open bowls were used as air fresheners, a practice that continues in modern potpourri blends. As they have for centuries, pet owners use aromatic cedar chips or shavings in their animals' bedding because the fragrance helps repel fleas. Everyone from dogs, birds and cats to people seem to relax and feel inspired when the room smells like apple pie or chocolate chip cookies. And the art of incense, from herbal smudges burned by Native American tribes to the medicinal incenses of Tibet, the sumptuous fragrances of India and the subtle, elegant incenses of Japan, are by themselves the topics of books.

Essential oils are so concentrated that they are rarely used full strength. They can be diluted in a "carrier" oil, such as almond oil, for use as massage oils or insect repellents. Pure or diluted essential oils can be sprayed in the air from a hand-held spray bottle, added to water in a humidifier or dispersed by a nebulizer, an electric pump that diffuses essential oils in a fine mist. Another air freshener is the candle diffuser, similar to a ceramic potpourri warmer, which heats essential oils in water and releases their fragrance slowly. Even simpler is the lightbulb technique: place a drop of essential oil on a cold lightbulb and turn it on. The resulting heat will release the oil's fragrance. Ceramic or paper lightbulb rings, which are sold by aromatherapy supply companies, work on the same principle. Or place a few drops of an essential oil on a radiator or any warm surface. Aromatherapy candles contain essential oils that release their fragrance when burned, or you can improvise your own by placing drops of essential oil on the outside of thin tapers, in the warm wax of a lit candle or near but not on the wick. If you have a fireplace or wood stove, place two or three drops of an essential oil such as pine, fir, cedar, cypress, thuja or sandalwood on a piece of firewood and let it stand a day or longer; then burn one treated log at a time. There are many ways to scent a room or the area surrounding your pet with a fragrance that will help him sleep through the night, relieve stress, speed healing or enhance his energy level.

Aromatherapists suggest that you begin with just a few essential oils and keep your first projects simple. Work with one fragrance at a time, or at most, combine two or three fragrances that share similar properties.

Warm, invigorating fragrances help reduce emotional stress, eliminate fatigue and inspire confidence. The invigorating herbs include eucalyptus, cinnamon, pine, rosemary and begamot. These same essential oils are useful in cases of respiratory congestion, low energy or poor circulation. Soothing, refreshing herbs that help balance energy, refresh the mind and strengthen the system include lavender, lemon, sage and lime. Chamomile is known for its calming influence and is recommended in the treatment of depression. Sandalwood is deeply relaxing. Basil, peppermint, rosemary and juniper are said to aid the memory.

Dilute, dilute, dilute — that's the key to using essential oils on animals. Essential oils are the most concentrated herbal products available, and such powerful substances can be dangerous to pets. For example, undiluted cinnamon oil can burn the skin and cause blisters, as can several other oils.

The external use of the undiluted essential oil of pennyroyal *(Mentha pulegium)* has been implicated in cases of liver damage in dogs and cats. In 1992 the *Journal of the American Veterinary Medical Association* reported the death of a dog who had been treated topically with 60 ml (almost 5 tablespoons) of undiluted pennyroyal oil as a flea repellent. Even though it's an effective insect repellent, this concentrated oil should never be applied full-strength to an animal's skin or coat, and, because pennyroyal oil is an abortifacient, it should not be used on pregnant animals. The essential oils of rue and wormwood are also potentially toxic. These oils, if used at all, are best applied to portions of a pet's bedding that do not touch the animal directly or greatly diluted.

Pennyroyal leaves, on the other hand, are safe to rub on an animal's coat, scatter on its bedding and plant around outdoor kennels. Pennyroyal tea can be used as an insect repellent, and many safe, effective repellents contain dilute solutions of pennyroyal oil. Rue and wormwood are ingredients in some highly regarded herbal tonics that repel fleas and mosquitoes by making the animal's blood "bitter," but these preparations use the leaves of the plants, not their essential oils. Rue in any form is not recommended for external application because it can cause skin irritation to those who touch the pet as well as the animal itself.

Tick and Flea Repellents

During tick season, everyone who lives with a dog or cat prays for a nontoxic, truly effective tick repellent. In the June/July 1994 issue of *The Herb Companion*, botanist Arthur O. Tucker reviewed the scientific literature on herbs that repel mosquitoes, flies, fleas, ticks, cockroaches and similar pests. He wrote that opopanax myrrh *(Commiphora erythraea)* has been shown in scientific tests to kill the larvae on contact and repel adults of the African brown ear, deer or black-footed, lone star and American dog ticks. Because opopanax oil is not widely sold, Tucker speculated that the more readily available common myrrh *(C. myrrha)* might likewise repel ticks. Other herbs indicated in the scientific literature as having tick-repellent properties include rose geranium, rosemary and California laurel.

After reading this article, Barbara Hall, a New York herbalist, began collecting live ticks from her cat. She gave them African (common) myrrh beads to play on, and play they did. She placed them on 3x5 cards, where they swam through drops of rosemary oil and laurel tincture with no sign of discomfort. Then she tried a drop of rose geranium oil. "You should have seen those ticks," she exclaimed. "They were practically turning summersaults, they were trying so hard to get away." Hall's insect spray is now a blend of 20 drops rose geranium oil, 3 drops citronella oil and a splash of bay leaf tincture (its alcohol dissolves the essential oils) in 10 ounces of water. She sprays this pleasant floral combination on herself, her clothes, her pets and anything else that needs protection.

According to essential oils importer Jim Dierking, true rose geranium *(Pelargonium graveolens)* is so rare and costly ($800 per ounce in 1997) that most of the essential oil sold as rose geranium is really palmarosa *(Cymbopogon martini motia)*, also known as East Indian geranium, Turkish geranium, Indian rosha or motia. A grassy-leaved relative of lemongrass, citronella and gingergrass, palmarosa has such a pronounced rose fragrance that for centuries it has been used to adulterate rose oil. Like true rose geranium, palmarosa is nontoxic, nonirritating and nonsensitizing.

Palmarosa ("rose geranium") is not without disadvantages: the fragrance is very strong, does not appeal to everyone and can briefly interfere with a dog's scent retrieval. The week we added it to our spray, Samantha and her friend Hobbes lost a dozen tennis balls and baseballs in the woods; in a few cases, they stood less than a yard from the ball they'd been chasing and couldn't find it. Hunting supply catalogs often mention that cedar oil and cedar bedding can interfere with scent retrieval. In fact, any strong fragrance can create problems for hunting and tracking dogs, though only temporarily. Most dogs adjust quickly, and scent-tracking experts claim that a focused tracking dog can work through just about anything, including a direct skunk spray, without losing the scent.

Another consideration is that your dog might not care for the fragrance you want it to wear. Hobbes so dislikes palmarosa that the first day we applied it he found some well-rotted mammal parts to roll in and the next day discovered a pile of green manure.

Opopanax, also known as bisabol myrrh or sweet myrrh, is more difficult to find than common myrrh, but some aromatherapy companies, such as Liberty Natural Products, carry the unadulterated essential oil. My substitution of opopanax for rose geranium in our tick spray is more to Hobbes's liking.

Rose geranium, palmarosa and opopanax are not the only effective tick repellents. Jungle Juice, a blend of the essential oils of clove, peppermint and lemon in a plant wax base, claims to be the most effective DEET-free insect and tick repellant available. Tested in the jungles of Cambodia and Brazil, it was shown to be effective for up to six hours against mosquitoes, flies, ticks and gnats, including the Brazilian sand fly "Borrachudo." Unlike most herbal repellents, it contains no citronella oil and has a pleasant, spicy aroma. For best results, apply frequently.

Certain skin-care products have a following, too. Samantha's breeder swears by a dilute solution of Avon's Skin-So-Soft lotion as a tick repellent and Juliette de Bairacli Levy claims that Old Spice after-shave cologne repels fleas.

In *The Complete Book of Essential Oils & Aromatherapy,* the English aromatherapist Valerie Ann Worwood, Ph.D., recommends a simple flea prevention strategy, which may also repel ticks and mosquitoes, and as a bonus it keeps the dog's coat in good condition. Wrap a wire brush with several layers of cheesecloth or a similar loosely woven fabric, so that the wire bristles protrude about 1 inch, more or less, depending on the length of your dog's coat. In a bowl of warm water combine 4 drops of cedarwood and pine oil, or, in keeping with the recommendations above, citronella, rose geranium, palmarosa, tea tree, clove, opopanax or eucalyptus oil or any favorite repellent combination. Dip the brush into this mixture, then brush the coat. This treatment disinfects the dog, conditions the fur and picks up parasites and their eggs. Thoroughly rinse the brush every few minutes, soak it in the essential oil mixture and continue brushing.

In her workshops around the world, Juliette de Bairacli Levy recommends adding several drops of eucalyptus oil to a liquid soap. She uses dishwashing products like Palmolive, but a gentler soap would be a liquid olive oil soap from the health food store, or simply add several drops of eucalyptus oil to a small amount of your favorite pet shampoo. Soap the dog thoroughly and use a flea comb or brush to dislodge eggs, larvae and adult fleas. Wait five minutes before rinsing thoroughly.

Maggie Tisserand wrote that lavender is highly regarded in parts of England as a flea repellent. In addition, it can be used to disguise the scent of an in-season bitch or the area in which an indoor pet has urinated or defecated to discourage repeat performances. A blend of lavender and peppermint oil can be applied to your cat's favorite unauthorized scratching post as well, for cats dislike strong fragrances.

Insect Repellent Oil for Use with Herbal Flea Collars

1 part French basil oil
1 part cedar oil
1 part cinnamon oil
1 part citronella oil
1 part clove oil
1 part lemon oil
1 part lavender oil
1 part pennyroyal oil
1 part rose geranium, palmarosa or opopanax oil
    for tick protection
Carrier oil (grapeseed, almond oil, etc.)

Warning: This combination is not suitable for pregnant animals, who should avoid the essential oils of pennyroyal, basil, cedar and citronella.

Substitutions: Use any three or more oils from the list above or substitute others (see list below). This is a forgiving recipe that encourages experimentation. Parts can be any quantity (1 drop, 10 drops, 1/8 tsp., etc.); simply use the same amount of each essential oil.

Dilute the resulting essential oil blend with an equal or slightly smaller amount of carrier oil. Pour the combination over a fabric collar and let it soak in a shallow bowl or plastic bag. Drain on a paper towel before using. Reapply the oil as often as needed, which may be every few days in summer. To refresh the collar, dab several drops of the oil on both sides; to recharge it, saturate again.

To apply this oil topically, double the amount of carrier oil and dab small amounts behind your pet's ears, under the tail and on the chest and abdomen. Brush the animal gently to distribute. Try the oil on yourself as well.

Change the recipe as desired, keeping track of your results until you find the most effective blend. Many essential oils are listed in aromatherapy guides as insect repellents, among them lemon balm, French basil, bergamot, borneol, white champhor, Virginia cedarwood, cinnamon, citronella, cloves, cypress, blue gum eucalyptus, lemon eucalyptus, geranium, lavender, lemongrass, litsea cubeba, mastic, patchouli, peppermint, rosemary, thyme and turpentine (the resin of longleaf pine and other pines).

Insect/Tick Repellent Spray

20 drops rose geranium, palmarosa or opopanax oil

3 drops citronella oil

3 drops rosemary or lavender oil

3 drops clove oil

1 Tbsp. bay rum or bay tincture (alcohol base)

1 Tbsp. black walnut hull tincture (alcohol base)

Mix together, then add to 1 cup water, aloe vera gel or a combination of water and aloe vera. The rose geranium, palmarosa or opopanax oil will help repel ticks, citronella repels mosquitoes, black walnut repels flies and fleas and rosemary, like lavender and clove, is an all-purpose repellent.

For best results, inspect your pet every day, combing for fleas and checking for ticks. (See page 393 for the best way to remove ticks.) Herbalists debate the effectiveness of insect-repelling herbs, such as eucalyptus, which some consider ineffective and overrated. Because essential oils vary according to plant species, growing conditions, chemical adulturation and other factors, as may the preferences of local parasites, try different combinations of the best-quality oils you can find. Label ingredients carefully and record the date used and effectiveness of each blend or individual oil.

How to Administer Essential Oils

Repelling fleas, ticks, mosquitoes and other insects is only one reason to use essential oils. In *Veterinary Aromatherapy*, Nelly Grosjean, a French naturopath and aromatherapist, recommends three methods of administering essential oils to pets: internally (give in food), by diffusion (spray in the air around them) or externally (direct application or massage). The last is not always appropriate for cats, warns Grosjean, for their skin and coat cannot tolerate all essential oils. For best results, use only gentle oils such as lavender for direct application, or dilute oils well before applying.

For internal use, Grosjean suggests a standard dose of 1 to 5 drops of essential oil mixed into food two to three times daily, depending on the animal and its size. As Grosjean's maximum doses are for dogs in the 110 to 120 pound range, this suggests 1 drop per 20 to 25 pounds of body weight. To divide 1 drop in half for a 10- to 15-pound dog, mix it into a small amount of food and divide the food, or dilute a measured number of drops in a quantity of almond oil that is easy to divide. For example, 1 drop of essential oil in 1 teaspoon almond oil can be divided into four 1/4 teaspoon servings, or eight 1/8 teaspoon servings.

Then, for conditions for three to seven days giving a single dose two to three times daily. For preventive or post-crisis use, give one dose per day for one to three weeks.

In *The Handbook of Aromatherapy*, Marcel Lavabre warns that any oil can be dangerous in high doses and that the most toxic essential oils, in decreasing order of toxicity, are rue, thuja, mugwort, sage, hyssop, anise and fennel. For pets, add wormwood, eucalyptus, pennyroyal, sweet basil and orange oils to his list. Among the safest essential oils for internal use are lavender, sandalwood and chamomile.

For example, lavender oil can be used internally to treat a number of conditions as it has antispasmodic, analgesic, antidepressive, antiseptic, carminative (gas relieving), diuretic and cardiotonic (heart-supporting) properties. The dosages above could be applied to an animal suffering from muscle spasms, irritability, insomnia, an infectious illness, flatulence, respiratory problems, fluid retention or a urinary tract infection.

For cats, kittens and birds, Grosjean recommends hydrosols, which are waters from the first stages of distillation. Lavender and orange blossom (neroli) waters are common examples. Hydrosols contain essential oil in suspension, and their use can be regarded as a type of "homeopathic aromatherapy" for all animals. The hydrosol of an oil that is not recommended for internal use because of its potential toxicity (wintergreen, eucalyptus, exotic or sweet basil, sweet orange, pennyroyal, wormwood or rue) can be safely used in place of the essential oil in, on and around all animals, including pregnant, nursing and infant pets. The standard dose of hydrosol for an animal of 110 pounds is 3 to 4 tablespoons hydrosol per quart of water. For smaller animals, use the same proportions and adjust the amount of solution.

"It should be remembered," wrote Grosjean, "that frequent, low doses repeated during the course of the day will be more effective than one strong dose once a day." Respiratory and antiseptic essential oils work well in an electric diffuser, which disperses essential oils into the air; for best results, let the diffuser run between one and two hours per day. According to Nelly Grosjean, essential oils used as sedatives or tonics are most effective when taken internally or applied topically. Essential oils that improve digestion or are used for draining or revitalizing should be taken with food.

Carrier or Fixed Oils

Carrier oils, also called fixed oils, are vegetable oils used to dilute and deliver essential oils. For aromatherapy, oils that do not have their own heavy fragrance are recommended. There are several effective carrier oils that can be purchased from health food stores or aromatherapy supply companies. Store them away from heat and light and refrigerate after opening.

Recommended Dosages for Essential Oils Used Internally

Check individual oil descriptions for safety; not all essential oils are safe for internal use, and some that are should not be used during pregnancy.

Treat acute conditions for three to seven days giving 1 dose two to three times daily. For preventive or postcrisis use, give 1 dose per day for one to three weeks. Serve in food.

Adolescent and Adult Dogs

1 to 4 lb. dog	= 1/4 drop (add 1 drop to food and divide for fractions of a drop)	33 to 44 lb. dog	= 2 drops
		45 to 56 lb. dog	= 2-1/2 drops
		57 to 68 lb. dog	= 3 drops
5 to 10 lb. dog	= 1/2 drop	69 to 80 lb. dog	= 3-1/2 drops
11 to 15 lb. dog	= 3/4 drop	81 to 92 lb. dog	= 4 drops
16 to 20 lb. dog	= 1 drop	93 to 104 lb. dog	= 4-1/2 drops
21 to 32 lb. dog	= 1-1/2 drops	105 to 120 lb. dog	= 5 drops

Cats, Rabbits, Puppies, Small Pets

1 to 4 lbs.	= 1/16 drop (divide in food)	6 to 10 lbs.	= 1/4 drop
		10 to 15 lbs.	= 1/2 drop
4 to 6 lbs.	= 1/8 drop	15 to 20 lbs.	= 3/4 drop

Schedule for Hydrosols
(Flower Waters)

Dilute 3 to 4 tablespoons hydrosol in 1 quart or liter of water. Give in small doses during the day; quantity recommended is the total for one day.

Kittens, Puppies, Cats, Dogs, Rabbits, Birds, etc.

1 lb. or less	= 2 tsp. dilute solution	21 to 25 lbs.	= 1 cup
1 to 3 lbs.	= 1 Tbsp. (3 tsp.)	26 to 35 lbs.	= 1-1/2 cup
3 to 5 lbs.	= 1/8 cup (1 oz. or 2 Tbsp.)	36 to 50 lbs.	= 2 cups
5 to 7 lbs.	= 1/4 cup (2 oz. or 4 Tbsp.)	51 to 65 lbs.	= 2-1/2 cups
8 to 10 lbs.	= 1/3 cup (2.6 oz.)	66 to 85 lbs.	= 3 cups
11 to 15 lbs.	= 1/2 cup (4 oz. or 8 Tbsp.)	85 to 100 lbs.	= 3-1/2 cups
16 to 20 lbs.	= 3/4 cup (6 oz.)	100+ lbs.	= 4 cups (1 quart)

Almond oil, often called sweet almond oil, is pale yellow in color with a light, mild fragrance. Rich in vitamins, minerals, glucosides and protein and one of the most widely used carrier oils, almond oil blends well with essential oils and other carrier oils. It helps relieve dry skin, itching and inflammation and can be used undiluted.

Apricot kernel oil, like peach kernel oil, is pale yellow, light in touch and fragrance and rich in vitamins and minerals. Both can be used undiluted.

Cooking oils. Canola, corn, grape seed, olive, peanut, safflower, sesame, soy and sunflower oils contain vitamins, minerals and proteins. All are moisturizing, easily absorbed and appropriate for full-strength topical application. Peanut, sesame and olive oils have distinct odors, so they are usually diluted with other oils for aromatherapy. Peanut oil should not be used on a person or animal allergic to peanuts. For best results, use organically grown oils that have not been chemically processed, and store them away from heat and light.

Castor oil. The intricately patterned bean or seed of the castor plant is so toxic that a single one can kill a child or small animal. Pharmaceutical-grade castor oil has been treated to remove the toxin. The oil, which is pale yellow, thick, viscous and very sticky, is a purgative laxative when taken internally. Externally, it can be used in massage oils in small quantities, and the blended oil requires shaking before using because castor oil is heavier than other carrier oils, causing it to sink. It is soothing, lubricating, rich in fatty acids and so penetrating that care should be taken when mixing it with other ingredients as they will be quickly absorbed. Never combine synthetic oils, ingredients of inferior quality or anything potentially allergenic or toxic with castor oil.

As a healing therapy for the liver, other internal organs and the immune system, few procedures are as effective in humans as the castor oil pack. A thick wool or flannel cloth is saturated with full-strength castor oil and applied to the abdomen or other appropriate body part, then covered with a heating pad or hot water bottle that is held in place for an hour. The effectiveness of castor oil packs has been repeatedly demonstrated in clinical use, and the one double-blind experiment so far conducted showed a significant increase in white blood cell counts following application.

Some holistic health guides recommend the use of castor oil packs on dogs, but I have never read a description of this advice put into practice. The healthcare professionals who recommend castor oil packs for people emphasize the importance of heat (not hot enough to blister, but almost) and duration (one hour minimum). However, castor oil is such a powerful healer that its undiluted application to a dog's abdomen may well have therapeutic benefits without involving a flannel pack, an uncomfortable heat source and an hour-long stay.

Sulfated castor oil, which used to be called Turkey red oil, is water soluble. It is the key ingredient in some luxury bath preparations containing only two ingredients, sulfated castor oil and an essential oil such as lavender or rosemary. Sulfated castor oil will make any essential oil water soluble for use in air sprays, insect repellent sprays and bath use. Simply add the essential oil to a small amount of sulfated castor oil, then dilute with water as desired. Sulfated castor oil is not recommended for internal or medicinal use.

Jojoba oil. Best known for its resemblance to the oil of sperm whales, this pale yellow oil is pressed from jojoba nuts or beans. It contains minerals, protein and a wax similar to collagen. Popular as a human skin and hair care emollient, jojoba oil (pronounced ho-ho-ba) is used in pet shampoos, insect repellents and other pet products and can be used to treat skin inflammations and dry skin. It is rapidly absorbed and blends well with other oils. Some aromatherapy guides recommend using up to 10 percent jojoba in oil blends, but it can be used full strength.

Jojoba's increasing popularity has produced at least one widely used synthetic, and some companies ferment the residue of pressed seeds and add the result to jojoba products. These substitutes should be avoided, for the unsaturated waxy esters that produce jojoba's benefits are present only in the natural oil. Jojoba is environmentally important because it grows well in arid regions, supports the Native American tribes that farm it in the arid Southwest and replaces spermaceti from sperm whales, which has many industrial applications.

Rose hip seed oil. The expressed oil of the seeds of *Rosa mosqueta,* which grows wild in the Andes, and *R. rubiginosa* have been shown to heal human conditions that have not responded to other therapies, including radiation burns, sun-damaged skin, chronic ulceration in paraplegics, bed sores, skin grafts, dry skin and serious scars over 20 years old. This is an appropriate oil for any scar, ulceration or healing wound in dogs, cats or other pets. For small burns, wounds and scars in dogs, apply the oil full-strength except near the eyes, which it can irritate. To treat large areas in dogs or any condition in puppies or small animals, dilute with a carrier oil. Rose hip seed oil can be added to shampoos and conditioners for an improved coat.

Other oils. Occasionally you may find an unusual vegetable or nut oil, such as pistachio, walnut, hazelnut or black currant seed oil sold as a salad dressing or health product. Any oil that is safe for human consumption is likely to be safe for external application on people and pets.

For instructions on using carrier oils in herbal infusions and salves, see page 129.

Liquid Measurements
(Approximate Conversions)

1 minim				= 1 drop
1 milliliter (ml)				= 1/5 tsp.
1 ml				= 12 drops
4 ml				= 1 fluid dram
5 ml				= 1 tsp.
1 fluid dram (drachm)				= 48 drops
1 fluid dram				= 4 cubic cc
1 fluid dram				= 3/4 tsp.
1 tsp.				= 60 drops
1 tsp.				= 1.3 fluid drams
3 tsp.				= 1 Tbsp.
1 Tbsp.				= 1/2 fluid oz.
1 Tbsp.				= 4 fluid drams
1 oz.	= 2 Tbsp.			= 30 ml
1 cup				= 8 oz.
1 pint	= 2 cups			= 16 oz.
1 quart	= 2 pints	= 4 cups		= 32 oz.
1 gallon	= 4 quarts	= 8 pints	= 16 cups	= 128 oz.

✥ Twelve Essential Oils for Animals ❧

M OST AROMATHERAPY counters in American department, cosmetic or health food stores offer dozens of essential oils; the catalogs of aromatherapy companies list hundreds. Any of the following oils or their hydrosols (flower waters) may be appropriate for use with your pet. Do not apply full-strength essential oils. Review the guidelines for veterinary application on page **xxx**.

Basil *(Ocimum basilicum or French basil, also called common basil; O. minimum or bush basil; O. sanctum or holy basil; but not including exotic basil, O. basilicum; see note below)*

French basil, also called common basil, is a tender culinary used in Eastern and Ayurvedic medicine. Its colorless or pale yellow essential oil, which has a light, sweet, fresh, spicy fragrance, is an antidepressant, antiseptic, antispasmodic, gas reliever, digestive aid, expectorant (it helps remove mucus congestion from the lungs), fever reducer, nerve tonic, adrenal cortex stimulant and general tonic. In addition, it stimulates the production of milk in nursing mothers. Applied to the skin or fur, basil repels insects; applied to joints and muscles, it helps relieve arthritis pain; inhaled, it treats respiratory infections; taken orally, it treats indigestion, nausea and flatulence; in all applications it helps relieve anxiety, depression, fatigue and insomnia.

As Julia Lawless notes in *The Encyclopedia of Essential Oils,* the gentler French basil and harsher exotic basil share the same Latin name, *Ocimum basilicum,* but exotic basil is a larger plant with a harsher odor and different constituents. Its actions are the same as those of French basil, above, but the plant contains methyl chaviocol, which is moderately toxic, irritating to the skin and possibly carcinogenic. Exotic basil is not recommended for internal or external use with animals. To avoid confusion, check with suppliers for positive identification.

All basil oils should be avoided during breeding and pregnancy.

Bergamot *(Citrus bergamia)*

Bergamot oil is distilled from the rind of an Italian citrus fruit and should not be confused with bee balm (*Monarda didyma*), which is commonly called bergamot because its fragrance resembles bergamot oil.

A traditional Italian folk medicine, bergamot oil was often used to treat fevers and worms. Recent Italian research has expanded its use to the treatment of mouth, skin, urinary and respiratory conditions. This oil has analgesic or pain-relieving, antiseptic, antispasmodic, antitoxic, gas-relieving, digestive, diuretic, deodorant, laxative, stimulant, tonic and worm killing properties. An appetite stimulant, it is useful in the treatment of anorexia. Taken internally, especially in combination with bee propolis tincture, it helps clear bladder infections. Bergamot also relieves colic, stomach or intestinal cramps and flatulence. Once important in the treatment of malaria, the oil helps reduce high fevers; it can be mixed with water and applied as a cold compress, diffused in the air or given internally for this purpose. An antidepressant, it relieves anxiety, stress and nervous tension.

Because it can make bare skin photosensitive, bergamot oil applied topically should be greatly diluted.

Chamomile *(Matricaria chamomilla,* known as German, true or annual chamomile and *Anthemis nobilis,* Roman or perennial chamomile*)*

The essential oil of annual German chamomile is thick and blue with an intense, sweet herbal fragrance. The oil of perennial Roman chamomile is clear and yellowish-green with a sweet, clean, fruity odor. Both are used in aromatherapy.

Chamomile is an anti-inflammatory, pain-relieving, antispasmodic, gas-relieving, fever-reducing, antiseptic, wound-healing digestive aid and calming herb of the highest order. Applied topically, it treats burns, cuts, infections and abscesses. Taken internally, chamomile is a specific for colitis, intestinal infections, gallbladder problems, colic, flatulence and gastritis. Sprayed in the air, it makes a spirit-lifting air freshener. Safe for kittens, puppies and nursing mothers as well as during pregnancy, chamomile is one of the most versatile and best-tolerated essential oils. Its calming influence relieves tension, depression and anxiety. I spray the house with chamomile or lavender whenever the kitty next door comes for a week-long visit, and it seems to help our cat adapt to her presence. In shampoos and conditioners, chamomile improves fur condition while highlighting red, yellow and light colored coats.

Cinnamon oil *(Cinnamomum zeylanicum* and other species*)*

Cinnamon oil is extracted by steam distillation from the leaves, twigs and dried inner bark of the tree. The result is a pale to dark yellow or brown oil with the familar fragrance of this popular culinary spice.

Cinnamon leaf oil is relatively nontoxic, though it should be used in moderation around mucous membranes. Cinnamon bark oil, a serious irritant to the skin as well as mucous membranes, is one of the most hazardous full-strength oils. It should not be used during pregnancy except in small amounts during labor or whelping, when it stimulates contractions. Cinnamon oil is obviously safe for internal consumption, for it is one of the food industry's most widely used flavoring agents.

Used externally to repel lice and other small parasites, diluted cinnamon leaf oil can be applied to warts, wasp stings and other skin conditions. Diluted cinnamon oil warms and relaxes arthritic muscles and joints. Taken internally, it stimulates the appetite, helps prevent colitis and heals intestinal infections. Sprayed around an animal, cinnamon helps improve circulation, combat fatigue and boost the immune system. This oil is considered an anthelmintic or vermifuge (worm killer), antidote to poisons, astringent, gas-relieving digestive aid and circulatory stimulant. The British Herbal Pharmacopoeia considers cinnamon a specific for flatulent colic and dyspepsia (indigestion) with nausea. Freshly ground cinnamon can be added to a pet's food as desired.

Clary sage *(Salvia sclarea)*

A close relative of garden sage and native to southern Europe, clary sage was highly regarded during the Middle Ages as a digestive aid and nerve tonic. Despite its effectiveness, the herb fell out of use and few people today have heard of it. Thanks to aromatherapists, clary is enjoying new popularity, for this clear, colorless oil with a warm, sweet, light, grassy fragrance eases cramps, stimulates digestion, reduces flatulence, treats respiratory infections, relaxes the spirit and reduces phychological tension, fear and nervousness. An effective deodorant and antiseptic, clary can be used in the treatment of skin infections. For respiratory problems, use in an aroma lamp, diffuser, humidifier or spray bottle.

The essential oil of garden sage *(Salvia officinalis)* is toxic in very small doses and should not be used on or in animals. Clary sage is much milder and is often used in place of sage oil for the treatment of physical ailments. Clary's reputation as an aphrodisiac stems, according to Susanne Fischer-Rizzi, from its relaxing influence combined with its ability to awaken curiosity and a spirit of adventure and optimism. Clary may be an appropriate oil to spray on and around dogs and cats during breeding. It is also an antidote to the stresses of travel, competition and performing.

Clove *(Eugenia caryophyllata, E. aromatica, E. caryophyllus)*

Clove oil, the traditional cure for toothache, can do more than numb the gums. This sweet, warm, spicy oil is an effective antiseptic that can be applied to infected wounds; in fact, when diluted to 1 percent, clove oil is up to four times more effective than phenol in killing bacteria. An effective insect repellent, clove oil can be used on herbal flea collars or added to herbal sprays. Taken internally, it helps prevent flatulence, digestive problems and diarrhea. As clove oil was traditionally recommended for strengthening the uterus and aiding in childbirth (some authorities recommend that women eat cloves during their last month of pregnancy and drink clove tea during labor), this essential oil may be helpful to dogs and cats in the week before giving birth. Clove oil is also an effective vermifuge or worm killer.

Three types of clove oil are available: clove bud, clove leaf and clove stem. All three can cause skin and mucous membrane irritation and should be greatly diluted when used topically. Clove bud oil has the lowest eugenol percentage and is the least toxic. All of the above oils are safe for internal consumption and are widely used flavoring agents.

Like cinnamon, cloves can be added to a pet's food. Use freshly ground cloves for this purpose because the spice's essential oils deteriorate rapidly after grinding. This is why freshly ground cloves smell so different from ground cloves that have been sitting on a shelf for months. The essential oils in whole cloves will dull the plastic parts of your spice grinder (clean it immediately after use with soap and water) and if you fill vegetarian gelatin capsules (Vegicaps) with ground cloves, their essential oil will cause the capsules to shatter within a few days. Regular gelatin capsules will not break.

Eucalpytus or Blue Gum *(Eucalyptus globulus)*

One of the world's most aromatic trees, eucalyptus is native to Tasmania and Australia, but now grows around the world. Its colorless oil, which turns yellow with age, has a harsh, woody, camphor smell. Externally, the oil is nontoxic and when diluted does not irritate the skin, but it can be toxic when swallowed. As little as 3.5 ml (less than a teaspoon) has been fatal to humans. Always dilute eucalyptus oil before applying it, and give it to your pet in food only in carefully measured doses, no more than 1 drop per 10 pounds of body weight per day. The amount of eucalyptus oil used in flavoring human cough lozenges is insignificant, and ingesting a similarly small amount of eucalyptus oil from an insect repellent blend will not harm your dog (it helps that eucalyptus is not their favorite flavor), but this is still an oil to treat with caution and respect. Do your blending away from animals to avoid accidental spills that could harm them, and store essential oils safely.

Eucalyptus oil is widely used as an insect repellent, applied topically to burns and wounds and dispersed in vaporizers to treat bronchial infections and improve breathing. Traditionally used in the treatment of malaria, eucalyptus can help reduce a fever or the elevated temperature of heat stroke when used in a cold water compress on the legs or abdomen. To prepare a compress, soak a cotton hand or dish towel in a bowl of cold water. Add 5 drops eucalyptus oil, stir well, saturate the compress, wring it enough to stop most of the dripping and apply. Every 5 or 10 minutes, or whenever the compress feels warm to the touch, soak it again. On a large dog, compresses can be wrapped around both hind legs as well as applied to the abdomen.

Lemon-scented eucalyptus *(Eucalyptus citriodora)* shares similar properties and is considered more effective in the treatment of fungal infections. The same precautions apply to all eucalyptus oils.

Lavender *(Lavandula latifolia* or spike lavender; *L. angustifolia* or *L. officinalis,* true lavender; and *Lavandula x intermedia* **or** *lavandin,* a cross between true and spike lavender)*

Among the most revered essential oils, lavender has a long history of medicinal and cosmetic uses. Originally from the Mediterranean, lavender is now grown around the world. There are many different types of lavender, but all share the same basic actions: analgesic or pain-relieving, anticonvulsive, antidepressant, antimicrobial, antirheumatic, antiseptic, antispasmodic, antitoxic, gas-relieving, bile-stimulating, deodorant, diuretic, insect-repelling, relaxing, circulation-stimulating, tonic and worm-repelling. Lavender is so effective against burns that it is a recommended treatment for most burns and scalds. For that reason and because it neutralizes the venom of insect bites and stings as well as some venomous snakes, it belongs in every first aid kit.

Distilled lavender oil is clear or pale yellow with a sweet, herby, woody scent. Inhaled or ingested, it treats respiratory conditions; taken orally, it relieves nausea, prevents flatulence, alleviates cramping, improves digestion and clears urinary tract infections; applied to the skin or coat, it helps repel insects and treats abscesses, fungal infections, ringworm, lice, scabies, sores, sunburn, dermatitis, earache, wounds and inflammation. In any application, lavender reduces anxiety and lifts the spirits.

By all the accounts I have read, full-strength lavender oil is safe for pets of all ages, but you may want to dilute it first with a small amount of carrier oil or vodka.

Lavender flower water is a familiar hydrosol. See page 173 for using hydrosols on birds, cats and other animals.

Myrrh *(Commiphora myrrha and other species)*

A hardened tree resin, myrrh was used by ancient Egyptians for embalming and perfumes. Myrrh resinoid is extracted by solvents; the essential oil is steam-distilled. Its actions are anti-inflammatory, antimicrobial, antiseptic, astringent, gas-relieving, expectorant, sedative, fungicidal and revitalizing. Myrrh oil has a spicy, medicinal odor that stimulates the lungs. Ringworm and other fungal infections respond to preparations containing myrrh. Because it may be toxic in high concentrations, myrrh is not recommended for internal use except when diluted.

Opopanax *(Commiphora erythraea),* also called bisobal or sweet myrrh and pronounced o-POP-a-nax, is a more expensive essential oil. Unfortunately, it is frequently adulterated, so buy from a reputable distributor. As noted on page 169, opopanax has been shown to be an effective tick repellent. Because it does not have common myrrh's medicinal scent, opopanax is used as a fixative and fragrance component in expensive perfumes; it is also an ingredient in some liqueurs.

Orange *(Citrus aurantium var. amara,* or bitter orange, and *Citrus sinensis,* or sweet orange)

The distilled essential oil of bitter orange is an anti-inflammatory, astringent, gas-reliever, digestive aid and tonic as well as an antiseptic that kills both fungi and bacteria. The oil of sweet orange shares these characteristics and is also a relaxing antidepressant. Orange and other citrus oils kill insects and are used in natural flea dip products, but these are of questionable effectiveness and safety. Veterinarians have reported toxic reactions in pets treated with citrus oil flea dips. Cats are more sensitive than dogs to the effects of citrus oil products, and they are particularly hazardous to kittens.

Both bitter and sweet orange oils are called phototoxic because treated skin reacts to sunlight, producing a rash or burn. This is true for pets as well as people. The essential oil of bitter orange is otherwise nontoxic and safe for internal use; the essential oil of sweet orange is toxic in large doses and has been fatal to children. Because of orange oil's safety issues, consider using either a hydrosol of orange or orange blossom oil, which is distilled from the tree's flowers instead of the fruit, for pet use.

The blossoms or flowers of the bitter orange, *Citrus aurantium var. amara,* are often called neroli after a princess of Nerola in Italy, who wore it as a perfume. Orange flower or neroli oil has a light, sweet, floral fragrance and has antidepressant, antispasmodic, deodorant, gas-relieving and mild sedative properties. It is a cardiac tonic, digestive aid and antiseptic. Widely used as a flavoring agent, neroli oil is neither toxic, irritating, sensitizing nor phototoxic. It can be applied to your pet's scars or wounds to stimulate healing. Given internally, it is a specific for chronic diarrhea, colic, flatulence and nervous indigestion. In all applications, neroli relieves anxiety, stress, shock, depression and nervous tension.

Orange flower water, also called orange blossom water or neroli water, is a familiar hydrosol used as a flavoring agent and cosmetic. Don't assume that every product labeled orange blossom water or neroli water is a true hydrosol, however; many are made by diluting synthetic neroli oil with water. A true hydrosol is the first product of steam distillation.

See page 173 for the use of hydrosols on birds, cats and other animals.

Sandalwood *(Santalum album)*

Its 4,000 years of uninterrupted use make sandalwood one of the oldest medicinal and aromatic plants. Its pale, viscous essential oil has a distinctive, soft, sweet, balsamic fragrance and is nontoxic, nonirritating and nonsensitizing. Like lavender and chamomile, sandalwood is usually well-tolerated by people and animals, even at full strength. Once used as a pharmaceutical disinfectant, sandalwood is an effective antidepressant, anti-inflammatory, antiseptic, antispasmodic, astringent, gas reliever, diuretic, expectorant, fungicide, sedative and tonic. Applied topically, sandalwood helps heal dry, cracked, chapped skin and, despite its moisturizing influence, it can be used to treat a greasy coat or skin. Diffused or sprayed in the air, it helps clear bronchial or respiratory infections and dry, persistent coughs. Taken internally, sandalwood is a specific for cystitis and urinary tract infections and it helps prevent diarrhea and nausea. In all applications, sandalwood lifts the spirits, relieves nervous tension and encourages restful sleep.

Tea Tree or Ti Tree *(Melaleuca alternafolia)*

Tea tree oil, also known as melaleuca, is a popular ingredient in pet shampoos, skin and coat products and herbal insect repellents. Tea tree oil is widely used to treat skin lesions, insect bites, rashes, burns, abscesses, cuts, abrasions, infected wounds and fungal infections in people and animals. Like eucalyptus oil, which it resembles, tea tree oil is a specific for the respiratory system as well as an all-purpose disinfectant. Although full-strength tea tree oil is an effective treatment for gingivitis in humans when massaged into the gums, this treatment is not recommended for dogs and cats; in addition to being potentially unsafe, the oil's numbing turpentine flavor is objectionable to all pets.

It is because of its unpleasant taste that some holistic pet guides recommend the application of tea tree oil to body parts that an animal chews or licks incessantly, such as the leg or tail. Such guides usually list full-strength tea tree oil as appropriate for use on insect bites, burns, infected wounds, cuts, ringworm and other fungal infections. However, the September 1994 issue of the veterinary journal *Small Animal Medicine and Surgery* warns, "Melaleuca toxicosis has been reported to the National Animal Poison Control Center when the oil has been applied topically in appropriately high doses to treat dermatological conditions in dogs and cats." Symptoms, which occurred within two to eight hours of application, included depression, weakness, incoordination and muscle tremors. The reaction disappeared within three to four days.

If you decide to use full-strength tea tree oil on your adult dog, do so sparingly, watch the animal carefully for adverse symptoms and, if they occur, discontinue use immediately. Full-strength essential oils should not be applied to cats, puppies or other small animals. Tea tree oil is not recommended for internal use. To treat ear infections, dilute the 15-percent solution with an equal amount of mullein or comfrey tea, aloe vera juice or water. Keep tea tree oil away from the eyes.

Like other essential oils, full-strength tea tree oil will remain fresh for more than ten years if stored in fully filled, tightly sealed glass bottles away from heat and light. High-grade plastics can be used for dilute solutions, shampoos and similar products, but glass containers are recommended for full-strength oil.

Diluting Tea Tree Oil

One of the claims made for tea tree oil is that a 15 percent solution is as effective as full-strength oil in killing yeast cells, mold, bacteria and viruses. This was demonstrated in research reported in the U.S. *Journal of the National Medical Association* and the *British Medical Journal* in the 1930s. Subsequent laboratory tests have shown that concentrations as low as 1 percent are effective against streptococcus and other gram-positive bacteria, *E. coli* and other gram-negative bacteria and several fungi.

To make a dilute solution of full-strength tea tree oil, take an intermediate step and prepare a water-soluble tea tree oil concentrate. The following recipe creates a water-soluble concentrate which is then diluted to a concentration of 15 percent tea tree oil.

15-Percent Tea Tree Oil Antiseptic Solution

2 Tbsp. full-strength tea tree oil
4 Tbsp. 80-proof vodka, vegetable glycerine or sulfated castor oil
Shake or stir well and let the mixture stand for 5 seconds. If a film of oil floats to the top, add more liquid and shake again. When no oil floats the surface, pour the solution into a measuring cup and add enough
- **aloe vera juice or gel**
- **herbal tea, such as comfrey or calendula**
- **pure water**
- **or any combination of aloe, tea and water**

to fill the cup to the 3/4 cup mark. At this point, your solution will be approximately 15-percent tea tree oil.

Note that this same procedure works with any essential oil, not just tea tree oil. Water-soluble solutions of essential oils are the foundation of many aromatherapy products, from soaks and lotions to air sprays.

The 15-percent tea tree oil solution can be sprayed on kitchen and bathroom surfaces, into air ducts and air conditioning units, on telephone receivers and mildewed shower walls, added to laundry wash water and simply sprayed into the air. If you prepare a raw-meat diet for your dog or cat, spraying the sink area, drawer knobs, refrigerator door handles and any surfaces you touched, including your hands, is a sensible precaution. Groomers, animal shelter workers, trainers and boarding kennel operators can guard against infectious diseases such as kennel cough with this spray. For even stronger disinfecting properties, add several drops of liquid grapefruit seed extract and/or full strength lavender oil.

20-Percent Oil Solution of Tea Tree Oil
2 Tbsp. full-strength tea tree oil
1/2 cup carrier oil
Stir to mix well.

This oil can be applied to your pet's ringworm infections, pustules between the toes, burns, cuts or other wounds, just like the water-soluble 15-percent solution. Use the oil wherever you want the solution to adhere without being washed or rinsed away. For example, this diluted oil can be added to ear oils used to treat ear mites and bacterial infections of the ear, or it can be applied to the skin of a dog who's going swimming.

Tea Tree Oil Soap or Shampoo
1-1/2 cups (12 fluid oz.) liquid soap or shampoo
(simple vegetable oil soap or natural pet shampoo)
1 Tbsp. full-strength tea tree oil

Stir to mix well. Use as a hand soap or pet shampoo. This blend is soothing to the skin of pets and people and is a mild disinfectant. Keep the soap away from your pet's eyes. Rinse well.

Concentrated Disinfectant
Liquid grapefruit seed extract already contains glycerine and can be mixed with a smaller amount of full-strength tea tree oil to make a concentrated disinfectant. In a 1-ounce eyedropper bottle, combine:
1 Tbsp. grapefruit seed extract
1 tsp. tea tree oil
1/2 tsp. lavender oil
1 tsp. 80-proof vodka
Shake well before using.

If your pet's bedding, food bowls or living areas need disinfecting, add 20 to 40 drops of concentrate to a load of laundry, bucket of floor wash water, automatic dishwasher or kitchen sink. To treat an animal's infected ears, cuts, wounds or hot spots, add up to 10 drops of the concentrate to 1 teaspoon or more of water, aloe vera gel or herbal tea. You can use a concentrated solution of tea tree oil without the addition of grapefruit seed extract or lavender oil for the same purposes. Simply dilute tea tree oil in enough vodka, glycerine or sulfated castor oil to dissolve it, as described for making a 15-percent solution.

Vinegar, Herbs and Essential Oils

Apple cider vinegar is an important food supplement, but it can be used externally as well. Applied to cuts, wounds, hot spots, dull fur, skin infections, calluses and itchy areas, it soothes the skin, improves the coat and repels fleas and ticks.

To make a fragrant astringent that doubles as a skin and coat tonic, make a cider vinegar tincture of fresh or dried leaves and flowers such as rosemary leaves, calendula blossoms, rose petals, lavender, lemon peel, sage, comfrey, plantain and/or chamomile. Chop fresh comfrey leaves and let them wilt to reduce their water content.

Arrange the plant materials loosely in a glass jar (fill the jar only one-third full if you are using dried herbs) and cover to the top with vinegar. Leave the jar in a warm place, in or out of the sun, for two weeks or longer. Gently shake the jar from time to time.

Strain the liquid through cheesecloth into a large measuring cup, adding several drops of essential oil such as rosemary or lavender to enhance the scent. Transfer to storage bottles and store in a cool, dark place.

To use as an insect repellent, pour a small amount onto a damp washcloth and wipe your pet's coat. To treat any itch, rash or irritated skin condition, apply it directly. Use this infused vinegar to disinfect cuts, abrasions and other wounds. Dilute it with an equal quantity of water for use as a final rinse after bathing your pet and let it air-dry.

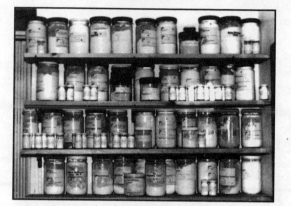

Homeopathy
for Pets

HOMEOPATHY IS A BRANCH of medicine that was developed in the early 1800s by the German physician Samuel Hahnemann. He wrote, "If a medicine administered to a healthy person causes a certain syndrome of symptoms, that medicine will cure a sick person who presents similar symptoms." He discovered this principle when he experimented with quinine from the bark of the Peruvian cinchona tree, which was widely used to treat malaria. Hahnemann, who did not have malaria, was surprised to develop the illness's symptoms for several hours each time he took the drug. He called this reaction "testing" the drug (the German word *prüf* is often mistranslated as "proving") and, for the next six years, Hahnemann administered different medicines to healthy volunteers and meticulously documented their responses, developing a detailed "drug picture" for each preparation.

Because so many of the preparations were toxic, he tried to minimize adverse side effects in his patients by giving them in very small doses, but in many cases, this made the reactions worse. This was because the patient was abnormally sensitive to the medicine causing similar symptoms. Diluting the preparations in stages, he discovered, maintained their effect while eliminating their toxicity. In fact, he found a greater dilution coupled with strong agitation of the mixture enhanced the medicine's effect. This discovery eventually led Hahnemann to call these medicines more potent and the medicines began to be called "potencies."

Hahnemann observed that his potent solutions of medicinal preparations triggered the body's healing mechanisms and that the more closely a patient's "symptom picture" matched the preparation's "drug picture," the more likely a cure. When he began to treat patients this way, that's exactly what happened, and for nearly two centuries, homeopaths have matched homeopathic remedies with patient symptoms to cure illnesses of every description.

Homeopathic drugs are produced from vegetable, mineral, animal and other sources, which are made from a crude substance or alcohol extract called the *mother tincture.* This material is diluted several times, and each dilution is vigorously shaken or *succussed.* Substances that are not soluble in water or alcohol are *triturated,* or ground to a powder using mortar and pestle, and then diluted with milk sugar. Once a substance is diluted to a one part per million ratio, it is considered soluble in water or alcohol. With each step, the liquid is diluted by a factor of 10 or 100, and the mixture is subjected to a series of sharp succussions, shakes or poundings. In Hahnemann's day the work was all done by hand; today it is partly mechanized, but prolonged trituration and succussion are still necessary. The system of potentizing is sometimes called *dymanization.*

During the course of treatment, one should avoid substances that *antidote* or interfere with the remedy. Hahnemann advised that several substances be avoided, especially by patients with chronic diseases; modern homeopaths usually suggest that patients avoid coffee, teas containing caffeine, whatever herbs or herb teas they consume on a regular basis, large doses of herbs, concentrated herbal extracts, such as tinctures, especially of herbs that affect the nervous system, strong-smelling essential oils such as tea tree, eucalyptus, peppermint, rosemary and thyme, all perfumes, strongly spiced or flavored foods and strong- smelling substances such as camphor and menthol. Mint, which contains menthol, is often prohibited for this reason. Lavender and some other essential oils can be used if diluted.

The potency of homeopathic medicines is measured according to the number of dilutions with succussion it has undergone. The *centesimal* scale measures dilution by 100 and uses the abbreviation "c." One drop of mother tincture diluted in 99 drops of water is a 1c preparation (1 in 100); 1 drop of 1c solution in 99 drops of water is a 2c preparation (1 in 10,000); 1 drop of 2c solution in 99 drops of water is a 3c preparation (1 in 1,000,000); and so on.

The *decimal* scale measures dilution by 10 and uses the abbreviation "x." One drop of mother tincture in nine drops of water is a 1x solution (1 in 10); one drop of 1x solution in nine drops of water is a 2x solution (1 in 100); one drop of 2x solution in nine drops of water is a 3x solution (1 in 1,000), and so on.

While the most common potencies (6x, 3c, 6c, 12c and 30c) are available over the counter in homeopathic pharmacies, health food stores, drugstores and by mail throughout the U.S., higher potencies are reserved for professional use. Very high homeopathic potencies, such as 1M strength (1M equals 1,000c), which have had this process done many times, are considered the most powerful and usually require a written prescription.

The alleged strength of such extremely dilute solutions is one of the paradoxes of homeopathic medicine. Critics argue that a solution so dilute that it contains no chemically measurable trace of the ingredient on the label can't have an effect on anything and that homeopathy must be a hoax and its cures are caused by the placebo effect or its satisfied patients are under the spell of a mass delusion. Laboratory research and clinical trials that support the theories and claims of homeopathy have been denounced by some scientists, medical journal editors and allopathic physicians as being biased, flawed and unscientific, although recent studies published in mainstream medical journals support their claims. Homeopathy remains suspect because its basic premise doesn't make sense to most American physicians and scientists.

In the 19th century, homeopathy was widely taught in the U.S. and Canada. In fact, it was the preferred system of medicine, being more effective and far safer than the techniques and procedures used by allopathic physicians. More than 200 homeopathic clinics in the U.S., run by several hundred graduates of the country's 40 homeopathic medical schools, treated all types of chronic and acute conditions, including infectious diseases. During yellow fever and cholera epidemics, for example, patients treated by homeopaths had a much higher survival rate than did those treated allopathically.

Despite its successes, homeopathy's popularity declined in this country, but not in Europe and Asia, where homeopathy has flourished all along. In the past 20 years, as growing numbers of Americans have rediscovered homeopathy's effectiveness and safety, it has been making a comeback. Most of America's licensed homeopaths are medical doctors (MDs) or doctors of veterinary medicine (DVMs) who learned homeopathy after receiving more orthodox medical credentials.

In the field of veterinary medicine, practitioners of homeopathy rely on the owner's observations to define a patient's complaints. Every veterinarian I interviewed for this book, including those who don't use homeopathy, stressed that the most important thing an owner can do when taking an animal to a healthcare practitioner is provide an accurate and thorough history. Allopathic veterinarians want to know about obvious symptoms, but homeopaths need all kinds of details. Consider keeping a journal of your pet's activities, diet, veterinary visits, appearance, normal temperature and unusual symptoms. Making weekly notes will help train you to become a more observant caretaker.

Does your dog, cat, rabbit, bird or other pet look or act different today? If so, how? Do you notice a change in appearance, behavior, sleep patterns, appetite, energy level or anything else? For example, does your affectionate rabbit suddenly dislike being held? Does your shy kitten suddenly climb into your lap and demand attention? Is your dog unusually thirsty, or not thirsty at all? Has your bird abruptly stopped talking or singing? Does the animal seek cool surfaces to lie on, or does he crave heat and warmth? Does your pet have obvious symptoms, like diarrhea, a cough, eye irritation, a discharge from any orifice, tremors or a fever? If so, when and how did these symptoms develop? If the animal vomits, is it soon after drinking water or eating food? What color is the discharge, and what does it look like? Does the vomited material or diarrhea contain blood? Is there an unusual or unpleasant smell from the skin, coat, ears or anything else? Is the animal itching, scratching, limping, fussing with his tail or chewing on his leg?

Handle and pet your companion every day, if possible, and check for fleas, ticks, dander, lumps, bumps and anything unusual. Pay attention to your pet's disposition. Does he seem depressed, lethargic, unresponsive or apathetic? Does she favor one side of the body, such as lying on her right side rather than her left? Does she crave anything, like a particular food or cold rather than room temperature water? Is anything different going on at home, like the introduction of a new pet, the departure of a child to summer camp or the installation of new carpeting? If you're in the habit of inspecting your animals every day, checking their eyes, ears, skin, feathers, fur and stools while paying close attention to their behavior, you will notice changes as soon as they begin to develop. A complete report from an observant owner is the first step in effective homeopathic diagnosis and treatment.

Veterinary Homeopathy in America
A Conversation with Richard Pitcairn, D.V.M., Ph.D.

Richard Pitcairn's name is synonymous with holistic veterinary care. His bestselling book, *Natural Health for Dogs and Cats,* has introduced hundreds of thousands of pet owners to alternative therapies. A doctor of veterinary medicine with a Ph.D. in immunology, Pitcairn has impressive academic credentials and experience with every conventional therapy used on America's dogs and cats. He seldom recommends them, however, preferring to treat his patients with improved nutrition and homeopathy.

For the past 19 years, Pitcairn has shared his knowledge of homeopathy with others. In 1992, he offered a series of classes to veterinarians, which led to the establishment of the Academy of Veterinary Homeopathy. Its professional course, offered annually, meets five times during the year, and graduates who submit cases from their practice and take an examination receive certification as veterinary homeopaths. In 1997, at the end of the fifth course, 175 veterinarians had completed the training. Altogether, an estimated 200 veterinarians practice classical homeopathy in the U.S. As the demand for homeopathy increases, so will this figure.

How can American pet owners use homeopathy for the benefit of their companion animals?

PITCAIRN: First of all, I recommend that they consult veterinarians who

have been trained and certified by the Academy of Veterinary Homeopathy
Homeopathy is undergoing a renaissance, and veterinarians of all stripes are
pulling together different methods of treatment. The approaches vary from person
to person. Our main purpose in establishing the academy is to educate veterinarians in the classical homeopathy developed by Samuel Hahnemann 200 years
ago, which has been widely practiced around the world with excellent results ever
since. Some people have come up with their own methods, styles or offshoots of
homeopathy, such as using energy transfer devices to prepare remedies or diagnosing with pendulums, electronic instruments, kinesiology muscle testing or
other subjective or intuitive methods, but our approach is based on Hahnemann's
teachings and writings, which we believe have stood the test of time and remain
unsurpassed.

In general, I would suggest that pet owners look to veterinarians trained in
homeopathy who don't combine homeopathic treatment with the use of conventional drugs, acupuncture or other methods of treatment that would possibly interfere with the therapy.

Are there any natural healing methods that do not interfere?

PITCAIRN: There are quite a few, actually. Homeopathy is something you
can apply to great advantage when there is an excellent program of nutrition in
place, such as superior food and nutritional supplements. Homeopathy seems to
go very well with chiropractic adjustments, as well as with naturopathic methods
such as fasting, grooming, exercise and some herbal therapies, but not herbs that
are very strong in their effects and that could interfere with the therapy. The milder
herbs used in small quantities are not usually a problem. Flower essences are
useful, too, such as the Bach flower remedies.

The main problem we see is with the use of allopathic drugs, which isn't
surprising, considering how strong they are, and with Chinese herbs, acupuncture
and some of the stronger-smelling essential oils, which seem to block the action
of homeopathic drugs.

Considering the scarcity of qualified, experienced veterinary homeopaths, how can someone who doesn't live near one use this therapy?

PITCAIRN: A number of credentialed veterinary homeopaths do consultations by phone with both veterinarians and pet owners. Homeopathy is based
on the detailed symptoms a patient presents, and the practitioner will ask many
questions about the behavior of the animal involved, the nature of the symptoms
and the progression of symptoms over time. With that information, one can often

find the appropriate treatment. Some veterinarians are comfortable diagnosing and prescribing without physically seeing the animal, and some are not. Those who do phone consultations usually suggest a homeopathic remedy as well as other appropriate therapies, such as improved nutrition.

How can pet owners obtain the recommended remedies?

PITCAIRN: The lower potencies, which go up to about a 30c strength, are usually available over the counter in health food stores and homeopathic pharmacies. Higher potencies, like 200c, 1M, 10M and so on, often require a prescription that can be filled at a homeopathic pharmacy, or the veterinarian may be able to provide it.

Are two dogs with the same disease likely to receive the same prescription?

PITCAIRN: Not necessarily. They might have the same disease but present different symptoms, just the way people do when they get the flu. For example, one person might have nausea and vomiting, while another has upper respiratory congestion and a headache. That situation results in two different treatments.

However, the same remedy is sometimes used for patients who share an illness. *Genus epidemicus* is a term used in homeopathy when an infectious disease sweeps through a community. After working with half a dozen or more patients, a practitioner will often find a pattern showing that a single preparation is appropriate for all or most of the patients.

In acute conditions, which usually appear quickly and are self-limiting in that they have a natural end or conclusion, the same homeopathic drug is often effective for most of the animals that develop the illness. The number of individual homeopathic remedies that can be considered in the treatment of acute conditions is very large, with the practitioner choosing from about 200 of the 1,000 or so remedies that have been described to one extent or another. Having found the remedy that tends to work for that particular epidemic, the practitioner would probably give that same remedy to most or all of the animals presenting the same clear symptoms.

The use of a single common remedy is less likely in the case of chronic conditions, which are ongoing and which tend to worsen with time, such as arthritis or hip dysplasia in dogs or feline leukemia in cats. Here the practitioner usually draws on a much smaller group of medicines, but they are selected more individually, depending on the animal involved.

What is a "healing crisis," and how can you tell one from an adverse side effect or an ineffective treatment?

PITCAIRN: A healing crisis is a temporary worsening of symptoms followed by overall improvement. In homeopathy, if a remedy is working, certain symptoms may increase for a few hours, but they shouldn't be severe or last long. If your pet's condition worsens or if new symptoms develop and these symptoms don't improve within a day or two, it is probably not a healing crisis, and the treatment should be reconsidered. Symptoms of healing include increased energy levels, playfulness, the return of the animal's normal disposition, normal appetite, self-grooming, especially in cats, restful sleep and the return of normal elimination. These improvements are seen at the same time or right after the aggravation, and that distinguishes it from a situation in which the disease becomes worse.

Are there any conditions for which you would use conventional therapy rather than homeopathy?

PITCAIRN: There would be if I had a more general practice. For example, if I treated animals injured in accidents, I would use homeopathic remedies but there would also be a need for suturing and anaesthesia. Most of my patients are those with chronic diseases, not emergencies. Once a year or so I'll prescribe antibiotics, such as for paralysis of the bladder, where the animal can't get rid of its urine because of an injury and bacterial infection is a continuing problem. Or sometimes if I can't figure out what's needed and nothing seems to be clearing a bacterial infection, then I'll recommend an antibiotic. But that's unusual.

Do all your patients improve?

PITCAIRN: Most of them do, but not all. I'm a last resort for some people, whose animals are near death when I see them for the first time. I can't help them if they're too sick or too damaged, but animals that are young rather than old and haven't had the disease for a long time usually get better. Homeopathy is my first choice because it's a complete system of medicine; in fact, it's broader in its coverage than conventional allopathic medicine.

For example, homeopathy can treat behavioral problems. Allopathic medicine attempts to do this with tranquilizers and drugs that alter the brain's chemistry, but homeopathy can actually cause the condition to improve permanently, without adverse side effects.

Or take a dog that's been hit by a car and has a broken leg. It goes through surgery, has a bone pin put in with a splint and receives antibiotics and other conventional treatment. At that point, all allopathic medicine can do is wait for the bone to heal. But in homeopathy, there are medicines that can be used to stimulate the healing of the fracture. You can treat for the initial injury with a homeopathic drug like *Arnica*; then you can treat with a preparation like *Ledum*, which would help remove the blood clot around the fracture; then you could use *Symphytum*, which is a homeopathic preparation of comfrey, to speed the bone's repair. Now the healing should only take two-thirds as long or maybe half as long as it would otherwise. There is nothing equivalent in allopathic medicine.

Homeopathy effectively treats bacterial infections such as abscesses or infected wounds, viral diseases, conditions caused by fungi and other common and uncommon problems.

What about intestinal parasites?

PITCAIRN: There isn't anything I know of that will act like a worm medicine, but if the patient is treated constitutionally to raise the level of its health in a general sense, then very often the animal will shed its parasites. In the case of a young animal that has a lot of worms, treatment with a worm medicine would be appropriate, followed by homeopathic medicines that support the overall health of the animal.

Homeopathic nosodes are promoted as an effective replacement for vaccinations. What are they?

PITCAIRN: Those are remedies made from the disease itself or from its products, really, and they can be quite useful both in prevention and treatment, but their use is very limited. They don't produce antibodies the way a vaccine would and they seem to be very specific, so that a nosode of parvovirus would not protect a dog from any other disease. I have used them off and on over the years, and they seem to be as effective as any of the conventional vaccines in that they provide as much protection from the incidence of disease as vaccines do. However, they're not perfect by any means.

They can be used to treat an active illness, and they seem to be most effective in the treatment of well-defined diseases such as distemper, kennel cough or parvovirus in dogs and panleukopenia in cats.

But homeopathic nosodes aren't always effective, and it would be helpful to keep in mind that homeopathy addresses specific symptoms. If you take two animals with the same disease, some of them will respond immediately to its homeopathic nosode, but there will always be some that won't because they have a different way of getting sick. Then you have to use a medicine that's suitable for treating their individual symptoms.

What do you think of over-the-counter homeopathic preparations for dogs, cats and other pets?

PITCAIRN: Some of them may be effective in treating acute conditions, but they aren't usually effective in treating chronic conditions. Also, many of these remedies are combinations of homeopathic drugs, and this violates a basic rule of homeopathy: you never combine remedies. There are companies that produce combination formulas, but this isn't ethical homeopathy because the combinations have never been tested to see what their effects are. Another consideration is that if you use these formulas for chronic diseases, you may confuse the situation so that a practitioner you consult later on can't figure out what to do because you changed the symptoms without curing them. That's why I wouldn't recommend using an over-the-counter combination formula for itching skin, arthritis, ear infections or any chronic condition. Chronic diseases should be treated very carefully.

I think these products are less of a problem with acute conditions, but they are not as effective as single remedies. In brief, combination remedies can act favorably but prevent a deeper response that results in cure. Another way of saying this is that they palliate or relieve symptoms just as drugs do. This may be helpful, but it is not the purpose of using homeopathy in treatment.

What does the word antidote mean in terms of homeopathy?

PITCAIRN: A patient is "antidoted" if something happens to stop his or her positive response to the homeopathic medicine given. It might happen right away or days or weeks later. The cause might be exposure to a fragrance, food, pharmaceutical drug or medical procedure that interferes, or it might be another homeopathic medicine. This happens easily and it's why remedies are never combined in homeopathy.

How do you reply to critics who say that homeopathy can't possibly work?

PITCAIRN: It's easy to criticize if one has no experience with something. I've spent 20 years using homeopathy and I see it working every day.

How to Use a Homeopathic Preparation

Homeopathic drugs are available in powders, tablets, pellets and liquids. Check product labels for exact dosages. In general,

1 dose = 1 tablet, or one of the following:

3 size #20 or size #35 pellets

5 to 10 granules

premeasured vial of powder or granules

specified amount of liquid, such as 10 to 20 drops,

or a quantity measured by dropper

Homeopathic dosages are not adjusted for the type, size, weight or age of the patient as they are in allopathic medicine and herbology. In homeopathy, it is not the size of the dose that matters, but rather its potency (strength) and the frequency of application. In most cases, as soon as the symptoms improve, the treatment is discontinued, for homeopathy works by stimulating the body's own healing processes.

Everything that touches the remedy should be scrupulously clean, dry and at room temperature.

If your pet will accept them this way, give tablets or pellets whole by placing them in his or her mouth from a paper cup, spoon, dispenser cap or a small sheet of paper curved to act as a funnel. Slide, pour, drop or lightly toss the tablet or pellets onto your pet's tongue, or place the tablet or pellets on a clean paper towel or sheet of paper held in your hand or set on the floor and let your pet help himself.

If your pet resists whole tablets or pellets, you can make them easier to swallow. To crush tablets or pellets into a powder, place them inside a folded piece of clean, previously unused heavy paper, such as a folded manila envelope, or use a sheet of paper folded in half and in half again. Holding the paper flat on a countertop or other hard surface, tap the tablet or pellets with the base of a cup or glass until crushed. Pour the crushed powder down the paper's fold line into the animal's mouth, let your pet lick it off or transfer the powder to a smaller piece of paper shaped into a funnel and dispense it from that. If some of the powder spills, don't worry. Whatever your pet swallows will have a therapeutic effect.

To make a pill or powder easier to dispense, you can dissolve it in distilled, filtered or spring water, preferably in a glass or clear (not opaque) plastic bottle. Do this by placing the tablet, pellet or crushed powder in a glass, ceramic cup, paper cup or small bottle. Add a teaspoon to a tablespoon of water, and the material will begin to dissolve. Stir gently with a clean spoon.

To dispense the liquid, pour it directly into your pet's mouth or use an eyedropper to squirt it onto the tongue or between the lip and gum line. After transferring all or most of the liquid, rinse the eyedropper before using it again.

If your pet isn't happy with these methods, you can pour the liquid into a small dish or his or her water bowl, though if your pet doesn't drink it all at once, it shouldn't be left where other pets might consume it.

Another method is to dilute tablets or pellets in milk. Because milk sugar is used in their production, this is the food most compatible with homeopathic remedies.

For as long as the treatment lasts, do not feed or expose your pet to strong flavors or fragrances, prescription drugs, full-strength herbal tinctures, Chinese herbs or tobacco smoke, as these may antidote or interfere with the remedy. For best results, give homeopathic preparations at least 30 minutes before giving your pet food or water or at least one hour after, although in acute conditions and emergencies, the time span can be shortened to five minutes on either side.

To avoid contamination, never return surplus tablets to a bottle or container. Store homeopathic drugs in their original containers away from heat, light and exposure to strong odors such as camphor, menthol, mothballs, scented soaps and perfumes. Open the container only when necessary, and don't open more than one container at a time.

Because of United States Food and Drug Administration requirements, homeopathic remedies sold in the U.S. are stamped with expiration dates, but these are usually meaningless. Homeopathic remedies that are stored away from heat, light, humidity and electromagnetic fields remain effective for decades, if not centuries.

Arnica and the Skeptical Medical Mind
by Deborah Gordon, M.D.

Many years ago I had a large, friendly, out-of-shape Golden Retriever who accompanied me on a strenuous backpacking trip in the Sawtooth Mountains. As we were hiking down and out the temperature rose uncomfortably, and we decided to combine a two days' hike into one. We all seemed to manage the hike, but the following morning my dog didn't get up with the rest of us. She lay barely breathing and certainly not moving, despite my most enthusiastic encouragement. I dribbled water into her mouth — nothing. I put some of her food, moistened with oil, into her mouth — nothing. If she wasn't eating I knew she was really sick. I remembered that strange little box of remedies I had brought along. I pulled out the homeopathy book I had intended to read at my leisure on the vacation. To the best of my reckoning, the dog needed *Arnica* (ailments from over-exertion). I had a bottle of *Arnica 30c* and placed a few pellets on her tongue. Within 30 seconds, I had my dog back, up and running around the room, licking my face and getting down to business — eagerly seeking her breakfast!

I learned something else that day. She continued to act normally until later in the afternoon when we all dunked ourselves in a natural sulfur hot spring in a creek. She dragged herself slowly to the car and once again collapsed, unresponsive. I let her sleep as we were planning a long drive, but I learned that in some cases, sulfur hot springs can antidote remedies! The dog was fine the next morning, and I was on my way to studying homeopathy.

Even as a skeptical medical doctor, there was no way I could deny that those little pellets had miraculously rescued my dog. No placebo effect at work, just a simple, gentle and effective cure.

— Reprinted with permission from *Better Health Through Homeopathy,*
Vol. 2, No. 3, September 1996.

Twelve Homeopathic Remedies for Pets

Courses of Treatment

Emergency schedule:

Give 1 pellet every 15 minutes for a total of three treatments, such as *Arnica 30c* for bleeding from a wound or cut, *Ledum 30c* for an insect bite or sting, or *Nux vomica 30c*, 2 pellets each dose, for poisoning.

For acute conditions:

Schedule 1: Give 1 pellet or tablet every 4 hours until symptoms are gone. If there is no improvement within 24 hours, try another remedy. If the animal improves, continue the treatment up to five days, discontinuing as soon as symptoms disappear. Withhold food for at least 10 minutes and water for 5 minutes before and after treatment.

Schedule 2: Give 1 pellet or tablet every 4 hours for a total of 3 treatments. Discontinue homeopathy for 24 hours, then evaluate the animal. If there is no improvement, try another remedy or one of the other treatment schedules. If the animal's condition has improved, there is no need for further treatment. Restrict food and water, as above.

Schedule 3: Give 1 pellet or tablet every 12 hours for three days for a total of 6 doses. If there is no improvement after this, try a different remedy. If a definite improvement has occurred, there is no need for further homeopathic treatment. Restrict food and water, as above.

For chronic conditions:

Schedule 4: Give only 1 treatment of 2 whole pellets or 3 crushed pellets placed on the tongue. Withhold food for 60 minutes before and after treatment, and withhold water for 10 minutes before and after. Wait for a full month before further treatment; do not repeat the remedy. If there is no improvement, select a different remedy. If the animal shows improvement, no further treatment is necessary.

Schedule 5: Give 3 doses, as described in Schedule 4, giving them 12 hours apart, withholding food for 30 minutes and water for 5 to 10 minutes before and after treatment. Wait one month. If there is no improvement, select a different remedy.

Schedule 6: Give the remedy for a total of four weeks, following a schedule of 1 tablet or pellet A) once a day, B) once every two days or C) once every three days, depending on the recommended option. These schedules are recommended for very low potency remedies, either 6x or 6c. Withhold food for 30 minutes and water for 5 minutes before and after each treatment. If the animal's condition improves, continue the treatment as long as it keeps helping for as long as several months.

— Adapted from *Dr. Pitcairn's Complete Guide to Natural Health for Dogs & Cats* ©1995
by Richard Pitcairn and Susan H. Pitcairn.
Permission granted by Rodale Press, Inc.

The following is only a small fraction of the hundreds of homeopathic remedies that make up the veterinarian's *Materia medica.* This introduction gives examples of remedies made from various parts of plants, animals, trees, rocks and minerals, some of them highly toxic in their normal state. The remedies are used in potencies ranging from 3x or 6x (the mildest) to 6c or 30c (stronger) to 1M (strongest). For those new to the subject, this brief overview shows homeopathy in action, treating a variety of canine, feline and avian conditions with detailed individual symptoms. For more information about homeopathy, and to use it effectively, see the Resources for this chapter in the Appendix.

Aconite

Aconitum napellus is the poisonous monkshood or wolfsbane, used throughout history on the tips of hunters' arrows; its name is derived from the Latin word for dart. Homeopathic *Aconite,* which is nontoxic because of its extreme dilution, is useful in treating fear, panic attacks, shock, burning pain, acute infections that develop suddenly and eye injuries that result in inflammation. Francis Hunter in *Homeopathic First Aid Treatment for Pets* considers *Aconite 30* the first remedy to give in any type of accident or injury, even if the patient is barely conscious. It can be repeated after 15 minutes; usually one to two doses are sufficient.

He also wrote that *Aconite 30c* can be given every 15 minutes for a few doses as part of the treatment for snakebite. When the bite is poisonous, immediate veterinary attention is required, but *Aconite* will help relieve shock. "Snakebites naturally alarm the owner as well as the animal involved," he added, "so take a dose or two of *Aconite* at the same time as you treat your pet!"

Richard Pitcairn recommends *Aconite 30c* according to dosage schedule 4 for corneal (eye) ulcers; the same remedy at schedule 3 is appropriate for the earliest stages of Lyme disease; and the same remedy at schedule 2 is recommended for metritis, a bacterial infection of the uterus occurring just after breeding or giving birth, as well as mastitis, an infection of the mammary glands in nursing mothers, and also feline viral rhinotracheitis (FVR), which resembles the common cold. If given when symptoms first appear, it may prevent further development of the illness.

In *Dogs: Homeopathic Remedies,* George Macleod devotes several pages to the treatment of canine distemper, calling *Aconite 30c* "the outstanding remedy for the early stages." It should be given as soon as possible when symptoms become apparent, especially anxiety, shivering or other signs of shock. "This remedy by itself might be capable of cutting short the development of further symptoms," he wrote. "It should be given at half-hourly intervals for a total of six doses."

In her *Homeopathic Treatment for Birds,* Beryl M. Chapman recommends *Aconite 30c* for birds chilled in cold, dry, windy weather, particularly if the bird is hot and

In *The Homeopathic Treatment of Small Animals* Christopher Day recommends *Aconite* for wing and toe injuries to improve circulation.

Apis

Apis mellifica is the Latin name for honeybee, and whole, live bees are used to prepare homeopathic Apis. It is used to treat insect bites that produce swelling or edema, blisterlike swellings that are sensitive to touch, fevers accompanied by a lack of thirst and burning, stinging pain, especially pain that is relieved more by the application of cold than by heat.

Pitcairn recommends *Apis 6c* at dosage schedule 1 for animals recovering from surgery, such as spaying or neutering. Chapman recommends *Apis 6c* every two hours for a total of two to three treatments for swollen abscesses in birds, and Hunter lists *Apis 30c* for abscesses in dogs and cats whenever there is much swelling and redness around a boil that looks shiny. Give 1 tablet every hour for up to 4 tablets, then 1 tablet three or four times daily until the abscess bursts or subsides.

In his book of homeopathic remedies for cats, Macleod recommends *Apis 30c,* 1 dose three times per day for three days, for laryngitis when inflammation is accompanied by swelling and edema, especially if the animal isn't thirsty and has an aversion to warmth. He suggested giving 1 dose of the same remedy daily for 14 days for glaucoma in cats as a support therapy to help reduce swelling.

Arnica

Arnica montana, well known as an herbal treatment for sprains and bruises, is excellent as a homeopathic first-aid remedy for physical and emotional shock and injury. It is useful in the treatment of burns, scalds, cuts, scrapes, eye injuries, sprains, strains, heart disease, arthritis, exhaustion and the discomfort that follows dental procedures. In addition, Macleod wrote that if given during pregnancy, it lessens the danger of difficult labor and, if given after parturition, it hastens the recovery of bruised tissue. Pitcairn recommends *Arnica 30c* given according to dosage schedule 2 during normal deliveries to strengthen the mother and prevent infection, for mouth pain resulting from accidents or injuries and for animals recovering from surgery. The same remedy at dosage schedule 5 is appropriate for animals suffering from seizures after head injuries.

Chapman recommends *Arnica 30* three or four times in one day for birds that suffer from blows and other injuries that produce pain, swelling, bruising and the shock that can kill a bird quickly. The time interval between doses can be shortened according to the bird's condition. For birds that suffer a concussion, she recommends *Arnica 200* every hour for a total of 3 to 4 doses, followed by *Arnica 30* four times per day for three days, if needed. *Arnica 200* given twice, two hours apart, aids healing after surgery and treats bloody diarrhea in birds.

Whenever a wild bird is stunned from hitting a window, herbalist Deb Soule dissolves a 30c *Arnica* pellet in a dropper bottle of water and places drops on the bird's beak every 5 to 10 minutes. "Sometimes I'm able to hold them," she says, "and sometimes I place them in a box for protection. It's amazing how quickly they recover."

Arsenicum

Arsenicum album is a homeopathic preparation of arsenic oxide. Infants and young animals suffering from fever, diarrhea and dehydration are helped by this remedy, which is also useful for anxiety, fear, insecurity, digestive disorders including food poisoning that causes burning vomiting and ailments that produce a burning pain that improves with the application of heat. Macleod recommends it for canine distemper, feline enteritis and dry eczema with dandruff-like skin flakes.

In her *Raystede Handbook,* M. Raymonde-Hawkins described a small Scottish Terrier with a chronically poor coat and dry, scaly skin. The dog, she wrote, "became completely presentable after three days treatment followed by three days rest over a period of one month" using *Arsenicum 6x.*

Pitcairn recommends *Arsenicum 6c* according to dosage schedule 6A for feline infectious peritonitis (FIP), especially in cats that are anxious, chilly, thirsty and restless. The same remedy at schedule 1 is appropriate for gastritis and indigestion caused by spoiled meat or spoiled food. For bright green, liquid diarrhea in birds, Chapman recommends *Arsenicum 30* given up to twice per day over two days.

Belladonna

Atropa belladonna, the deadly nightshade, is the source of homeopathy's *Belladonna.* It treats acute conditions that begin suddenly or violently, such as high fevers, and ailments that produce sensitivity to noise, light, touch, pressure or pain. It can be used for boils, earaches, fever in young animals, nursing problems, such as red, swollen breasts, and the discomfort young animals feel while teething.

Macleod recommends it for fits of various kinds in dogs, including eclampsia in bitches and canine distemper, as well as heat stroke. Pitcairn recommends *Belladonna 6c,* 1 pellet every 15 minutes until symptoms are relieved for eclampsia, and *Belladonna 6x* according to dosage schedule 1 for the stage of liver disease in which fever, restless agitation, a hot head and dilated pupils are symptoms. For metritis that does not respond to treatment with Aconite, treat with *Belladonna 30c* using dosage schedule 2. The same therapy is appropriate for mastitis in dogs with fever, dilated pupils and excitability.

~~Belladonna (for an individual) is recommended for gastritis in feverish, excitable animals~~ with dilated pupils. Chapman recommends *Belladonna 30,* 1 dose every two hours for a total of 2 to 3 doses, if needed, for abscesses in birds that produce redness and pain but little swelling. Discontinue as soon as improvement occurs.

Carbo. veg.

Carbo. vegetabilis is homeopathic charcoal made from beech, silver birch or poplar trees. It is recommended for low vitality, exhaustion, weakness or shock, especially after surgery, and for poor circulation, indigestion, flatulence and bloating. Pitcairn recommends *Carbo. veg. 30c,* 1 dose of 3 crushed capsules every 15 minutes for a total of 3 treatments for dogs with bloat, especially if they are greatly distended with gas, look very ill, have cold legs and ears and have a bluish color in the tongue and gums. A dog that has had at least one serious episode from which it has not fully recovered can be treated with dosage schedule 4.

For birds that collapse, Beryl Chapman writes, "There is one remedy in homeopathy that is known affectionately as the 'corpse reviver.' Always have this on hand. As you must have a fast response, it has to be *Carbo. veg. 200c* as the 30c would not be quick enough." If the bird is cold and barely breathing, she recommends 1 dose every 30 minutes until improvement occurs; then, when the bird can open its eyes and hold up its head, change to *Sulfur 200c* for up to 3 doses, three hours apart.

Ledum

Ledum palustre, also known as Labrador tea, wild rosemary or marsh tea, is the source of homeopathic *Ledum,* one of the most widely used first aid remedies for animals. Taken internally, it is recommended for insect bites, stings, bruises, eye injuries, conjunctivitis, corneal ulcers, cuts, scrapes and puncture wounds. It is also recommended for rheumatic pain, swollen joints and stiff tendons. After trying various homeopathic preparations for Lyme disease with limited success, Dr. Stephen Tobin, a Connecticut veterinarian, found that *Ledum 1M* (a prescription-strength potency) is "about as close as you can get to a specific cure." Tobin has tested this remedy in several hundred cats, dogs and horses, giving 1 pellet three times daily for three days.

For puncture wounds in birds over which the skin has closed and where the skin is also cold, Chapman recommends *Ledum 12c* three or four times per day for two days.

Merc. Sol.

Mercurius solubilis hahnemanni is homeopathic mercury or quicksilver. Although highly toxic, mercury has a long history of medicinal application, especially in the treatment of syphilis. Its key homeopathic uses are for ailments that produce strong-smelling, profuse, burning bodily discharges, throat and mouth complaints, bad breath, gingivitis, chronic conjunctivitis and nasal mucus. It also treats skin or scalp lesions, blisters and open sores or skin ulcers. According to Macleod, this is an indispensable remedy for dogs, treating ear infections, dysentery, liver problems and kidney disease. "A strong guiding symptom for its consideration," wrote Macleod, "is an abundance of slimy saliva." In his book *Cats: Homeopathic Remedies,* Macleod prescribes *Merc. sol. 6c* in one dose daily for 10 days for gingivitis in cats, especially simple inflammations with excessive saliva, a dirty look to the mouth and a worsening of the condition at night.

Richard Pitcairn recommends *Merc. sol. 30c* according to dosage schedule 2 for cats with bladder problems who act annoyed with their rear ends, licking after urination and thrashing the tail while straining to urinate. The same remedy at schedule 3 is appropriate for dogs with Lyme disease with other symptoms, such as red, inflamed gums, bad breath and a tendency to drool or salivate as well as for cats with feline calicivirus (FCV) in which they have ulcers in the mouth, a bad mouth odor, excessive saliva and the tongue coated with a yellow film. *Merc. sol. 6x* at schedule 1 is appropriate for hot spots with a yellowish or greenish puslike discharge and hair loss that leaves raw, bleeding patches of skin, especially if the condition is worse in hot weather or very warm living quarters. For abscesses in birds which do not respond to *Belladonna* or *Apis,* Chapman recommends *Merc. sol. 6c,* 1 dose every two hours until improvement occurs, for a maximum of 2 to 3 doses.

Nux Vomica

Strychnos nux vomica is a small seed called poison nut or Quaker buttons that grows in Asia and Australia. Although highly toxic, strychnine extracted from these seeds was used in the Middle Ages to treat bubonic plague. *Nux vomica's* primary uses in homeopathy are to treat insomnia, digestive complaints such as indigestion, vomiting, diarrhea with painful intestinal cramps, nausea with colicky pain and constipation. Urinary tract infections such as cystitis, frequent urination, morning sickness in pregnancy, labor pains and irritability respond as well. In addition, Macleod lists it for the treatment of umbilical hernias in young patients.

Pitcairn suggests *Nux vomica 6c* according to dosage schedule 6A for anemia and *Nux vomica 30c,* 1 pellet every 15 minutes for a total of 3 treatments for acute bladder infections in cats and for acute gastric dilation or bloat in dogs with a greatly enlarged abdomen. The same remedy given according to schedule 3 is recommended for cats with feline leukemia (FeLV), especially cats that become irritable and withdraw to a quiet place; the same remedy at schedule 4 is recommended as an occasional treatment for uremia or kidney failure; the same remedy at schedule 2 is recommended for dogs with pancreatitis, especially if they are irritable, withdrawn, prefer to be alone and are easily chilled, and for cats with feline viral rhinotracheitis (FVR), especially if they are irritable and prefer not to be held. For constipation in dogs caused by poor quality food, eating too many bones or emotional upset, or for cats that strain ineffectually or pass only small amounts without relief, he suggests *Nux vomica 6c* at schedule 3. The same remedy at schedule 1 is recommended for animals with acute gastritis and vomiting that is not caused by swallowing a foreign object, especially if the dog or cat wants to be alone; this treatment is also appropriate for indigestion caused by overeating. *Nux vomica 3x* can be given, 1 tablet before each meal, to dogs with greasy, malodorous coats.

According to Pitcairn, *Nux vomica 6x* is appropriate for animals with back pain, muscle tightness, lower back spasms and weakness or paralysis of the hind legs; give 1 tablet three times daily when symptoms first appear or during attacks. Taper off when improvement occurs; discontinue until needed again if constipation develops after two or three weeks of treatment. This therapy works best when the disorder is caught early; dogs with long-standing intervertebral disk problems should follow schedule 6A.

Sepia

Sepia officinalis is a soft mollusk called cuttlefish, a relative of the squid and octopus. Like those deep sea animals, it produces a brownish black ink that it ejects when disturbed. Homeopathic *Sepia* is made from this ink's pigments.

Best known for its gynecological applications in women, *Sepia* treats the reproductive systems of female dogs and other animals as well as exhaustion, muscle weakness, indigestion from milk or fatty foods, gas and tenderness in the abdomen, nausea, circulatory problems, hair loss and itchy, discolored patches of skin in animals of both sexes. Macleod recommends *Sepia* for the treatment of infertility and pyometra in females and as an aid to whelping and postpartum discharges, as well as skin conditions such as alopecia and ringworm. "It is capable of promoting the maternal instinct in those animals which are indifferent to their young," he writes.

For pyometra, Pitcairn recommends *Sepia 30* according to schedule 3 if treating with *Pulsatilla 30c* on the same schedule has not produced results. *Sepia 30c* at schedule 2 is appropriate for cats with recurring bladder infections, especially those who are finicky, aggressive toward other cats and difficult to handle or medicate. They may produce "crystals" in their urine. For cats, *Sepia 30c* according to dosage schedule 4 is his choice for the most severe and persistent constipation; the same therapy is appropriate for treating animals that suffer hair loss after giving birth. The same remedy at dosage schedule 5 is appropriate for cats with waxy, dirty, itchy ears and for dogs and cats that lose hair after giving birth and nursing their young. *Sepia 6c* at schedule 6A is recommended for cats with feline leukemia and very red or inflamed gums as well as cats with kidney failure combined with nausea, vomiting or loss of appetite.

Silicea or Silica

Silicea terra, more familiar as quartz or rock crystal, was the original source of homeopathic *Silicea,* sometimes called *Silica.* The remedy, one of homeopathy's tissue salts, is now prepared chemically. Its main uses are the correction of undernourishment, leading to recurring infections, skin and bone complaints, the ejection of foreign objects such as splinters or thorns, and ear infections. According to Macleod, this widely used formula is indicated for infections producing pus after acute symptoms have passed and a chronic state develops. Certain forms of anemia respond to infrequent, high-potency doses, and *Silicea* is also recommended for corneal ulcers of the eye, cysts in dogs, the absorption of scar tissue and the regression of some forms of tumor. Pitcairn recommends a treatment of *Thuja 30c* according to dosage schedule 5, followed one month later by *Silicea 30c,* for the treatment of breast tumors. For other cancers, such as solid tumors in dogs or lymphosarcoma, especially if associated with rapid weight loss and a ravenous appetite, he recommends *Silicea 30c* according to schedule 6B. The same remedy at schedule 4 is appropriate for animals that get small pimples, discharge pus or have inflammation around the nails as well as those with large warts, especially warts that develop over a vaccination site.

For dogs with constipation associated with weak rectal muscles that do not expel the stool, he recommends *Silicea 6c* according to schedule 3. The same remedy at schedule 6A is appropriate for dogs and cats with foxtails, wild oat seeds and other stickers that won't leave. *Silicea 30c* at schedule 5 is appropriate for recurring ear inflammation in dogs accompanied by excessive wax production or accumulating fluid. *Silicea 6x,* widely sold as a tissue salt, can be given to dogs with disc problems, back pain and partial paralysis; use dosage schedule 6A. The same remedy at schedule 6B is appropriate for use between attacks of bloat in dogs, especially those with a history of skin or ear eruptions with itching and discomfort. Pitcairn warns that when this therapy is successful, it is accompanied by a healing crisis in which the skin eruptions return temporarily.

For hard cysts in birds, Chapman recommends *Silicea 30c* twice daily for two days, then once a day for a week, then once a week until there is improvement.

Thuja

Thuja occidentalis, the familiar landscaping evergreen arbor vitae or white cedar, is the source of homeopathy's *Thuja,* which is pronounced THOO-ya and sometimes spelled *Thuya.* It is used in the treatment of warts and other skin complaints, claws and nails, genitourinary tract infections, ailments characterized by green or greenish yellow phlegm, exhaustion from overexcitement and a loss of appetite in the morning. Some veterinarians administer *Thuja* as a support therapy for Lyme disease and as an antidote to vaccine reactions. Pitcairn recommends *Thuja 30c* according to dosage schedule 5 for dogs with kidney or bladder stones, followed one month later with *Calc. carb. 30c.* "This treatment program will not be effective in every case," he wrote, "but will with many and is worth trying." *Calc. carb.* is the tissue salt calcium carbonate.

For breast tumors, Pitcairn recommends *Thuja 30c* according to dosage schedule 5, followed one month later by *Silicea 30c;* at the onset of other cancers, *Thuja 30c* given according to dosage schedule 4 is appropriate, for it removes the influence of prior vaccinations that may stimulate tumor growth. The same remedy is an antidote to vaccination-caused skin and coat problems. "Many of the animals I treat developed their skin problems within a few weeks after being vaccinated," says Pitcairn. "I find that giving this remedy occasionally during treatment for improved skin and coat really helps such dogs recover." The same therapy is appropriate for the prevention of warts in dogs and older pets, which are sometimes an expression of vaccinosis. It is also recommended for epilepsy in dogs or cats, followed one month later by *Silicea 30c. Thuja 30c* at schedule 3 is recommended for cats with cold symptoms, including nasal discharge that develop three to four weeks after vaccination.

Nosodes

In addition to remedies like those above, some veterinarians use homeopathic nosodes either as an alternative to vaccinations or to treat an active illness. A nosode is a homeopathic remedy made from the products of the disease itself. These preparations require a prescription from a veterinary homeopath.

Steven Tobin uses the Lyme disease nosode, a homeopathic preparation of the spirochete bacteria *Borrellia burgdorferi* as a preventive in dogs. Beverly Cappel-King reports, "We've treated dogs who have kennel cough with the kennel cough nosode and, within 24 hours, they stop coughing. There are nosodes for just about every condition, including leukemia nosodes for cats. I'm amazed that the FIP nosodes have turned around close to 75 percent of the FIP cases we've treated. That's very impressive. The feline leukemia nosode works well, but its cure rate in our practice hasn't been as high as the FIP cure rate. Still, it's worth trying.

"Over in Westchester County we have a cat who has had feline leukemia for years. He's an outdoor cat and, thanks to the nosode, he's still doing well at 14. In Manhattan there is another cat who's had feline leukemia since the owner got her, along with lymphoma of the kidneys, and we've kept her going with the nosodes. Her kidneys aren't great, they're borderline, and every now and then she has a crisis, but she's still alive six years after all the expert predictions said she would be dead in a matter of months."

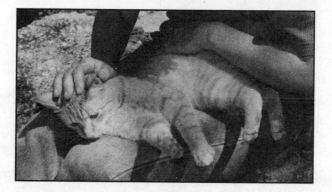

Hands-On Therapies:
Acupuncture, Acupressure, Massage, Chiropractic and Related Therapies

TOUCH IS THE OLDEST, most universal healing therapy. Humans, dogs, oceanic mammals, wild animals, farm animals, cats and birds use touch to soothe, reassure, groom and bond with their offspring, mates, friends and relatives.

With techniques as simple as the laying on of hands and as complicated as acupuncture or chiropractic adjustments, people have experimented with healing touch for millennia. In recent years the application of these methods for pets has become increasingly accepted, as reflected by the growing number of orthodox veterinarians and other healthcare practitioners who have become trained in their use.

A Convincing Demonstration

When my friend Dolores Schaub took Java, her arthritic Doberman Pinscher, for his monthly acupuncture treatment and chiropractic adjustment, I went along to watch.

Java, a rescued dog, was never socialized as a puppy, and to call him dog-aggressive is an understatement. As we waited, Java alternated between climbing into our laps for hugs and leaping, snarling, growling, lurching and lunging at the elderly sheepdog who slept quietly with her back to us at the other end of the waiting room. Whenever new patients arrived, he did his best to terrify them. By the time his name was called, we were almost as frazzled as he was.

In the examining room, Java stood like a tightly coiled spring, every muscle tense. Beverly Cappel-King pulled out a box of acupuncture needles and began inserting them along his spine, explaining as she did so which acupressure points she was stimulating. I was almost too distracted to listen, for in less than five minutes, Java transformed himself, first into a calm Dobie standing politely, and then, with head down and eyes glazed, into a brown puddle stretched flat at my feet. I knew acupuncture was supposed to work fast, but this was amazing.

Java strolled leisurely across the hall to his chiropractic adjustment, which sent him into even deeper states of bliss. When we left, the waiting room was far more crowded than it had been, and not just with snoozing geriatrics. Here were alert, young Rottweilers and other large dogs who watched us intently. Java ignored them and floated by on a pink cloud. He slept all the way home and through the next afternoon, and his relaxed, laid-back attitude continued for days.

Veterinary Acupuncture

Acupuncture is the 3,500-year-old Chinese technique of inserting small, sharp needles into specific points on the body to stimulate healing. According to traditional Chinese medicine, energy imbalances cause illnesses, and correcting those imbalances cures them. Acupuncture points can be stimulated by needles, the application of heat (moxibustion), massage (finger or thumb pressure, called acupressure) or, more recently, techniques that utilize electrical or ultrasound stimulation, the implantation of substances such as small gold beads or the application of laser light.

The term "auricular medicine" is used to describe the application of acupuncture to the ears of a person or animal, for the ears are said to contain energy points that correspond to all parts of the body. Hand and foot reflexology, widely used on humans, has application in dogs and cats, too, for there are important energy points on the paws.

Western practitioners explain acupuncture's effectiveness by saying that it stimulates nerves, increases blood circulation, relieves muscle spasms and releases hormones, all of which assist the body's self-healing. Java's response reflected his body's release of endorphins, which are mood-elevating pain-control chemicals, and cortisol, a natural steroid. Acupuncture can be used to treat behavioral disorders, skin problems such as lick granuloma or allergic dermatitis, respiratory problems such as feline asthma or kennel cough, gastrointestinal problems such as diarrhea or colic, reproductive problems, musculoskeletal disorders such as arthritis and injuries, inflammation, burns, trauma, edema and shock.

In small animals, as in human beings, the needles are so thin and sharp that their insertion is virtually painless. Larger needles are used on large animals, such as cows and horses, and their insertion may cause brief pain as the needle passes through the skin, but correctly positioned needles seldom hurt. Most animals respond as Java did, by becoming very relaxed or sleepy. In fact, most animals on a regular schedule of treatments enjoy the procedure so much that as soon as they see the acupuncturist and watch the needles being unwrapped, their posture changes and they go limp in anticipation.

Side effects other than relaxation, a feeling of euphoria and sound sleep are unusual, although an animal's condition may seem to worsen for one to two days following treatment. Like Java's lethargy, this reaction is considered an indication of deep physiological changes that mark the beginning of the body's self-healing process. They are usually followed by improvement in the animal's condition. Infection at the needle site is extremely rare.

Treatment time varies from 10 seconds to half an hour. For a simple acute problem, such as a sprain or infection, a single treatment may be all that's needed; for well-established chronic conditions, such as arthritis, one to three treatments per week may be necessary. According to the International Veterinary Acupuncture Society, "A positive response is usually seen after the first to third treatment. Once a maximum positive response is achieved (usually after four to eight treatments), treatments are tapered off so that the greatest amount of symptom-free time elapses between them." For most animals with chronic conditions, this results in a maintenance program of two to four treatments per year. Animals involved in intense athletic training or exercise may benefit from treatments once or twice weekly or monthly, depending on the activity involved and the animal's condition.

In the U.S., veterinary acupuncturists are licensed veterinarians. At this time, the International Veterinary Acupuncture Society offers the only accredited certification program for veterinary acupuncturists. Most countries, states and provinces consider veterinary acupuncture a surgical procedure.

Acupuncture, like acupressure, is a fascinating and complicated subject. It involves the study of energy meridians, such as the lung, large intestine, stomach, heart, small intestine, bladder, kidney, pericardium, triple heater, gall bladder, liver, spleen, conception vessel and governing vessel meridians, each of which contains up to 67 acupuncture points, as well as their yin and yang natures and association points. No wonder it takes years to become an expert.

But one needn't become a professional acupuncturist to use this healing art. Veterinarian Alan Schoen wants people to know about the acupuncture point called Governing Vessel 26 (GV26), which is located halfway between the nose and upper lip. In his best-selling *Love, Miracles and Animal Healing*, Schoen recounts a visit to a major veterinary hospital, during which he gave a talk about acupuncture and described this vital point, saying that an animal could suffer cardiac arrest and lose all vital signs, yet be brought back to consciousness by its stimuation. One prominent veterinary surgeon denounced his claims as nonsense and walked out, leaving an embarrassed silence and a demoralized Schoen behind. A few minutes later, fate intervened, for as Schoen walked with a friend to the clinic's emergency room, technicians rushed in with a 12-year-old

German Shepherd whose heart had stopped after surgery. The nine veterinarians on duty inserted a tube down the dog's throat, administered manual cardiac massage, injected the dog with epinephrine and bicarbonate, then wired him to electrodes and gave him electric shocks. The dog's electrocardiogram traced a flat line and he was pronounced dead. A technician was about to disconnect the oxygen when Schoen asked if he could try. As the artificial respiration continued, he pulled out an acupuncture needle and applied it to point GV26 in a series of short jabs to the cartilage. Within seconds, the dog began breathing and his heartbeat resumed.

In his book, Schoen recounts his use of acupuncture to treat arthritis in dogs, colic in a horse, allergies in a Siamese cat, neck stiffness in a llama, epilepsy in an Alaskan Malamute, labor problems in a Burmese cat and a low sperm count in a stud bull, illustrating well the versatility and effectiveness of this ancient art.

Acupuncture in Action
A Conversation with Beverly Cappel-King, D.V.M.

Dr. Beverly Cappel-King uses acupuncture in combination with medicinal herbs, chiropractic treatments, nutritional supplements and other therapies. She applied the needles that sent Java into his altered state.

What are the main uses of veterinary acupuncture?

CAPPEL-KING: Most of our patients come in for arthritis pain, hip dysplasia, mobility problems, back pain, disc problems and things of that nature. But it works just as well for degenerative diseases, like kidney or liver disease. Here's a good example. About three years ago a shepherd was brought in with chronic red eyes. The dog had already seen two vets and two ophthalmologists, and those doctors prescribed antibiotics, cortisone, antihistamines and other conventional things. Nothing worked, and the eyes were still red.

When I saw the dog, there was something that just didn't seem right, something that didn't fit. I told the owners that I couldn't explain why, but I didn't think it was an eye problem. The owners said, "No, he's been checked, it's definitely an eye problem." I ran my hands over him, going gently down his spine, and his liver points on the spine felt very hot. When I applied gentle pressure to those points, the dog winced and buckled.

I showed the owners a chart and explained that according to Chinese medicine, the liver and the eyes are on the same meridian, and the liver is directly related to the eyes. Any time you have a liver problem, it will show up in the eyes.

"No, no," they said, "he's fine, we just want something holistic for his eyes."

I said, "It doesn't work that way. Holistic means the whole animal, and any time I treat an animal, I treat the whole animal. I'd really like to see some blood work on this dog."

"No, no," they said, and we argued back and forth. Finally I said, "Look, I am so convinced that this dog has a liver disease that if the blood work shows he doesn't, I'll pay for the test."

That convinced them. We ran the blood test, and the liver was so bad that the results were what you'd expect to see in a case of chronic liver failure or cancer. I did an acupuncture treatment on the dog after I had the owners touch the area so they could feel how hot it was. When I put the needles in, the dog cried out, which almost never happens because acupuncture is so painless. I worked on the liver points and on some associated organs because I knew that would stimulate healing.

Minutes later his liver points were cool to the touch. The acupuncture treatment had relieved the heat, it was completely gone, and I knew we had taken the inflammation out of the area. I gave the owner some supplements and herbal tonics and said to call me in a week.

When she did, the owner said that the dog's eyes looked much better, but more than that, he had much more energy. Two or three weeks after that, she called to say that his eyes were completely clear and looked great and that he had shed his entire coat and was now growing the most incredible, shiny, fluffy coat, the kind he hadn't had since he was a puppy. She said his energy, appetite and appearance were so different, it was like having a new dog. All those veterinarians and specialists had tried to treat the red eyes, but it's never just one thing like that, it's always something systemic.

Six Important Acupuncture/ Acupressure Points in Dogs and Cats

Acupuncture won't always work on an ailing dog, cat, rabbit or other pet, but the clinical results and research support for this procedure are so unambiguous that acupuncture should always be considered, even if all other attempts at treatment have failed.

Although you should consult a veterinary acupuncture expert to deal with serious illness, there are simple acupressure techniques every pet owner can apply to help the healing process. Allen Schoen teaches his clients and readers how to use the following six

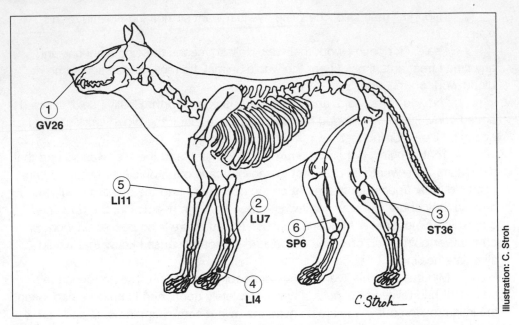

Illustration: C. Stroh

acupoints to relieve temporary distress and give first aid in a crisis. Two of these are emergency points, while the other four are called "master points" which have general, beneficial effects on the body and which can help treat specific illnesses.

These points are easy to locate on your own body. Find them first on yourself, then locate them on your dog or cat. You will know you've found the right spot when you feel tenderness. In *Canine Acupressure: A Treatment Workbook*, Nancy Zidonis and Marie Soderberg recommend positioning the ball of the thumb at the acupressure point; they prefer the thumb because of its neutral polarity. Schoen suggests using the tip of your index finger, middle finger or thumb. If your nails are long, try the knuckle of your bent index finger. Begin by pressing gently, then increase the pressure as your pet allows. Keep both hands on the animal, one to apply pressure and the other to soothe the pet and check for reactions such as muscle spasms. If working on a large dog, straighten your arm at the elbow and lean into the point with partial body weight. The pressure can be simple and direct, or you can use a pulsing motion or rotate your thumb or finger in a circular motion. To energize or stimulate your pet, use a clockwise motion; to relax her, rub counterclockwise. Complete at least three to nine full revolutions.

1. Emergency Point for Cardiac Arrest (GV26)

The stimulation of Governing Vessel 26 (GV26) can speed the recovery of a pet or person who has gone into cardiac arrest or a state of shock. It is just below the base of the nose and above the upper lip, in front of the front teeth. A series of sharp jabs with your fingernail or a needle will stimulate the production of adrenalin (epinephrine), the body's fight-or-flight hormone, improving the animal's chances of survival. Do not stimulate this point on a conscious animal (Schoen warns that you might get bit) but it can be used on newborn pups or kittens that have difficulty breathing.

2. Emergency Point for Respiratory Problems (LU7)
A critical emergency point for any animal suffering respiratory distress is Lung 7, or LU7, called "Broken Sequence" in Chinese medicine. Located above the wrist (front leg) on the side closest to the body in a depression just above the wrist bone in people and just above the corresponding small protuberance in pets, this point can be massaged in an up, down and circular motion. It is traditionally used to treat dry coughs, such as kennel cough in dogs, and it can interrupt a wheezing attack in which the animal pants and gasps for breath, such as asthma in cats. In *Four Paws, Five Directions,* Cheryl Schwartz recommends stimulating this point to help treat constipation, dry or itchy skin, dry and red inflamed ears and bronchitis. Because this acupoint moistens the upper body, it is recommended for dry conditions.

3. Master Point for Gastrointestinal Complaints (ST36)
This point, which the Chinese call "Three Mile Run" or "Walk Three Miles," boosts the energy and relieves gastrointestinal symptoms. It is located just below the knee (hind leg) on the outside of the shinbone in a depression where muscles of the lower leg join the knee. In one case, Schoen treated a three-year-old Bull Mastiff for inflammatory bowel disease (IBS) and taught his owner how to treat recurring symptoms by massaging ST36 in a counterclockwise direction for five minutes on each hind leg. The next time he overate and had an attack of indigestion, this treatment relieved his distress.

According to Schwartz, acupoint ST36 stimulates circulation and strength in the lower legs, improves the digestion and absorption of food and is an appropriate point to work in cases of chronic hepatitis, cirrhosis, the vomiting of water, bloating, coldness, watery diarrhea containing undigested food, dry constipation, arthritis resulting in weakness and immune system disorders. It stimulates the appetite, white blood cell production and resistance to disease. Schwartz warns against using ST36 if fever is present.

4. Master Point for the Head (LI4)
The acupoint known as Large Intestine 4 (LI4) is on the human hand or animal paw at the intersection of thumb (dew claw) and index finger (first long toe). Known in Chinese as "Adjoining Valleys," this is the master point for the head; it helps circulate blood and energy around the eyes, and it is appropriate for treating every condition involving the head, face, eyes, ears, nose, mouth and throat. As Schwartz notes, because the large intestine meridian ends at the nose, acupoints along this meridian affect upper

respiratory conditions, sinus congestion, sore throats and difficulty swallowing. This is a "longevity point" that increases microcirculation and contributes to a long, healthy life. Massaging this point on yourself or your pet can soothe neck aches and pains of the front leg and shoulder; in addition, it treats conjunctivitis, kennel cough and ear infections, and it may even help improve vision.

Because many dogs and cats dislike having their paws touched, Schoen suggests approaching this point gingerly. Don't use it if your pet becomes aggressive or upset. Otherwise, hold either side of this point with your thumb and index finger and massage the webbing in a back and forth motion.

5. Master Point for the Immune System, Allergies and Metabolic Imbalances (LI11)

The acupoint Large Intestine 11 (LI11), known as "Crooked Pool" or "Pond-in-the-Curve" because it is a depression at the curve of the elbow, clears heat from the upper body and regulates the immune system. To find it, bend your arm and look at the outside corner of the elbow for the end of the elbow crease. Feel there for a slight depression.

Applying pressure there can reduce pain in the shoulder and elbow, and massaging the point can help alleviate arthritis discomfort. Schoen used this acupuncture point to treat a Bernese Mountain Dog for severe arthritis of the elbows, and the dog became a puppy again. One day while running, he twisted his elbow and had a spasm. His owner massaged LI11, the spasm subsided immediately and the dog resumed his active play. According to Schwartz, the same acupoint can be used in the treatment of fever, conjunctivitis, upper respiratory infections with mouth sores in cats, chronic ear wax buildup, chronic moist ear problems, acute ear infections, acute mouth sores, diarrhea, colitis, skin scabs accompanied by a "doggy" smell, allergic dermatitis, flea allergies, food allergies, fungal and bacterial infections and any disorder that would benefit from the increased production of white blood cells.

6. Master Point for Endocrine Disorders (SP6)

Spleen point 6 (SP6), known as "Three Yin Junction," moistens and tonifies the blood and fluid. It is located on the inside of the leg (hind leg in pets), just above and to the front of the ankle or heel.

Schoen demonstrated this acupoint to a woman whose cat had diabetes, which was difficult to regulate with insulin. She massaged the point on each leg daily for five minutes in a counterclockwise direction. At their next visit, she reported that for the first time in a year, the cat's blood sugar and insulin levels were approaching normal.

Schwartz recommends stimulating SP6 in cats and toy breed dogs that develop light and wind sensitivity, which causes their eyes to tear in windy weather; she also recommends it for early heart imbalances, cardiomyopathy in cats, liver blood deficiencies or imbalances, skin rashes that itch, kidney disorders, thirst, constipation, dry or itchy skin, anemia, insecurity, an intolerance of heat and noise, diarrhea, colitis and all stress-related disorders.

The Acupressure Treatment

In *Canine Acupuncture: A Treatment Workbook,* Nancy Zidonis and Marie K. Soderberg provide detailed maps of acupuncture/acupressure points in dogs, which are identical to those in cats. If you're interested in massage, an understanding of acupuncture/acupressure points will multiply the benefits of your hands-on work. The *Canine Acupressure* workbook gives detailed step-by-step procedures for locating and stimulating about 150 major points as well as treatment programs for commonly seen problems, such as lower back soreness, neck stiffness and hip problems. "These treatments are based on our work with show and pet dogs over a period of several years," they explain. "Where the owner has been consistent in giving the dog treatment, each dog presented to us has shown significant improvement."

Among their recommendations: To prepare for an acupressure treatment for your pet, start by clearing the day's activities from your mind. Get in touch with your own Chi energy by focusing on your breath. Inhale and feel it move through your lungs and into your abdomen. Hold the breath in your abdomen for several seconds and feel its balancing, healing properties. Exhale and follow the vibration of your breath as it moves across the room. Repeat this exercise for 10 to 15 breaths. Finally, focus your energy on your pet and think of the fun you have had with her.

Work in a room or area familiar and comfortable to you and your pet. If your pet has long hair, brush him thoroughly before beginning your treatment. This will help you feel the energy meridians and give your thumbs more direct access to the skin.

Adjust the pressure you apply according to the size and condition of your pet. For example, use more pressure on a young, sturdy, athletic dog than on his arthritic, elderly or fragile relatives.

Allow ample time so you aren't rushed. In general, a complete treatment takes from 20 minutes to an hour, beginning with opening work (centering yourself, positioning the animal and gliding the palms of your hands over the animal's body), followed by point work (stimulating individual pressure points), closing (all-over massage with a smooth, light touch) and five to ten minutes of gentle stretching exercises.

Do not give your pet a full acupressure treatment if:

• She is pregnant.

• The animal has just been fed. Wait three to four hours before beginning a treatment.

- Your pet is fatigued from strenuous exercise. Wait until his breathing returns to normal and he has cooled down.

- Your pet has just bred or been bred. Wait 12 hours before treating a stud. Before doing a full acupressure treatment on your bitch or queen, determine whether she is pregnant. If so, wait until she delivers before doing a full acupressure treatment.

- Your pet has a high fever or an infectious disease. Call your veterinarian for help. While the appropriate emergency or master point can be stimulated, this is not the time to give a complete treatment.

Otherwise, you can safely administer acupressure to your pet at any time. Carefully watch the animal's responses, noting obvious symptoms like muscle spasms, excessive licking or yawning and more subtle reactions, such as changes of facial expression, relaxation of the eye, neck twisting, stretching, chewing, intestinal sounds, changes in breathing, leg stretching and moving into or away from the point pressure. Your pet may be tender following a full treatment; this is normal, for it takes about 24 hours for Chi energy to cycle throughout the body. The animal should show improvement within 24 to 36 hours. For complete instructions on giving an acupressure treatment, study *Canine Acupressure: A Treatment Workbook* (see the Resources for this chapter in the Appendix).

Tellington TTouch

When Moishe Feldenkrais was hit by a bus and lost the use of his legs, he refused surgery and ignored his doctors' pessimistic predictions. The Israeli physicist and athlete instead developed a program to reeducate his legs by bypassing the habitual way in which he had moved. He did this by utilizing every alternative motion that he could discover, from gross muscle movement to the smallest and most subtle flexing. Within two years, he was walking again, and his discoveries improved the lives of not only those with obvious disabilities but athletes, dancers and others who wanted to enhance their performance.

Feldenkrais trained these people in what he called Awareness through Movement or the Feldenkrais Method of Functional Integration. He believed that as we learn to walk, talk or ride a bicycle, our movements become habitual because every motion involves a pattern of neural responses between brain cells and muscles. Feldenkrais introduced new movements and manipulations that awaken unused brain cells and activate unused neural pathways, breaking old habit patterns and establishing new, more efficient ones. He taught his clients how to walk, run, speak, think and move in entirely new ways.

The practitioners he trained spent hundreds of hours lying on the floor, studying and experiencing the minute muscle movements that activate this process. One of them was Linda Tellington-Jones, who realized that horses and other animals could, like people, learn new responses very quickly if their old habit patterns were disrupted in a non-threatening manner. Her method, Tellington TTouch (pronounced Tee-Touch), has transformed dogs, cats, cows, goats, birds, reptiles and zoo animals, as well as their owners, companions and caretakers.

Like all of the methods described here, TTouch could fill a book by itself, and it has. *Tellington TTouch* by Linda Tellington-Jones and Sybil Taylor has generated study guides, videotapes and a network of practitioners and teachers. TTouch deserves the following it has attracted, for its methods work, and they work fast. With a minimum of equipment (wooden dowel rods, her fingertips and in some cases a wooden labyrinth made of sticks or boards), Tellington-Jones has befriended and calmed wild lynxes, African servals, snow leopards, coyotes, owls, bears, foxes, elephants, chimpanzees, giraffes, pythons, feral cats, unhappy cockatoos, hyperactive dogs, uncooperative or injured horses and a host of other animals in zoos, rehabilitation centers, clinics, ranches and private homes, training them to accept medication, correcting behavioral problems, treating physical or neurological ailments or helping them learn new ways of moving, acting and learning.

TTouch borrows some of its techniques from auricular medicine, described in the preceding section on acupuncture. According to this theory of Chinese medicine, the ears contain points that correspond to different parts of the body. If you massage and stimulate the entire ear, you stimulate the entire body, while specific points on the ear stimulate specific parts of the body.

Thanks to the demonstrations of TTouch practitioners, thousands of people who know nothing about acupuncture or TTouch know that one of the best ways to calm a restless animal or speed its healing is by rubbing its ears. An all-over ear massage is helpful almost any time, but treating an animal for shock after an injury by working the tips of the ears can make the difference between life and death. Ears can be worked by making tiny circles with a forefinger inside the ear or sliding fingers from the base of the ear to the tip while holding the ear between thumb and forefinger. Begin gently and apply pressure as appropriate. The shock point is found at the tip of the ear at its center or point, which makes it easy to locate in cats, dogs and rabbits that have pointed ears.

The most often-used motion in TTouch massage is the circle, specifically one and one-quarter circles made in a clockwise direction with relaxed fingers. That is, go one quarter turn past the starting point, then stop. Begin with fairly fast circles that take about one second to complete, then, as the animal relaxes, slow the circles to about two seconds each. On small or fragile animals, use only the lightest touch; on larger, heavier animals, begin with gentle pressure and increase it only if the animal responds positively.

TTouch massage strokes are named for animals. The Clouded Leopard, for example, involves the pads of the fingers when the hand is held gently cupped or curved. This is the basic TTouch. Its close relative, the Lying Leopard, uses more surface area of the fingers and palm; it can be used to reduce the pain and possibility of swelling in fresh injuries. The Raccoon, which uses the lightest possible pressure and the very tips of the fingers, is recommended for small animals and delicate work. It speeds healing, reduces swelling, increases circulation and activates neural impulses in the lower legs. Other maneuvers are called the Snail's Pace, Bear, Abalone, Lick of the Cow's Tongue, Tiger TTouch, Noah's Arc and Python Lift.

For information about Tellington TTouch training videos, workshops and equipment, see the Resources for this chapter in the Appendix.

Veterinary Chiropractic

When people go to chiropractors, it's usually because of back pain, muscle stiffness, sciatica, sports injuries or restricted movement. Dogs and horses are the primary patients of veterinary chiropractors, and they go for the same reasons.

The term subluxation describes the misalignment of vertebrae resulting in a disturbance of normal function. Subluxations cause animals, like people, to compensate for the resulting pain with changes in posture or movement, such as shifting weight or avoiding certain motions. Secondary subluxations can occur in other parts of the spine as a result, causing complications.

Subluxations are often the cause of abnormal or uneasy posture while standing or sitting, a refusal or unwillingness to go over jumps, the development of unusual behavior patterns such as biting or growling in a previously gentle animal, unusual sensitivity to touch, a lack of coordination or gait abnormality, stiffness on rising, stiffness in lateral movements of the back or neck, muscle atrophy, lameness in hindquarters, abnormal biting or chewing of the coat or tail, increased sensitivity to heat or cold and a limited range of motion.

In a chiropractic examination, the major muscle groups are checked for atrophy, hypertrophy, tone, symmetry, heat, tenderness and pain. In addition, the spine is palpated and examined for abnormal protuberances and other unusual features.

When a vertebral subluxation is diagnosed, the animal chiropractor performs an adjustment consisting of a short, rapid thrust on the affected vertebrae. When properly performed, this mobilizes or frees the vertebrae and restores normal function. Spinal adjustments can reverse a variety of nerve, muscle and motion problems.

Marc L. Sommer is the chiropractor who worked on Java, the acupuncture-sedated Doberman Pinscher described earlier. "Adjusting is an art as well as a science," he says. "It requires a knowledge of anatomy, biomechanics and physics as well as the manual skill to move specific, individual spinal segments."

You might take a dog to the chiropractor because of mobility problems or arthritis, but the treatment of specific symptoms is not the purpose of chiropractic. "Chiropractic adjustments are made to correct subluxations," explains Sommer. "It's the subluxation that causes problems, and those problems might be visible and obvious, or they may still be developing. We think of the subluxation as the problem, its adjustment as the cure and the improvement of symptoms as a desired side effect. Most animals show significant improvement after one to four adjustments."

While some doctors use a small impacting device called an activator to move the vertebrae, large and unwieldy devices like mallets or hammers are not needed to adjust even the largest animals and can create more acute and serious conditions, he says. Other procedures Sommer warns against include the use of excessive force and jerking on the legs or tail. "These practices do not constitute a chiropractic adjustment," he says, "and they may exacerbate an already existing injury. Remember that skill, not extreme force, is the key to successful adjustments."

For information about the American Veterinary Chiropractic Association, on whose board of directors Dr. Sommer serves, see the Resources for this chapter in the Appendix.

Therapeutic Touch and Energy Balancing for Animals
A Conversation with Carol Robin, D.C.

Therapeutic Touch is an energy healing method developed from the traditional laying-on of hands by theosophist Dora Kunz in the early 1970s. Her most enthusiastic student was Dolores Krieger, a registered nurse, Ph.D. and professor of nursing at New York University who has taught Therapeutic Touch to thousands of nurses, doctors and other health workers. Thanks to Dr. Krieger's efforts, Therapeutic Touch is an accepted medical practice in many hospitals and healthcare facilities. Her books *The Therapeutic Touch* and *Accepting Your Power to Heal* have taught it to millions more.

Carol Robin, a New York chiropractor, learned Therapeutic Touch as an adjunct to her professional practice. When she tried it on her dog and three cats, they responded as well as her human clients. Robin studied the effects of this simple technique on animals of all sizes and species and now teaches Therapeutic Touch and Energy Balancing to pet owners.

What are the benefits of Therapeutic Touch for our dogs, cats and other pets?

ROBIN: It's a powerful tool for centering, relaxing and grounding, and it helps with both behavior problems and physical ailments. If animals are hyper or nervous, it calms them down; if they're afraid of thunderstorms or strange noises, it can help them be less fearful; in cases of injury or illness, it helps them relax and gets their energy flowing more freely to speed up the healing process. In fact, I can't think of a condition where Therapeutic Touch wouldn't be helpful. It is completely safe and has no side effects. It works by increasing or improving the flow of energy through the body, and that stimulates healing.

What exactly do you do?

ROBIN: When I work on a dog or cat, I begin by placing one hand on the head and one on the base of the spine, right above the tail, over the sacrum. I touch very lightly with the palms of my hands or, on a small animal, with the ends of my fingers. Then I imagine energy flowing from the animal's head, down the spine and out the end of the tail, as though water were flowing down the body. I hold that position for one or two minutes, until I feel a sense of balance under my hands and the animal begins to relax.

How do you know when it's balanced? Is it something you feel, like a vibration or a change in temperature?

ROBIN: Everyone perceives energy differently. Some sense it as warmth or coolness; others feel a tingling, a feeling of density or a vibration. It's a very individual thing and it doesn't matter how you perceive it. What matters is noticing changes when they occur. Imagine that your hands are in bowls of water of different temperature and that you can add heat to one and cold to the other. When the bowls are the same temperature, you notice their balance, you notice that they feel the same. This is similar to what balanced energy feels like. The sensation in one hand, whether it's a temperature, a tingling, a buzz, a sense of heaviness, a sound, a color or whatever you feel, matches the sensation in your other hand.

Four-legged animals have a horizontal axis, which is convenient for this type of work. After holding the head and sacrum, lightly stroke from the head down the spine and tail. On the head, always move from the nose back. If an animal is nervous, applying a little more pressure is usually reassuring, but remember that this is **not petting**. Let your touch be slow and gentle but very intentional, not casual. Intention, imagination and focus are essential to successful energy balancing. You are feeling for any area that feels different. It may feel hot or cold, tight or loose, hard or soft, thick or thin, light or heavy, tingly or dull, bright or dark, loud or soft, smooth or disturbed — what you're looking for is an area where the energy feels different. When you find one, just lightly brush your hand over it, as though you were ever so gently brushing off some dust from the animal's fur. Do this several times, then run your hand down the body again to determine whether the area feels like the rest of the body. If it does, it means that the blocked energy is flowing again and the area is in balance. If it doesn't, repeat the procedure two or three times. Often the change happens quickly, but if it doesn't, move on and come back to it in your next session.

After working the spine, move to the animal's front legs. Place one hand on the right or left shoulder and lightly stroke down to the corresponding paw, feeling for differences in the energy and brushing them away. Repeat this process on the other side, then on the hind legs from hip to paw. After you have done all four limbs, complete the session by running your hands lightly from head to tail again, and you are done. Let the animal rest or get up as she wishes, but don't pet her yet; give her time to absorb the treatment.

How do you prepare for a Therapeutic Touch session?

ROBIN: The most important thing to do before you begin is take a few deep breaths and center yourself. If you're upset or distracted, you'll only agitate the animal. Be clear about your intention to help him or her and let go of your preconceptions about what "should" happen. This allows you to really listen to your animal's body and what it needs, rather than imposing your ideas on it. Remember that if your intention is loving and healing, you will be helpful to your animal companion.

Work in a quiet place where you won't be interrupted. Breathe and relax. Work slowly and meditatively. Trying hard only gets in your way. For Therapeutic Touch to work, you have to be relaxed and centered. In my workshops, I teach a simple breathing exercise to help people quickly become more calm, centered and focused.

Imagine a tall tree or a mountain in the distance. Take three long, slow, deep breaths, imagining that as you inhale, you are drawing your breath from the top of the tree or mountain. As you exhale, send the breath back there. Even if you are using Therapeutic Touch in an emergency to calm a sick or injured animal, take the time to center yourself first.

What position should the animal be in while you work?

ROBIN: He or she can be sitting, lying down or even standing. Animals often lie down during the session as they become more relaxed.

As you're learning, it's best to practice frequently, so you and your animals become comfortable with the process and you learn what's normal for them. Practice for five to ten minutes on each pet, several times a week. Most sessions take less than ten minutes, but pay attention to your animals. They will usually tell you when they're done. As they become more accustomed to being touched in this way, they usually love it and feel very relaxed. If you're dealing with a sick or injured animal, you can do several short treatments over the course of the day. If you work with your animals every few days, you'll be better able to notice when something is out of balance and you'll know how to treat it.

What if you're working with a bird or other type of animal?

ROBIN: I've used this work on birds, snakes, mice and a turtle. With an injured animal, I just run my hand lightly a little bit above the body rather than touching it directly. I once lived in a place with a large picture window, and periodically birds would fly into it. I'd hear a loud thud and run outside to find an unconscious bird on the ground. I would just run my hand over its body from head to tail, over and over, until the bird opened its eyes. Most of them quickly hopped up and flew away.

Is there any conventional or alternative therapy that is not compatible with Therapeutic Touch?

ROBIN: No. It's really the all-purpose support therapy; it doesn't interfere with conventional or alternative treatments and it supports the body's own innate healing abilities. All it takes is a clear intention to help, a calm, focused attention and a willingness to listen to the body and let its energy guide your hands. Therapeutic Touch is based on practices we do instinctively. Mothers sit by their sick children stroking their heads without knowing anything about energy fields. Combine the laying on of hands with a loving intention and you stimulate healing. Therapeutic Touch is simply an organized, well-tested way of doing that.

Myotherapy for Animals
A Conversation with Margie Amster-Herr

Myotherapy, which is also called trigger point massage, compression massage or myofacial compression, was developed in the United States by Dr. Janet Travell, who was President Kennedy's back physician. Travell treated human patients but applied the same methods to her own animals with good results.

Myotherapy's success in treating back and muscle pain resulted in the establishment of pain clinics and training schools. Margie Amster-Herr studied the technique at the Academy of Myotherapy and Physical Fitness in Lenox, Mass., where she pioneered the treatment of horses and dogs. Since 1988, when she established Equi-Myo in Connecticut, Amster-Herr has trained approximately 100 canine and equine myotherapists who practice in the U.S. and Europe.

Can myotherapy be used on animals other than dogs or horses?

AMSTER-HERR: Absolutely. It is safe and effective for cats, kittens, puppies and every other large or tiny animal. One of our graduates is a circus trainer who uses it on elephants. If the animal has muscles, it can be treated.

How does a myotherapist work?

AMSTER-HERR: At the first session, the myotherapist takes a complete history of the animal, examines the gait, measures mobility and documents any health problems. Then the practitioner maps the entire body by gently pressing the muscles, following a grid pattern across and down the back and sides, then across and down the legs and tail. Although some of the areas being pressed are acupuncture or acupressure points, myotherapy is completely different. While pressing, the therapist checks for responses or reactions from the animal, anything from the most subtle muscle tightening to a twitch or something more obvious, like the animal glancing back to see what's going on or shifting position.

Any point that produces a reaction is a trigger point. Trigger points are specific to the individual, and they vary from one session to the next. In other words, there is no single map of trigger points. They can occur at any time in any muscle. Applying further pressure to trigger points with an appropriate method of compression, such as with the fingertips or a knuckle, relieves pain and improves mobility by interrupting and then increasing blood supply to the area and by triggering the release of endorphins and other hormones. This type of compression is called ischemic, which means that it is held or sustained for several seconds. Then the practitioner stretches the affected muscle to interrupt its tendency to return to its previous condition. Muscles have their own memory, so releasing tension in the muscle is only part of the treatment; without follow-up stretches, freed muscles can go back where they were.

At the end of the treatment, which usually lasts about an hour, the myotherapist teaches the owner stretching exercises that should be done with the animal on a daily basis in order to prolong the benefits.

What are some of the benefits of myotherapy?

AMSTER-HERR: It's an effective therapy to use in the treatment of arthritis, physical injury or surgery, for it improves mobility and speeds healing. It's also used as a preventive treatment to keep the animal in excellent shape and for more subtle things, like improving a dog's gait in the show ring. The position of an animal's tail often changes with myotherapy along with its sense of balance and coordination.

An observant owner will notice when a dog experiences stiffness when rising or has a little trouble jumping into the car or climbing stairs. It's not always the last thing you ate that makes you sick, and it's not always the most recent exertion that causes an animal to develop an obvious limp. If minor symptoms are treated with myotherapy, they usually improve quickly and prevent more serious symptoms. Myotherapy helps the animal use its own healing processes, including the elimination of toxins and the increase of circulation, to improve its own health.

What is a typical course of treatment?

AMSTER-HERR: It depends on the condition. A minor sports injury in a young, athletic dog might require only one treatment, while chronic arthritis or lameness in an older dog may require several, although obvious improvement should occur even in the older dog after the first or second session. The older dog's treatment schedule might involve weekly visits for a month or so, then every two weeks or every month; it all depends on the animal's progress and the owner's willingness to continue the recommended stretching exercises. Joints are surrounded by muscle, and if we can loosen up the muscle and improve circulation in the area, the animal's mobility and flexibility usually improve.

What is the background of people who become canine myotherapists?

AMSTER-HERR: Most of them are involved with horses as well as dogs, so they take the equine myotherapy training as well as canine myotherapy. Many of our canine practitioners are groomers, trainers, veterinary staff, human health-care professionals or simply dog lovers. It's an intensive course of study involving anatomy and hands-on practice, but it's inspiring work because its effects are so immediate and lasting. And even though I have focused on dogs in this conversation, your readers should remember that myotherapy can be used to treat cats, rabbits and other animals with the same excellent results.

Exercise and Your Pet

Although every animal needs regular exercise for good health, dogs are the pet kingdom's star athletes. They work outdoors as herding and hunting dogs, in the frozen north as sled dogs, in all terrains as rescue, military and police dogs and in all circumstances as guiding eye, hearing ear and assistance dogs. Millions of America's purebred and mixed-breed dogs participate in obedience, agility, scent tracking, retrieving and other sports.

The physical therapists featured in this chapter know all too well the damage that these activities cause when owners and handlers are not aware of their animals' physical limitations. A motivated dog will do everything she can to please her handler, even when it means moving in pain. Ignoring a minor injury or insisting that a dog hold her head in a certain position or jump when her body is out of alignment can cause lasting problems.

When you hurt yourself, observant friends notice right away. Your body moves differently. Some joints and muscles are restricted or frozen while others move in exaggerated ways to compensate. No one insists that you move a piano, paint the house or compete in a tennis tournament.

But if your dog injures herself, you might ignore her limp and instruct her to work on, assuming or hoping it will go away. If she doesn't hold her head correctly or is reluctant to go over jumps, you might not realize she has pulled a muscle or bruised her shoulder. Some owners punish their dogs for what they perceive as disobedience when, if they would stand back and look at their animals objectively, they would understand the physical cause of unwanted behavior.

Standing back and looking at your dog objectively is exactly what Suzanne Clothier wants you to do. Clothier, an accomplished dog trainer and prolific author, has worked with Sue Ann Lesser, D.V.M., to develop a system of physical therapy for canine athletes. In seminars, books and a well-produced video tape, Clothier teaches owners, handlers and trainers how to recognize, analyze, document and treat injuries, how to condition dogs to prevent injuries and how to improve a dog's overall condition with simple hands-on therapy.

In their handbook *Physical Therapy for the Canine Athlete,* Clothier and Lesser explain that accurate observation and records are essential for the proper veterinary treatment of injuries. When and how did your dog hurt herself? Don't assume you'll remember; write it down. A dog limping because of a single bruising injury needs entirely different care from a dog who's limping because of prolonged inflammation and irritation.

Clothier's most important advice: Whenever you're in doubt about your dog's ability to perform, stop. Never force an injured animal to work or compete, no matter how important the event. When is an injury serious enough to require attention and therapy? The minute it interferes with your dog's ability to perform at her peak.

An injured, lame or limping dog may improve on her own so that the symptom disappears, but this does not mean her body has fully recovered. Just as people feel their football injuries and automobile accidents decades later, the physical traumas experienced by dogs, cats and other animals affect their mobility long after the event.

To become an expert on your pet's physical condition, learn how to give a visual examination. Clothier's video *Your Athletic Dog: A Functional Approach* is an excellent guide to monitoring your own animals' normal traits and noticing problems in others. Even if you know nothing about canine or feline anatomy, your eye will be drawn to whatever is out of alignment.

By noticing and documenting changes in your pet's gait or range of motion, you will be more aware of her needs and limitations. All of the hands-on therapies described in this chapter can improve your pet's mobility, coordination and flexibility. The simple stretching exercises recommended by canine myotherapists and physical therapists like Clothier help condition dogs and cats to prevent injury. In addition, regular massage and Therapeutic Touch release tension, improve muscle response and help return the body to its normal equilibrium.

Active physical exercise improves the health of any animal, whether dog, cat, bird, rabbit, horse or human. Exercise strengthens muscles, limbers joints, increases blood circulation, stimulates the flow of lymph, tones all of the body's systems, relieves stress, alleviates boredom, burns calories, strengthens bones and bolsters the body's resistance to disease and infection.

Healthy puppies, kittens, baby rabbits and young birds are naturally energetic and active. All they need for a physical workout is room to move. Older animals may be less rambunctious but they too need regular workouts. Observant, imaginative owners let their pets teach them favorite games and inspire them to invent new ones. Combine training with play to make physical activity fun and interesting. All the while, observe how your animal moves. Make simple stretching exercises part of your daily routine. For example, stand beside your dog to keep his back legs from moving, hold a treat or toy in one hand and slowly move it from under his nose out to the side and in toward his hip. To reach the treat, he will turn his head as far as he can. A flexible dog will shape himself like a U to get the pelue, but if he isn't able to reach that far, reward him for turn ing as far as he did. Do this on the other side and compare his range of motion.

Physical therapy books and videos can teach you how to test your pet's range of motion in other areas, such as in the joints and tail. These tests serve a dual purpose, for they are therapeutic exercises as well. If your dog turns his head far to the left as he follows your moving hand but is unable to reach all the way to the right, use any of the physical therapies described in this chapter to improve his flexibility and use treats or a toy to encourage longer stretches every day.

Another easy exercise is the bow. Dogs bow when they stretch and yawn with front legs extended and hindquarters up. This same posture, called the play bow, is an invitation to romp. "The bow," says canine myotherapist Christiane Wolski, "stretches the abdominal muscles, which are otherwise difficult to manipulate. Dogs like to bow, so this trick is easy for them to learn. The front legs can be extended straight out or bent, with elbows on the ground. What matters is a high reach up with the back legs and hindquarters; that's what makes this an effective exercise."

Some of Wolski's clients have taught their dogs full body stretches, with the dog standing vertically with front paws on the owner's shoulders, or they make the stretch horizontal by lifting the hind legs so the body and front feet form a wheelbarrow. "Not many dogs are this flexible," says Wolski, "but if your dog enjoys these positions, doing them every day will keep the abdominal muscles stretched and toned."

Some dogs, especially small breeds, sit up and beg without anyone showing them how; others have to be held in position before they catch on. Sitting with both front paws in the air is an exercise in balance that also strengthens the back muscles. Start your dog in a corner for support. Use a toy, treat or other reward to encourage longer stays in this position once or twice a day.

Waving one paw in the air, as high as the dog can reach, tones the muscles of the sides and shoulders. Teach your dog to wave with either paw so that both sides receive the stretch. If she can't balance on her haunches with both paws in the air, teach this command from your dog's normal sitting position.

Crawling is another good exercise. You can teach the crawl as a trick by combining "down" and "come," or lure the dog under an obstacle such as a low table.

"Many of these commands and others, such as jumping through hoops and over obstacles, balancing on beams, climbing over A frames, crawling through fabric tunnels and weaving around poles, are part of agility training," says Wolski, who teaches this popular canine sport. "If you want to keep your dog well-toned and flexible as well as mentally challenged, join an agility class. But you don't need a class or special equipment to give your dog an all-over workout. Running or hiking over uneven surfaces, climbing up hills, jumping over logs or benches, crawling under things, swimming, going up and down stairs, playing tag, doing tricks and stretching are all activities that keep a dog in shape. A myotherapist, massage therapist, veterinary chiropractor or other physical therapist can help repair injuries and release tight muscles, but no amount of physical therapy can compensate for a lack of exercise."

When is exercise dangerous? When it's overdone, either because of age, infirmity, the dog's physical limitations or the weather. Long hikes and prolonged jumping games, like leaping high for a ball or Frisbee, can damage the growing bones of a young dog; according to most experts, puppies should be 14 months old before their joints are stressed by vigorous endurance exercise. Owners who aren't aware of their dogs' physical limitations can push them from minor to major injuries, which is why range of motion tests, visual examination and careful monitoring are important. Monotonous exercise like jogging around the flat track of an athletic field overuses some muscles and underuses others; variety is as important in physical activity as it is in diet. Temperature extremes make any exercise potentially dangerous; schedule your summer workouts for early morning or evening, not midday.

There are many reasons to postpone or modify ambitious activities, but a lack of exercise can be just as damaging as too much exercise. Owners of dogs whose breeds are known for disc problems, hip dysplasia or bone and growth disorders are often warned not to do anything athletic because of the risk of injury. On the contrary, this approach increases the risk. Your dog's ability to prevent and recover from injuries depends in large part on the tone and condition of his bones and muscles.

To appreciate the effects of gradually increased daily exercise, consider Orient, the German Shepherd seeing eye dog who accompanied his blind owner, Bill Irwin, on the Appalachian trail in 1990. Before they began training for the hike, which covered over 2,000 miles and took them from Georgia to Maine, Orient was in good shape by American pet standards but no endurance athlete. At the beginning of their eight-month journey, they made frequent stops so Orient could rest. But the longer they climbed over rocks, up steep hills and down the long trail, the stronger he became. At one point on their journey, some people who assumed the dog was abused and overworked took a veterinarian onto the trail to inspect him. By then, Orient was so strong and fit that the veterinarian declared he had never seen a healthier animal.

Before beginning an exercise program, check with your veterinarian and, if the animal has any physical limitations, illness or injury, work with a trainer or physical therapist to create a program that will correct imbalances and prevent injury. Be sure the activities you plan are appropriate for your dog's size and age. Separate large meals and physical activity by at least an hour. Give him unlimited access to water before and after exercise and provide it during your walk, hike or run. Let your dog drink from your hand, water bottle or portable dish, then pour water over his neck and back to help him stay cool. Follow the same common-sense guidelines that apply to people. Start with a gentle warmup, move slowly into more demanding activity and follow vigorous exercise with a gradual cool down. Then let your dog rest uninterrupted for as long as he likes. Increase your dog's activity in small increments; don't expect an overweight couch potato to run several miles, but do expect him to walk longer distances each day. Walk on different surfaces, such as gravel, concrete, grass and bare soil, which will toughen your dog's paw pads and help prevent foot injuries; avoid hot pavement, broken glass and sharp rocks.

If your dog enjoys the company of other dogs, arrange for play visits or shared hikes or swims. Exercise should be fun and interesting, not boring. Think of new places, new faces, new toys and whatever will reward and motivate your canine athlete.

For notes on exercising cats, rabbits and birds, see pages 358 and 462.

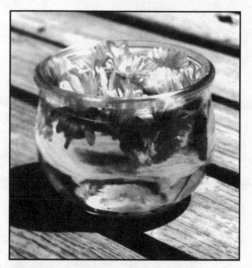

Flower Essences

A PUPPY CRIES AT BEING LEFT ALONE, but after drops from a brown glass bottle are rubbed into her gums, she relaxes and sleeps peacefully. A cat who usually hisses and growls in the veterinarian's waiting room is sprayed with a dilute solution before leaving the house, and so is his carrier. This time, his trip to the vet is noticeably calmer. A dog competing in an obedience trial senses her handler's anxiety and is distracted by the sights, smells and other dogs all around her. But after drinking several drops mixed with water, she focuses her attention and wins a ribbon.

What are these animals taking?

Flower remedies, which are also called flower essences, are a rapidly growing segment of the natural health movement, and enthusiasts credit their human use with everything from relief of migraine headaches to stress reduction, courage, optimism and the end of chronic depression. In pets, they treat conditions as varied as anxiety, skin and coat problems, eating disorders and misbehavior.

What no one can explain is how or why these preparations work. Like homeopathic medications, they are so greatly diluted that they contain little, if any, of the blossom on the label. Yet credible health care professionals, psychologists, veterinarians, parents and pet owners swear they are effective. Flower essences are part of vibrational medicine, the study of high-frequency subtle energies, which includes homeopathy, gemstones, crystals, aromatherapy, color work, hands-on healing and healing through thought or prayer.

In an interview in the summer 1995 *Flower Essence Society Newsletter,* physician Stephen Nezezon, who attended medical school after receiving undergraduate and graduate degrees in physics and astrophysics, was asked how something so subtle can have such powerful effects. He replied, "I'm grateful for my original training in physics. If modern physics were truly understood by the medical community, we would have a different scientific basis for evaluating healing." On the atomic level, tiny amounts of matter contain subtle but powerful forces, and this is how he regards flower essences. "When I say they are subtle, it does *not* mean that they are weak," he explained, for subtle forces working on the atomic level can have profound effects on living organisms.

In the early years of the 20th century, Edward Bach, an English physician and homeopath, discovered flower remedies. He filled small glass bowls with pure spring water, placed freshly picked blossoms on the water's surface and left the bowls in direct sunlight for three hours. During this time, according to his theory, the water became impregnated with the plants' healing powers.

The blossoms or flower heads were then discarded, and the activated water preserved in brandy. This mixture was called the "mother tincture." When a tree rather than a flower was the active ingredient, Bach boiled its twigs for half an hour, then left the tea to cool before adding brandy.

The next stage of preparation was to dilute the mother tincture with additional brandy, the result of which was called the "stock" remedy.

Today, this simple procedure is followed by flower essence practitioners, herbalists and ordinary people around the world. They gather flowers from organic gardens or unpolluted wild habitats at the peak of blossoming and place them in glass bowls of pure water. In some cases, bottles of the resulting liquid are rhythmically succussed, a procedure similar to the succussion method used in homeopathy to make a therapy more effective.

The most famous flower preparation is a formulation for emergency and stress, a blend of five of the 38 remedies developed by Edward Bach, which is sold today under the brand names Rescue Remedy, Calming Essence or Five Flower Formula, depending on the manufacturer. To avoid brand name confusion, the term "Dr. Bach's emergency formula" is used throughout this book to refer to the different commercial preparations of his original blend.

As its name suggests, this formula is appropriate for all emergencies; it combats shock, panic and mental paralysis. It does not replace medical attention but alleviates mental anguish and helps the body begin its own healing process.

In her book *The Bach Flower Remedies Step by Step*, Judy Howard described how Edward Bach selected the ingredients: star of Bethlehem for shock, rock rose for fear and panic, impatiens for tension and mental agitation, cherry plum for lack of emotional control and clematis for the sensation one experiences just before fainting. Dr. Bach first used Rescue Remedy in the early 1930s, when he gave it to a young fisherman who was being lifted from the sea after a shipwreck. As he was carried unconscious up the beach,

Bach moistened the mans lips, wrists and the skin behind his ears, and he soon revived.

As these ingredients suggest, every blossom, leaf or twig used in flower remedies has its own unique significance. There are 38 original Bach Flower Remedies and in the years since their development, flower enthusiasts have added herbs and blossoms of every description. Thanks to practitioners in Australia, the Americas, Europe, Asia and around the world, new and experimental remedies abound.

The bewildering assortment of remedies and their unusual application makes the study of flower essences confusing at first. But there are several built-in safeguards. The remedies are completely safe and it's impossible to harm yourself even if you overdose — unless, of course, you are sensitive to alcohol and drink several bottles of brandy-laced stock or mother tincture. Remedies can be blended together, as they are in the emergency formula, or taken separately. A course of treatment may last only a few hours or several months. Each person is different and everything depends on the individual's response.

If a remedy is not appropriate for the condition being treated, it will have no adverse effect. Remedies with different actions never contradict or interfere with each other. There are few healing practices so free from risk.

To understand how remedies are organized, consider Bach's seven groups. His 38 Bach remedies, organized by category, are: rock rose, mimulus, cherry plum, aspen and red chestnut for fear; cerato, scleranthus, gentian, gorse, hornbeam and wild oat for uncertainty; clematis, honeysuckle, wild rose, olive, white chestnut, mustard and chestnut bud for insufficient interest in present circumstances; water violet, impatiens and heather for loneliness; agrimony, centaury, walnut and holly for oversensitivity to influences and ideas; larch, pine, elm, sweet chestnut, star of Bethlehem, willow, oak and crab apple for despondency or despair; and chicory, vervaine, vine, beech and rock water for excessive concern for the welfare of others.

Here in the United States, the Flower Essence Society is the most ambitious organization researching and testing flower essences. Its preparations will sound more familiar to Americans than the Bach remedies, for they include such common plants as aloe vera, basil, black-eyed Susan, blackberry, bleeding heart, California poppy, dandelion and lavender among dozens of others.

For every imaginable condition or state, there is a compensating flower or combination of flowers.

Potency is increased not by taking more drops at one time but by giving the remedy more often, especially in an emergency or acute situation. When treating animals for most conditions, start with one or two applications daily and observe the results. The easiest way to administer a flower essence is by placing the drops on your finger and massaging the animal's gums or by diluting several drops in water and spraying the solution on and around the animal. They can be applied topically, behind the animal's ears, on the bare skin of the abdomen, on the upper thigh or underarm area, on the paw pads or wherever seems appropriate.

As for results, in some cases they are dramatic. The stories told about Rescue Remedy alone number in the thousands. Any flower remedy or combination of remedies can bring an immediate, dramatic change, though this reaction is unusual. In some cases, the animal may not display any noticeable difference, even after weeks of daily doses. The most typical pattern is to realize gradual effects over a period of time. Flower essences are not cure-alls or panaceas. Rather, they stimulate transformation in subtle ways and are most effective when used as part of a holistic program of health maintenance and improvement, which they support by stimulating a greater awareness of one's inner life and a unifying bridge connecting body, mind, soul and spirit.

Generally, according to those who train flower essence practitioners, it is best to work with no more than three to five essences at one time. Often two remedies combine to form the perfect custom blend. Working with only a few remedies makes it easier to focus on the main issues without distraction. Of course, someone with complex issues to resolve will obtain best results by working with a health care professional who has experience with flower remedies. A growing number of holistic veterinarians are flower essence practitioners.

How to Make Your Own Flower Essences

At the peak of its blooming, on a sunny morning, harvest the flower you want to use. Be sure to use blossoms from healthy plants that have been organically grown or that you gather from your garden or in the wild from a clean, unpolluted area far from busy highways.

Fill a glass bowl with pure water (distilled, bottled, spring or filtered water) and cover its surface with freshly picked blossoms. If you don't have enough blossoms to fill the bowl, don't worry; a single flower will work if that's all you have. Let the bowl stand in the morning sun in a quiet, undisturbed outdoor location for at least three hours, or longer if the weather turns cloudy. Because the preparer's state of mind is as important as the blossoms and water, keep your mind on the flowers you're working with and away from any negative thoughts or worries.

If you are making more than one essence at a time, wash your hands before handling each bowl. Remove the blossoms from the water and measure the liquid. Add an equal amount of brandy and pour the brandy-diluted mother tincture into storage bottles. For best results, use amber glass bottles.

Understanding Flower Essences
A Conversation with Patricia Kaminski

Patricia Kaminski is codirector of the Flower Essence Society, which has 60,000 members worldwide. She is one of the most widely published, best-known experts in the field; her *Flower Essence Repertory*, written with codirector Richard Katz, is a comprehensive guide to North American and English flower essences. Kaminski has worked with flower essences for over 20 years, documenting their effects on people and pets of all ages and teaching others how to make and use them.

How do flower essences compare with homeopathy?

  KAMINSKI: Both are energy or vibrational medicines that extend the range of known matter through the process of potentization. Dr. Bach was himself an accomplished homeopath, and in his early research he developed homeopathic nosodes that are still used to this day. It's important to understand that he did not want to replace homeopathy. However, he closed his practice to look for a therapeutic approach that would work more directly with the feeling life and emotions. While seeking it, he realized that a different method of preparation was necessary. Instead of grinding dried herbs with a mortar and pestle, which is what's required in most homeopathic preparations, he went to the source, walking long distances to observe plants in their natural habitat. This led to his experiments with dew and his development of the methods we use today. The method of preparation, including both raw materials and procedures, is the most obvious difference between homeopathy and flower essences.

  One of the rules of classical homeopathy is that you never combine remedies. Dr. Bach used both single and combined flower essences, so that's another difference. Remedies don't have to be combined — some of the great cases in flower essence literature are single remedy cases — but they can be and they work well together.

  Another difference is that flower essences are not as easily antidoted as homeopathic remedies. We don't recommend that they be taken with food, but I think they are more stable and less likely to be adversely affected by essential oils and other things. In homeopathic terms, flower essences are 3x remedies, which is a very low potency. I think that's what gives them their stability.

  All holistic therapies have a valuable role to play in healing. I see them as forming a spectrum, and there are certain niches that each modality fits into. Flower essences fill the emotional niche.

Are the methods for using flower essences on dogs, cats, birds, rabbits and other pets basically the same as for people?

KAMINSKI: Yes, and in many cases people become interested in studying flower essences because they try them first on their pets and get good results. They realize that the change wasn't due to a placebo effect. I think the placebo effect is a good thing because it stimulates healing, but it does introduce an element of confusion. Was it the remedy that worked or just the power of suggestion? With animals, that's not an issue.

Why do people turn to flower essences for their pets?

KAMINSKI: It's usually for two reasons. First, they're desperate. They've tried everything and nothing has worked and the only thing left is flower essences. As you can imagine, these are really challenging cases and flower essences can't always help. However, when the underlying cause is primarily emotional and contributing factors such as nutrition, the progress of the disease, the effects of previous medical treatments and the animal's environment are not in themselves insurmountable, flower essences can make a dramatic difference.

The second reason people turn to flower essences is because they're familiar with holistic methods and this is a logical extension of what they're already using or doing. Flower essences are entirely compatible with homeopathy, acupuncture, acupressure, herbs, healing touch, chiropractic, massage, color therapies, nutrition, aromatherapy and conventional medicine. Also, there is a growing awareness in our culture of animals as sentient, conscious, feeling, intelligent beings. This awareness is reflected by all the books that have been published in the last several years on this topic. With that whole paradigm shift, we're seeing animals in a totally different way, and as a result, many people make flower essences their first choice among healing therapies.

Flower essences can be used not just to treat existing conditions but to prevent problems from developing. When you recognize a potentially damaging emotional trait, you can use flower essences to transform it into something positive instead of letting it develop into an out-of-control behavior or a physical condition.

When we accept animals as partners and think with our hearts as well as our heads, we're able to get inside and see how an animal perceives the world. Really good animal trainers, people who have a special talent for working with horses or dogs or other animals, have this quality. When we develop it, we're more likely to diagnose conditions correctly, choose the right remedy and have a positive outcome.

The first step is to develop a meditative approach, clearing the mind and allowing for deep relaxation and breathing. The second step is to allow the gradual unfolding of an imaginary conversation with your animal. Actually allow the animal to speak in a dialogue with you. This practice will become easier as you cultivate it. Take notes of the outcome of this conversation. Although it may sound fantastic, this exercise is extremely potent and can reveal many clues to the solution of the puzzle. Thirdly, you can construct a list of your animal's symptoms and behaviors. Group these together and free-associate until you can perceive a larger picture or overall Gestalt which speaks to you about your animal's condition.

For example, your cat might have no appetite in the morning, be hyperactive in the evening and hide under the bed whenever the doorbell rings. Most people would see these as unrelated behaviors, but if we consider them carefully, there may be one common theme connecting all of them, such as fear and nervous hypersensitivity. The point of the exercise is to find the common denominator linking seemingly unrelated behaviors, and this in turn will lead to an effective selection of flower essences.

If the key to using flower essences is understanding an animal's emotions, then are psychological symptoms more important than physical conditions?

KAMINSKI: Yes. We get about 20 calls a week from people who say their dog or their cat has arthritis or hot spots or a thyroid condition or some other ailment and they want to know which flower essences to use. Or they might focus on behavior and ask, "What do you have for a cat that hides under the bed?" It's useful to note these symptoms and behaviors, but we have to go a step further and define the feelings behind them. More meaningful questions from the flower essence perspective are, "Why is my animal afraid? How can I understand what she needs? And what can transform the situation?"

There are several major ways flower essence can help pets. The first is to calm the animal down and restore his sense of place. While this is important in humans, it's absolutely essential in animals because of their territorial instinct. The second is to dispel fear, which is a very big emotion in our animal population. It is the emotion behind hostility, aggression, separation anxiety and all kinds of behavior problems.

When you administer an essence to an animal, it's important to do so in a way that is calming and not frightening, so the animal can be receptive to it. Many animals have been over-handled, especially sick animals that have been to the vet. You want to use a reassuring, calm tone of voice and gentle motions. It is more difficult to get good results if you yank your cat up, stick a dropper in her mouth and toss her back down.

Assuming that you take the time to make this a pleasant experience, the most successful method of application is to place the drops directly in the animal's mouth. If she isn't receptive to this, place the essence in a misting bottle and lightly spray it around her or apply it to your finger and rub it into her gums or apply it behind the ears, on her feet and slightly under her nostrils so she can lick it off. The other obvious application method is in drinking water, but the problem is that flower essences evaporate. Unless you know for sure that the animal will drink the water in a short time, within an hour or so, this method is unreliable. All the same, some people have done nothing more than add flower essences to drinking water and they've gotten good results. And while we don't recommend giving essences in food, some people drop the essences on dog biscuits and administer them 15 to 30 minutes prior to feeding other foods with good results.

In general, the more often you give a remedy, the better, so you could apply it topically, spray it in the air, rub it into the gums, squirt it into the mouth, put it in the water bowl and add it to food. Different applications work on different parts of the body/mind complex and can speed the healing process. But most people don't have time to do all these things, so we try to streamline the process and suggest giving flower essences first thing in the morning and last thing at night.

You can use flower essences in combination with hands-on healing, such as Tellington TTouch, massage therapy, chiropractic, therapeutic touch or myotherapy and the results are fabulous. Whenever you treat an area of disrupted energy, apply a flower essence and you should notice even greater improvement. If you want the most impressive results, include an affirmation or use the model that Larry Dossey and others have developed and pray or hold a positive picture for the outcome. If you combine sensitive and meditative work with actual physical application, you can develop a very efficacious and synergistic healing outcome.

Seventeen Flower Essences for Dogs, Cats and Other Pets

All of the flower essence descriptions in handbooks are written from the human perspective, and applying that information to animals requires some creative extrapolation. To provide more meaningful information, Patricia Kaminski reviewed Flower Essence Society records and compiled a list of the remedies that have been most helpful to animals treated by the organization's members. "If your readers decide to experiment with flower essences, and I hope they will," she told me, "these remedies are an excellent place to begin. There are literally dozens of remedies that work for animals, but the following are those that work exceptionally well. They have brought profound and positive change to dogs, cats, horses, birds, rabbits and other animals around the world."

I am grateful to Patricia Kaminski for so generously sharing this important and previously unpublished information.

Emergency Formula

Hands down, Rescue Remedy, also known as Five Flower Remedy and Calming Essence, is the most widely known, widely used flower essence blend. It has introduced more people to flower remedies than any other product. Dr. Bach's emergency formula addresses an animal's fears and has a calming effect. It's appropriate for treating any kind of stress, trauma, panic or disorientation and can be given whether the animal is conscious or unconscious. It has revived birds trapped in chimneys, helped pets and farm animals relax while giving birth, calmed frightened pets, made injured animals more comfortable and reduced anxiety in animals of every description.

"We have more reports on this single remedy than anything else," says Kaminski. "Without exaggeration, you could write a book about all the dogs, cats, horses, birds and other animals it has helped." Many holistic veterinarians use it daily; so do dog trainers, horse trainers and pet groomers. If you're going to keep one flower essence in your pocket or backpack, make it this one. For a description of the remedy's ingredients, see page 242.

Yarrow or Yarrow Special Formula *(Achillea millefolium)*

While the remedies that follow are arranged alphabetically, Dr. Bach's emergency formula and the yarrow formulas deserve their place at the top of the list. White or pink yarrow by itself and in blends have become best-sellers in animal circles. According to Kaminski, "Some animal caretakers and vets are saying that yarrow essences are as important as, if not more important than, Dr. Bach's emergency formula."

The first Yarrow Special Formula was developed after Dr. Aubrey Westlake of England experimented with combinations of English flower remedies in salt water as a possible treatment for those exposed to nuclear radiation. At Kaminski's suggestion, Westlake endorsed the idea of using yarrow, an American flower remedy, in radiation formulas two years before the 1986 Chernobyl nuclear accident. Following that event, a blend of yarrow essence and salt water was used in the Ukraine and Europe with many favorable results.

In 1995, a combination of yarrow, arnica and echinacea replaced the original formula. Arnica and echinacea were added to help the body withstand shock and trauma while strengthening the entire system and stimulating its survival mechanisms. Yarrow Special Formula has been helpful to people and animals exposed to video-display terminals, X-rays, radiation therapy, the high altitude radiation of airplane travel and other sources of invasive electromagnetic fields.

"There is a weakened condition in animals that is almost endemic," says Kaminski. "On a genetic level, their lives have been so disrupted that they aren't as strong as their ancestors were, and they are exposed to stresses that didn't exist 25 or 50 years ago. In addition, animals have tremendous emotional sensitivity and they are often psychic reservoirs of whatever is negative in their environment. These factors are complicated by the powerful bonds they have with people and places. Dogs, cats and other animals do what they can to protect the living beings and places they love, but they also need our protection in order to thrive in conditions that are in many ways unnatural. I think of yarrow by itself and in combination formulas as a protection or countershield against all of these levels of stress and depletion."

Yarrow and blends containing yarrow are appropriate for all pets in almost all situations. It is difficult to imagine a physical or behavioral condition that won't respond in some way to yarrow's protective influence.

Borage *(Borago officinalis)* for Depression

This remedy, which uses the star-shaped blue flowers of medicinal borage, was developed for humans dealing with grief and depression. According to Kaminski, it has a special affinity for animals. "We don't know why," she says. "There are lots of different flower essences for depression, but this is the big one for lifting the spirits of animals. We use it on older animals that lose their enthusiasm for life and kind of mope about. For animals who have moved from one place to another and are still adjusting, we combine it with walnut. Borage is an excellent remedy for a grieving animal, one who has lost a companion, either human or another animal. As I said, we don't know why borage is an effective with pets. There are seven or eight other depression remedies that work very well for humans, but borage is the remedy we have the largest amount of animal cases on. There must be something in it that's particularly valuable for them."

Chamomile *(Matricaria recutita)*
for Digestive Problems and Agitation

For centuries, chamomile has been one of the world's most widely used and loved herbs, and its flower essence acts much the way its teas and tinctures do. Chamomile calms, soothes and balances. "In animals," says Kaminski, "chamomile essence works well for those that operate from the stomach, which is appropriate because medicinally, chamomile is a digestive aid. What I mean by operating from the stomach is having an out-of-control appetite caused by a disturbed emotional center or having personality upsets that are linked to digestive upsets. Herbally, chamomile is a specific for fussy, colicky babies. Their fussiness, discomfort and crying all stem from muscle spasms and distention in their immature digestive systems, and these are conditions that chamomile calms and soothes very quickly. Puppies and kittens can experience digestive problems when they are weaned from their mothers and move onto solid foods. Chamomile flower essence is very helpful then.

"In people, eating can be a displacement activity and the same is true in our pets. Chamomile helps reduce the compulsion to overeat. This flower essence also helps animals who eat because they're nutritionally starved, that is, they're hungry all the time but they don't digest their food well so they aren't absorbing nutrients. It also calms hyperactivity. We use chamomile for children with attention deficit disorder, or ADD, and for equivalent hyperactive behaviors in dogs, cats and other animals. They can't sit still, they can't relax, they're hyper-alert, agitated all the time and easily distracted. Chamomile helps them slow down and focus their attention."

Chestnut Bud *(Aesculus hippocastanum)*
to Encourage Positive Behavioral Changes

The green buds of chestnut trees make a flower essence that Dr. Bach associated with wisdom and the ability to learn from life's lessons. Or, as Kaminski puts it, "This is the remedy that Dr. Bach developed for people who just don't get it. They keep repeating the same experiences over and over; they can't seem to learn from those experiences and move on. This is true for some of our friends in the animal world. They just can't seem to get a behavior under control, learn from it, get past it and move on. We combine this remedy with cosmos because the blend opens up channels of communication on one hand and increases learning receptivity on the other.

"In general, we use chestnut bud for animals that are fixed in old behaviors. I don't want to suggest that chestnut bud will transform every problem behavior or that it will work by itself. It's important to combine it with new training methods or other techniques to help the animal move from old behaviors to positive new ones. Chestnut bud can be a catalyst that helps the animal move in a new direction, but it doesn't define or provide that new direction."

Cosmos *(Cosmos bipinnatus)* to Enhance Communication

"Cosmos is one flower essence that we can't forget to mention," states Kaminski, "because it's the big human-animal communicator remedy. It opens up all kinds of channels, helping us listen to our animals and helping them listen to us. Some of our letters are from dog trainers who report that their ability to convey information and their animals' ability to understand it are enhanced when both take the remedy. For training purposes, cosmos is often combined with chestnut bud. But even if we're not in a training situation and just want to know what our pets are thinking or what they're trying to explain to us, cosmos enhances communication and focus."

This is also a remedy to take when you're puzzling over which flower essences to use for a particular condition. "Take it yourself, give it to your pet and try the conversation again," Kaminski suggests. "It will help you understand your animal's emotions and it will help remove the confusion that often accompanies flower essence diagnosis."

Dill *(Anethum graveolens)* for Overstimulation

The yellow blossoms of this familiar culinary herb treat hypersensitivity to the environment. "This is the remedy we use for animals who are overstimulated," Kaminski reports. "There's just too much going on in their lives. Either they're coming and going to too many activities or their households are chaotic, with people arriving and departing and something happening all the time. You can use a remedy like chamomile to help animals calm down, but dill addresses the overstimulation that overwhelms them. It helps an animal make sense of what's happening by building inner strength and tranquility. Dill is a great traveling remedy; we recommend it for any animal that's being shipped from one place to another or for pets who aren't used to riding in cars. It helps dogs who are going to obedience class or puppy kindergarten for the first time, where the whole experience of going to a new place, encountering other dogs, smelling all the smells and dealing with dozens of sensory distractions is just too much. In situations like this, dill combines well with Dr. Bach's emergency formula."

Holly *(Ilex aquifolium)* to Foster Trust

Universal compassion is the key word for holly; this is the remedy most synonymous with an open heart and love for others. As one of Dr. Bach's original remedies, it has been tested for more than 60 years, longer than most of the essences now in use, and practitioners around the world have verified his description of it. "This is a good remedy for animals to help them develop trust," says Kaminski. "It's recommended for animals being introduced to each other and it combines well with quaking grass on that level."

Holly helps eliminate the insecure emotions that cut an animal off from loving feelings; it helps prevent jealousy, envy and suspicion. This is an appropriate remedy to give to an entire family, including small children and pets, whenever a dog, cat, puppy, kitten or other animal is the focus of household stress. While it doesn't necessarily generate patience, it does promote a forgiving attitude, which is often the first step in developing patience.

Mariposa Lily *(Calochortus leichtlinii)*
for New Puppies or Kittens and Abandoned Animals

The Mariposa lily is white with a yellow center and purple spots. Of the remedies defined by the Flower Essence Society, it has one of the shortest research histories. In most cases, reports are collected for a decade or more before the society publishes descriptions of any new remedy, but within a few years of its listing, practitioners all over the world reported the same basic findings for Mariposa lily: it addresses maternal issues, heals the inner child and helps one overcome feelings of abandonment or estrangement from the mother.

"The Mariposa lily is used a lot for younger animals," Kaminski reports, "especially puppies and kittens that have just left their mothers and are adjusting to new homes. Mariposa lily helps them realize that they can have a new source of loving and nurturing. We also use it at a deeper level for animals that were abandoned, either by their natural mothers or their first human caretakers. Mariposa lily animals are not usually hostile or aggressive; instead, they're needy, like small children that haven't completed their maturation. These are the kitties who meow for attention all the time or suck on your buttons because they were weaned too early or dogs that crave a lot of cuddling and babying. Mariposa lily helps them grow up."

Mimulus *(Mimulus guttatus)* for Fear and Anxiety

The yellow mimulus with red spots is the universal flower remedy for fear. "This remedy treats what Dr. Bach called the everyday fears," says Kaminski. "These are known fears, the little things. We can and should use other fear remedies for animals, too, but if I'm going to choose one, it would be mimulus. This is an excellent remedy for animals that startle easily or have a nervous, anxious quality."

Mimulus is often combined with yarrow for pets, joining the themes of fear and protection. Mimulus helps build courage and confidence.

Oregon Grape *(Berberis aquifolium)* for Hostility

The yellow blossoms of the Oregon grape make an essence revered for its ability to replace feelings of fear and apprehension with optimistic and positive expectations of others. "In humans," explains Kaminski, "we use the Oregon grape for paranoia. In pets it has a similar application. Let's say an animal has been abused or neglected in the past or has just become wary of humans and expects the worst. We use the Oregon grape not for the nervous, hypersensitive fears some animals have but rather for the more active hostility and suspicion they display in the presence of people or other animals. When a dog or cat automatically growls and snarls or hisses at anyone who approaches or quakes in fear when someone raises a hand or a voice, its reaction is an old habit that has nothing to do with present circumstances. Dogs labeled people-aggressive or dog-aggressive are good examples. So are homeless animals in shelters. So are animals that have been abused or harshly punished. Oregon grape helps them overcome their negative expectations and deal with people and other animals more realistically."

Quaking Grass *(Briza maxima)* for Multiple-Pet Households

"In humans," Kaminski says, "quaking grass is the remedy we use to develop group bonding. For example, therapists working in family systems therapy use this flower essence to help the members of the household all begin to hear and listen to each other. We use quaking grass a lot in multiple-pet households, where there are two or three or more animals living together. It helps these animals get along and care for each other, and it's especially helpful when a new animal is introduced into the family. Quaking grass helps build group harmony."

Red Clover *(Trifolium pratense)* for Trauma

The flower essence made from the lovely pink-red blossoms of medicinal clover promotes a calm and steady presence, especially in emergencies. It helps prevent hysteria, panic and anxiety. "Red clover," says Kaminski, "is one of the remedies that belongs in that basic, primordial fear category. This is the remedy for panic. It's what you want to use when taking animals to the vet for surgery or subjecting them to a trauma or when helping them recover from a trauma. Of course, Dr. Bach's emergency formula is a specific for these conditions, but you can add red clover to it, especially if the animal is really out of control with fear and hysteria. Or if a kitty is caught somewhere, like up in a tree, and is so freaked it can't think straight. Wild animal rescue people use red clover a lot because the animals they treat are often in this condition. You could also use it for pets who are afraid of thunder or the loud noises and disruption of home remodeling and things like that."

Self-Heal *(Prunella vulgaris)* for Recovery

The light purple or violet self-heal, also known as heal-all, got its name from its multiple uses in herbal medicine. It has similar connotations as a flower essence. "This is an overall remedy for any animal who's been sick and is in recovery," says Kaminski. "It is appropriate for animals recovering from surgery or from an acute illness as well as any animal in a debilitated state. In one of our cases, a litter of orphaned kittens was brought to an animal rescue shelter when they were nearly lifeless, starving and dehydrated. The person who treated them has a lot of experience with orphaned kitties and fully expected them to die, but she gave them a combination of self-heal and Mariposa lily, the mothering remedy, and hoped for the best. Within hours, the kittens responded and they were nursed back to good health. As part of the holistic treatment of an active illness, self-heal really has earned its name by stimulating the animal's self-healing mechanisms."

Snapdragon *(Antirrhinum majus)*, the Mouth Remedy

The yellow snapdragon, like the tiger lily, is often used in combination with Oregon grape. "The snapdragon essence has an interesting history," says Kaminski, "because it was developed after a horse trainer discovered its benefits. Instead of being a human remedy that has since been used for animals, it started as an animal remedy that is now used for people. We call this the mouth remedy because it's so helpful for those who hold a lot of tension in the jaw and mouth. For example, people who grind their teeth or who have TMJ (temperomandibular joint syndrome) respond well to it, and so do animals that tend to bite or nip as well as teething puppies and kittens and any animal that's constantly biting, crunching, chewing on things and barking or vocalizing."

Tiger Lily *(Lilium humboldtii)* for Wild or Untamed Animals

The festive orange tiger lily with brown spots encourages cooperation with others. It is often combined with snapdragon and Oregon grape for use with animals. "This is the remedy that is most recommended for wild or untamed animals," Kaminski reports, "especially those whose wild or untamed tendencies work in a negative way. Most of our reports come from its use in dogs considered difficult to train, especially breeds with pronounced traits in that direction, and in feral cats. It will help any animal making the transition from the wild."

Walnut *(Juglans regia)* to Ease Transitions

Dr. Bach used the green flowers of the English walnut to help people overcome limiting influences and develop the courage to follow their own path or destiny. Walnut is especially helpful for those who are strongly influenced by family ties, the expectations of others and past habits. In animals, where territorial instincts are strong, walnut aids the adjustment to new places and new experiences. "Walnut is especially good for animals that are subjected to travel," says Kaminski. "It helps them make transitions. Also, whenever a family moves from one house to another, it's a time of stress. In this respect, animals suffer more than people because no matter how much we're attached to a place, dogs and cats are usually more so. Several years ago when we first moved here, my kitty started spraying all through the house. He'd never done this before, and I realized that he was marking out territory, making this new place smell and feel familiar. I gave him walnut to help him realize that this was his home now and he belonged here. It helped him break the link to his old home and settle into his new one. He has never sprayed since."

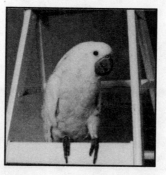

Healing with Light and Color

WHILE A HIGH SCHOOL STUDENT in the 1930s, photobiologist John Ott experimented with what is now known as time-lapse photography. This painstaking technique involves positioning cameras so that single exposures of slowly changing subjects such as blossoming plants can be taken at regular intervals. When played back, the images run at such accelerated speed that months or years of growth take only a minute or two to watch.

While filming the life of a pumpkin for Walt Disney's *Secrets of Life*, a feature movie released in 1956, he photographed pumpkin vines growing under fluorescent lights. All went well until the female blossoms turned brown and fell off the vine. No baby pumpkins. The following year under different fluorescent tubes, his replacement vines flourished until all of the male flowers turned brown and fell off. Ott realized that the light emitted by fluorescent tubes must interfere with normal plant growth just as glass does when it blocks ultraviolet light. Ott found that whenever electric lights or clear glass replaced or interfered with natural sunlight, buds refused to open, fruit refused to ripen or plants were spindly and unhealthy. These observations led him to create the first plastic greenhouse, for plastic allows nearly all of the sun's ultraviolet and full-spectrum rays to pass through.

On a visit to a seawater aquarium in Miami, Ott noticed "black-light" ultraviolet tubes over some of the fish aquarium tanks. He learned that the lights had been installed for decorative purposes, to give the fish an eerie and attractive appearance, but the added light had solved a common health problem in aquarium fish (*exophthalmus,* or pop-eye), and fin-nipping had disappeared. The aquarium's curators later wrote articles reporting that fish considered too fragile to keep in tanks thrive under black-light ultraviolet, and similar reports are now common regarding birds, reptiles and other animals in zoos around the world.

Ott coined the term "malillumination" to describe the health-damaging light deficiencies he observed in plants, pets, captive animals and humans, including himself. When he stopped wearing sunglasses and exposed his eyes to unfiltered natural light for several hours a day, his severe arthritis disappeared and X-rays showed new bone growth in his hip. Malillumination is now known to contribute to sterility and other breeding problems, depression, hostility, suppressed immune function, fur loss, skin damage, cancer, fatigue and a loss of strength and muscle tone in domesticated animals.

Light enters the eyes not only to facilitate vision but to activate the hypothalamus, which in turn controls the nervous and endocrine systems, which regulate functions throughout the body. The pineal, pituitary, adrenal, thyroid, thymus and sex glands are all directly or indirectly dependent on the eyes' exposure to natural light. Their health in turn affects body temperature, sleep patterns, growth, the immune system, emotions, fluid balance, energy balance, circulation, blood pressure, breathing, reproduction and aging. Exposure to natural light is crucial to the health of your pet's hormone and immune systems.

The Ultraviolet Debate

Wait a minute. Isn't ultraviolet light dangerous? Aren't we supposed to protect ourselves and our pets from it as much as possible?

In *Light, Medicine of the Future,* Jacob Liberman, O.D., Ph.D., reviewed the benefits and hazards of ultraviolet light. The medical literature shows that ultraviolet light activates the synthesis of vitamin D in the body, lowers blood pressure, increases the efficiency of the heart, improves electrocardiogram readings and blood profiles of patients with atherosclerosis, reduces cholesterol, assists in weight loss, effectively treats psoriasis and asthma, kills infectious bacteria and increases hormone levels.

At the same time, everyone agrees, too much ultraviolet light can be harmful. No one, including John Ott, recommends that people stare directly at the sun or limit their outdoor activities to the middle of the day, when its rays are hottest and brightest. But in recent years, the definition of "too much exposure" has become "any exposure at all," and doctors warn their patients to avoid all sun exposure and to wear sunglasses that block 100 percent of the ultraviolet spectrum.

Many scientists argue that ultraviolet light causes cataracts, but their conclusions are based on studies in which extremely high doses of ultraviolet light from highly concentrated sources were directed at close range into the clamped-open eyes of physically restrained animals in laboratories. Retinal damage, cataracts and skin cancers did result but, as Lieberman observes, the only scientific association that the abuse of animals in laboratories causes cancer, blindness and death. To date, no one has proved that daily exposure to unfiltered natural light under natural conditions in the U.S. and similar latitudes causes retinal damage, cataracts or skin cancer in humans or other animals.

What does all of this have to do with your dog, cat, bird and rabbit? Exposure to natural light, preferably for several hours per day, is necessary for good health. Whenever possible, give your indoor pets this essential nutrient. Natural light is any type of outdoor light, not necessarily direct sunlight. A shady screened porch, the shelter of a large tree, even an open northern exposure window or doorway gives the body what it needs. Remember that there is no substitute for natural light, not even fixtures advertised as full-spectrum lights. Take your dog for leisurely walks and provide a safe and comfortable place for her to rest outdoors. Cats love open windows. Be sure your screens are securely attached and, if the sill is narrow, expand it with a feline window shelf; check catalogs, cat magazines and pet supply stores.

Although several companies advertise full-spectrum light bulbs or tubes, none of these products exactly duplicate natural light — and, if you read their product literature or contact the manufacturers, none of them claim to. When outdoor activity isn't possible, consider combining cool white fluorescent tubes or regular incandescent bulbs with a black-light ultraviolet fixture installed near the ceiling of the room where your pet stays during daylight hours. See notes in the Resources for this chapter in the Appendix.

Harming and Healing with Color

WHEN HE PHOTOGRAPHED living cells under microscopes, Ott noticed that changing the color filters on his camera lens often changed the cells' behavior. When pharmaceutical companies hired him to document the effect of different drugs on living cells, lens color changes had a more dramatic effect than the drugs did.

These effects have been demonstrated in many countries on many types of animals. In all cases, prolonged exposure to a single color caused reproductive problems, fur loss, toxic symptoms, digestive disorders, sterility, abnormal bone development, abnormal body weight or cataracts.

On the other hand, short-term exposure to certain colors can have the opposite effect. In the late 19th century, several English physicians found that exposure to light of different colors caused measurable changes in their patients. Since then, researchers in Europe and other countries have explored the ways in which exposure to color influences health. In the U.S., color was a popular healing therapy until conventional doctors and the U.S. Food and Drug Administration made the use and sale of medical color projection equipment illegal.

William Campbell Douglass, M.D., is one of several American physicians who have rediscovered color therapy. In his book *Color Me Healthy*, Douglass describes one of his first color patients, a Croatian women with a large ulcer on the side of her leg that was five years old, half an inch deep and full of pus. She had tried salves, potions, antibiotics and a year of surgery (debridement or scraping) with no improvement. Douglass treated the ulcer by shining indigo light on it and taught the woman's son how to apply this therapy at home. She was treated twice per day, one hour at a time. Within a few days, new skin began to cover the open sore; within a week she was free from pain for the first time since the ulcer developed. Six weeks after her initial treatment, the patient returned to show Douglass a leg that had almost completely healed.

"I know it's hard to believe," he wrote, "but color therapy really works. And not just for external wounds. It also works for many internal ailments at which modern medicine just throws useless drugs and surgery."

Most of the American veterinarians, ophthalmologists and other healthcare professionals who treat patients with color follow the guidelines of the Dinshah Health Society, which publishes books and instructions for constructing and using color therapy equipment at home. One method is to project colors with a slide projector using color filter material held in photo slide mounts, adjusting the projector so its heat doesn't damage the filters. Another is to construct a projector box with a lamp, cardboard and large pieces of filter material. William Douglass illuminates small filters with a hand-held flashlight. Nearly any method can be used so long as the color shines directly on the patient, either completely (this is called a front systemic or back systemic, depending on the side being treated) or a more narrowly focused area, such as the throat or abdomen.

The filter material is theater gel, sold by theatrical supply companies to color floodlights and spotlights, and by scientific instrument companies. For instructions on building a simple projector or adapting a slide projector for this purpose, see the Resources for this chapter in the Appendix.

The Veterinary Applications of Color Therapy
A Conversation with Joanne Stefanatos, D.V.M.

Joanne Stefanatos became a veterinarian in 1972 and, after six years of conventional practice, began pursuing alternative therapies, primarily acupuncture, homeopathy and color therapy. Stefanatos uses colors in combination with methods not described here, such as radionics, magnetism, applied kinesiology and Interro Electrodiagnostic computer technology. The following interview describes her use of traditional color therapies.

How does color affect animals?

STEFANATOS: In ways that are profound and powerful. Color is energy, it's just a different way of applying energy, and different colors cause the body to respond in different ways.

Often when animals are being hospitalized, we shine red, green, blue or other colors on them. We also make color-treated water for them by filling a glass gallon jug with pure distilled water and leaving it in the sun. We used colored cellophane for this in shades that match the standard colors recommended by the Dinshah Health Society. This is the type of cellophane you can buy at party stores or hobby shops for decorating gift baskets. We wrap the gallon jug with the appropriate color and leave it in the sun during the hottest part of the day, from 10:00 in the morning until 2:00 in the afternoon. This water is then given to the animals as drinking water.

For intestinal problems we make orange water, for certain thyroid problems we make indigo water and for immune problems or leukemias we make red water. Those are just a few examples. The water itself does not change color; it looks just like regular water. What it does is obtain the Angstrom energy level of the color it was exposed to and then it's a therapeutic water. We do that here at the clinic and we have the owners do it at home.

How much water do you give the animal?

STEFANATOS: As much as it wants. This water replaces its normal drinking water. We also have owners put it in a spray bottle and finely mist their pets. This works especially well for birds. You just spray them all over.

We use the Dinshah projector on some of our patients, and some of the owners have built their own or borrow one so they can continue this therapy at home. We always tell them how long a tonation should last and how often it should be given, depending on the animal's condition.

Also, we recommend surrounding the animal as much as possible with the appropriate color — its bedding, its collar, whatever you can match to the healing color. We usually suggest using the prescribed color for about a week, then we reevaluate the animal.

Do you use color as a primary or support therapy?

STEFANATOS: I seldom use just one therapy. I probably could use color by itself, it's such powerful medicine, but I prefer to combine it with other holistic methods. I always go for whatever will work the best and the fastest, and I think the combination of color and homeopathy is often the best treatment.

Is color a therapy you would recommend that those who have read* Let There Be Light *experiment with on their own?

STEFANATOS: Absolutely, because it's easy to do and it works. Tonations (color treatments) work especially fast with birds. With dogs and cats, they work but it takes a little longer. By that I mean it may be a day or two before you really see results. The therapeutic water works right away when the animals drink it and so does spraying them with it. The Dinshah Society guidelines for specific conditions work well, especially with acute conditions. Those usually respond very fast, while the chronic conditions tend to take a while. You still see improvement, but not as quickly.

Often we get birds that have fatty livers and they have lipomas, which are benign fatty-cell tumors, all over their bodies. Usually, during the first week, we shine yellow on them every day for around an hour, and that helps the bile flow, increases peristalsis, stimulates the lymphatics and decreases the swelling of the lipomas because the body begins to resorb them.

Or let's say your dog or cat has a high fever and you want to bring it down. The animal is petrified to be put in the tub, so you can't cool him down that way. Well, the color blue has an immediate cooling effect, so shine blue light on him. Make blue water and spray it on him or dampen him as much as you can with a towel soaked in blue water. Wrap it around his neck, put it on the back of his head, soak his feet in it and he'll feel better right away. The color blue works on burns, too. You can use other treatments for burns as well, but blue light and blue water have a cooling effect that quickly takes away heat and pain.

Or let's say you have a bird that's hyperventilating from an anxiety attack and you want her to calm down fast because her heart is racing. Shining violet on the bird will make a difference right away. Violet sedates the heart; it's very calming.

Red stimulates the immune system. We use red on all deathly sick animals with viruses, heavy bacterial infections, hepatitis and illnesses like that. The first thing you have to do is subdue the infectious agent, and red does that. It really stimulates the immune system to fight off any foreign invasion.

Green is your stabilizer. Usually an animal goes from another color to green. You use green when the animal has reached a point of stability or equilibrium again. It completes the healing process.

What advice do you have for people who are interested in color and light but don't know where to begin?

STEFANATOS: The first thing to do is get rid of all the fluorescent lights in your house and put in full-spectrum tubes. We did this throughout our hospital and it makes a significant difference. Read Let There Be Light and start learning your basic colors and what they do. Lots of times you won't have a medicine or homeopathic remedy on hand and if you don't do acupuncture, you're kind of stuck, especially in an emergency. But if you have color, you always have something to start with. Color stimulates detoxification of the body, normal health and equilibrium.

Healing Colors: A Brief Review

Red

Stimulates the sensory nervous system, liver and blood, energizes the five senses. A detoxification color whose use may cause skin redness, itching or small eruptions until the cleansing process is complete. Counter-agent for burns from X-rays and sunlight.

Orange

Stimulates the lungs, respiratory system, stomach, skeletal system, bones, mammary glands and thyroid. Relieves cramps and muscle spasms. A decongestant.

Yellow

Nerve builder for the sensory and motor systems. Stimulates the lymph system, intestines, pancreas, digestive fluids and bowel movements. A depressant for the spleen, helps lift melancholy, used to expel worms and parasites.

Lemon

Dissolves blood clots and improves the body's ability to assimilate nutrients. Promotes coughing to expel mucus and fluids from the respiratory system. Stimulates the brain, thymus, digestion and bone growth. Treats chronic disorders and helps the body gradually repair itself by improving internal nutrition.

Green

Brings the body into balance. Activates the pituitary gland, stimulates the rebuilding of muscle and tissue. General antiseptic, germicide and disinfectant, helps destroy pathogens and prevent decay.

Turquoise

Improves nutrient assimilation and the repair of acute disorders. Slows excess activity of the brain, rebuilds burned skin, acts as a skin tonic, has a cooling influence.

Blue

Cools, relieves itching and irritation, encourages perspiration, mild sedative, reduces or removes fever and inflammation, stimulates the pineal gland.

Indigo

Stimulates parathyroid, calms or slows the thyroid, respiration and mammary milk production. Controls abscesses, reduces secretions, arrests discharges, stops bleeding. Promotes the production of phagocytes which destroy harmful micro-organisms. Eases suffering, lessens excitement, has a sedative effect.

Violet

Spleen stimulant, decreases muscular activity, including the heart, calms the central nervous system, promotes the production of white blood cells.

Purple

Induces deep relaxation, decreases pain sensitivity, increases functional activity of the blood veins, lowers blood pressure, dilates blood vessels, reduces heart rate, decreases activity in the kidneys and adrenal glands, lowers body temperature, controls fevers, calms the emotions. A sleeping color.

Magenta

Balances emotions, strengthens and balances the heart, circulatory system, kidneys, adrenals and reproductive organs.

Scarlet

General stimulant. Increases functional activity of the arteries, kidneys, adrenal glands, reproductive organs, circulatory system. Emotional stimulant.

Theses descriptions are based on Dinshah Health Society guidelines. For complete information, see Let There Be Light *by Darius Dinshah.*

Color Elixirs
How to Make Sun-charged Waters

There are several ways to make sun-charged waters or solar elixirs, and you may want to try all of them.

Many kitchen supply stores, antique shops and markets sell glass bottles in a rainbow of colors. For best results, use those that match the Dinshah Health Society's recommended colors or buy colored cellophane at party stores and use it to wrap clear glass bottles. In some cases, layering two or three different colors of cellophane is necessary to create the desired color. Or you can place a clear glass bottle in a cardboard box and use a color filter on top. Cut the cardboard top so that only colored light shines through.

Fill your glass jar or jug with pure filtered, distilled, bottled or spring water. If desired, treat it first with Willard Water concentrate, a splash of liquid trace minerals and/or a pinch of unrefined sea salt. Cover and position the bottle for maximum exposure to sunlight outdoors or in a sunny window. Leave it in the sun for at least one hour in the middle of the day or as long as desired. Water can be charged with light sources other than the sun, such as a standard incandescent bulb with the appropriate color filter. When tonating several colors at once, keep the bottles sufficiently far apart to keep their colors separate, so that light passing through one does not enter another. Sun-charged water should be used promptly. Be sure to label clear glass bottles with their appropriate colors after tonation.

Some color therapists tonate herbal remedies such as tinctures or nutritional supplements before taking or feeding them. Anything that will be ingested can be light-charged as described above.

How to Give a Tonation

For best results, have your animal on a natural diet as commercially prepared foods containing inferior ingredients, chemical preservatives, artificial colors and synthetic vitamins can interfere with healing. Use filtered, distilled or purified water, not city tap water, in your pet's bowl, which should be glass, stainless steel or ceramic, not plastic. As much as possible, expose your pet to natural light. Prevent the animal's exposure to tobacco smoke, automobile exhaust, pesticides and other environmental pollutants. Give your pet active daily exercise to maintain healthy blood and lymph circulation.

Give the tonation in a room or area that is comfortable for your pet, such as the animal's cage, crate or bed. Darken the room as much as possible, although total darkness is not necessary. Using a projector, lamp, flashlight or other light source, shine light through the appropriate color filter onto the animal's entire body (called a systemic treatment) or onto a narrowly focused area, such as a leg, the abdomen or other affected body part.

Dark colors, such as magenta, are difficult to see, especially if a large area is to be covered. To make focusing the color easier, use a more visible color to position the light, then change to the darker filter for treatment. Color therapy works whether the subject is awake or asleep, conscious or unconscious, but it is most effective when the room is quiet or if soothing music is played in the background. Keep nearby TV sets turned off. The brightness of the light source is not important; small lamps and flashlights work well.

The usual recommendation is two tonations per day, each lasting one hour. Often one is given in the morning and the other in the evening, but they can be given whenever convenient and separated by as little as two hours. The Dinshah Health Society publishes an annual calendar of recommended tonation times.

Wait at least an hour after feeding before beginning a tonation. The exception to this rule is any condition relating to digestion, in which case tonate after feeding and keep the tonation short, such as 10 to 15 minutes.

Let There Be Light provides detailed schedules for specific conditions in people, and while author Darius Dinshah makes no claims regarding their application to animals other than humans, veterinarians have obtained excellent results from these guidelines.

Most tonation schedules involve two or more colors. To follow the schedule, tonate twice per day using the colors in their recommended sequence, and when the series is complete, begin again. For example, to treat thyroid underactivity or hypothyroidism, a condition common in dogs, *Let There Be Light* recommends a) an orange and lemon systemic front and b) green on the face. Begin with a full-body tonation of orange light on the front of the animal (as much as possible) for one hour; wait two or more hours and give a full-body front tonation with lemon. The following day, tonate the face and head with green light. Two or more hours later, begin the cycle again with a full-body orange tonation. On the third day, begin with a full-body treatment with lemon and, later in the day, tonate the face with green. Continue the series for as long as desired. Because hypothyroidism is a chronic condition, treatment may take several weeks.

To treat thyroid overactivity or hyperthyroidism, which is common in cats, the recommended procedure is: a) lemon and indigo systemic front, b) green on the face and c) purple on the chest. Begin with a one-hour full-front lemon tonation, followed two or more hours later with a full-front indigo tonation. The following day, tonate the face with green, followed two or more hours later with a purple tonation over the chest area. Begin the sequence again the following day.

Experienced users, as Dinshah explains, can follow any sequence of recommended colors or repeat colors, using a color once, another color twice, a third color several times, etc. "For those who are first learning about the technique," he says, "it is advisable to simply use the colors in rotation."

When treating long standing chronic conditions that improve slowly or acute conditions that do not respond within a few days, interrupt the sequence with a color from the other side of the spectrum, then resume as before. Red, orange, yellow and lemon are on one side of the spectrum; turquoise, blue, indigo and violet are on the other. Green, in the middle, is called the physical equilibrating color.

When the animal is improving and convalescing, the recommended colors are a lemon systemic front followed by yellow and concluding with turquoise. In cases involving hemorrhage, the recommended convalescent treatment is magenta followed by lemon and yellow; conclude with turquoise.

At the end of each tonation, if possible, offer the animal sun-charged water that has been treated with the same color as the tonation. Let the animal rest for 10 to 15 minutes after the treatment before feeding or going out for exercise.

If it is not possible to give two tonations on the same day, give one; if it's necessary to skip a day, resume when you can. Color-charged water can be given in place of a tonation as necessary.

It is not uncommon for the cleansing colors lemon, green or turquoise to produce a rash or diarrhea as they activate the body's detoxification. These symptoms are usually mild and disappear within a day or two.

"It is impossible to harm yourself or your pet with the recommended doses of colored light," Darius Dinshah assured me. "If you use the wrong color you may cause discomfort, but it isn't like giving the wrong drug. This therapy is so simple that people underestimate it or assume it can't possibly work, but it is a powerful healer. While I cannot make specific claims for the use of color on animals, I can't think of any reason why it wouldn't work on pets exactly as it does on people. I hope your readers will consider using color to improve their own health and that of their companion animals."

Exact color matches are important. For best results, follow the Dinshah Health Society's recommendations and use filters from its recommended sources. See the Resources for this chapter in the Appendix. ❧

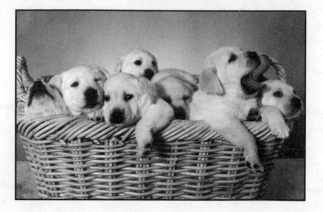

The Vaccine
Controversy

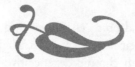

DO PUPPIES AND KITTENS need the vaccinations commonly prescribed for them? Do adult dogs and cats require annual booster shots? Conventional veterinarians say yes to both questions. Vaccines save lives by preventing disease and the more often an animal is vaccinated, the better, they say. Vaccines work by stimulating the immune system in response to specific viruses or bacteria. The vaccines are scientifically tested, FDA-approved and proven safe. If a few dogs and cats die from adverse reactions caused by vaccines, that's acceptable because the greater good is served. Just as smallpox, polio and measles vaccines have eliminated those human diseases in much of the world, so have vaccines for animals prevented large numbers of deaths in our pets.

That, at least, is the allopathic perspective. Is it correct? A growing number of immunologists and health experts say no. Public health historians have always noted that epidemic rates of contagious diseases around the world decreased more as a result of public sanitation measures than any medical treatment program. In fact, the incidence of most of the diseases for which children are vaccinated had dropped by more than 95 percent because of improvements in local water supplies and sewage treatment before their vaccines were perfected.

Veterinary researchers struggle with the same issues as their counterparts in human medicine. Do live vaccines cause more problems than killed virus vaccines? Are the illnesses for which animals are routinely vaccinated so rare that their vaccines cause more infection than natural exposure would? Does infant vaccination compromise adult health?

A growing body of veterinary evidence suggests that polyvalent or combination vaccines, which contain several viruses, suppress the animal's immune response by interfering with lymphocyte responsiveness and reducing platelet count. Immunologists and veterinarians have documented vaccination-related side effects in dogs and cats ranging from paralysis, convulsive seizures, blindness and death to less dramatic but still serious conditions such as tissue damage, cysts, allergies and chronic diseases. Some immunologists suggest that feline leukemia evolved as a result of mass vaccinations for feline panleukopenia and that subsequent vaccinations for feline leukemia produced the epidemic called feline AIDS.

In 1979, veterinarians (and brothers) Robert and Marty Goldstein wrote an article opposing the blanket use of vaccinations in animals. Their clinical observations and research linked annual revaccinations to chronic degenerative diseases such as arthritis, cancer, chronic skin problems, diabetes and autoimmune diseases. The conventional veterinary community ignored them. Now the mainstream veterinary literature has recognized vaccine-induced fibrosarcoma, a serious and often fatal cancer in cats that develops at the site of vaccine injections and which is often more aggressive and more resistant to treatment than other cancers of this type. "Finally, researchers and veterinarians are using *vaccination* and *cancer* in the same sentence!" exclaimed Bob Goldstein in the October 1996 edition of his *Love of Animals* newsletter. "The veterinary community is beginning to accept that suppression of the immune system can lead to cancer."

Nowhere in the world, except possibly Japan, is the germ theory of disease so alive and well as in the United States and Canada. Louis Pasteur, the famous 19th century French chemist, taught that germs invade the body and cause disease. His name is synonymous with his method of heating milk and other liquids to destroy their microorganisms.

But Pasteur owed his theory to a contemporary, the French physician Antoine Béchamp who, from 1853 to 1905, researched the causes of disease. Béchamp accused Pasteur of misunderstanding, distorting and plagiarizing his theory, and, at the end of his life, Pasteur renounced his germ theory and agreed with Béchamp. By that time, pasteurization and germ theory were so widely accepted that few took him seriously. Most Americans today believe that germs are the sole cause of disease and that the only way to prevent sickness is to kill germs before they can invade and infect the body.

Béchamp taught that what matters is not the germ but its host. If a person or animal is in poor health, he or she may be a good host for opportunistic microorganisms; animals and people in excellent health are poor hosts. As Sandra Priest, D.V.M., explained in the January 1996 issue of *Dog World,* exposure does not equal disease. Exposure to infectious bacteria, viruses and parasites takes place daily in backyards, on walks, at dog shows, at veterinary offices and in obedience schools. "We are rarely aware of this exposure because most of the time the animal's immune system eliminates the infective agent without noticeable symptoms," wrote Priest. It is only when the animal is a good host to pathogens because of low resistance that illness is likely to follow exposure.

Vaccinations and the Immune System
A Conversation with Susan Wynn, D.V.M.

S USAN WYNN received her Doctorate in Veterinary Medicine from the University of Georgia in 1987. She has just completed a four year post-doctoral fellowship researching viral immunology. President of the Georgia Holistic Veterinary Medical Association, Wynn is a board member of the American Holistic Veterinary Medical Association, national secretary of the International Association for Veterinary Homeopathy and coeditor with Allen Schoen of the veterinary textbook *Complementary and Alternative Therapies in Veterinary Medicine: Principles and Practice.*

There is a great deal of controversy and confusion about vaccinations and immunizations. What is your position?

WYNN: The holistic viewpoint is that vaccinations are bad because they sometimes cause the diseases they're supposed to prevent in addition to other, less recognized syndromes. This is well demonstrated in practice; we've seen it with distemper and kennel cough in dogs, possibly *calici* virus in cats and things like polio in humans. In addition, vaccines are sometimes ineffective and simply don't work. Animals can and do contract the same diseases for which they were vaccinated months before.

Another complaint is that vaccinations cause chronic, long term immune system disorders. The homeopathic term "vaccinosis" was coined to describe these conditions. There have never, ever been any studies done anywhere to support what veterinarians do these days with annual revaccinations. No one has ever proved that immunity only lasts a year. Veterinarians tend to treat vaccines as harmless, as though they are injecting water, but that's simply not true. Immunologists now recognize that viruses, whether they're vaccine viruses or viruses in the environment, can cause autoimmune disease, worsen allergies and disrupt the immune system. As a result, we have a lot of sick pets.

This is the dilemma. Conventional veterinarians don't recognize that vaccines can cause problems and believe they are essential for good health, holistic doctors say vaccines cause every problem and you should never use them and I think the truth lies somewhere in between. Probably puppies and kittens should be vaccinated, but judiciously and carefully. After that, there is less reason to focus primarily on vaccines in preventive medicine.

Rabies is the only exception to this rule, and that is a matter of law. Some states require an annual rabies vaccination, others once every three years. It's a legal requirement and there's nothing we can do to get around it.

What is the immunization schedule you would recommend for a puppy or kitten?

WYNN: I prefer not to recommend a specific schedule because it varies from case to case. If I were vaccinating my own puppy or kitten, there are certain things I would avoid. I think that the FIP vaccine (feline infectious peritonitis) is far from being safe and well proven. That's a controversial statement, but I base it on my study of the literature. I feel ambivalent about the feline leukemia vaccine. Most veterinarians in practice truly believe that we see less feline leukemia when most cats are vaccinated, and I thought the same thing when the vaccine first came out. On the other hand, the data just don't support this, and I've seen several cats that contracted feline leukemia after being vaccinated for it. If it were my cat, I would not vaccinate for feline leukemia and I'd keep the cat indoors.

I think leptospirosis is a regional problem and not every dog should be vaccinated for it. Coronavirus is not a fatal disease, so I would not use its vaccine. Ronald Schultz at the University of Wisconsin vet school, who is one of the nation's leading experts on veterinary vaccines, calls canine hepatitis an exotic disease that we haven't seen in the U.S. for years, so I wouldn't use the adenovirus vaccine that protects against it. The Lyme disease vaccine is so questionable that I wouldn't use it, either, or kennel cough unless the animal is going to be exposed to it.

I think distemper and parvovirus are the most important for dogs. I would probably vaccinate my puppy or kitten starting at age six or seven weeks, once every three weeks until about fifteen weeks, and I would use a modified live virus. This is controversial because a lot of people say modified live viruses are strongest and cause the most problems, but I believe they result in stronger and longer lasting immunity. However, in animals that are genetically predisposed to react adversely to vaccines, modified live virus vaccines are potentially dangerous, so I would use a killed virus for them.

How can you predict whether an animal is at risk for a bad reaction?

WYNN: You have to research the line and that can be a problem if the breeder isn't honest or doesn't know of vaccine-related problems in the line or if you have no way of knowing the animal's background. However, we know of certain families of certain breeds that absolutely have vaccine-related problems.

There's no doubt about it. Not everyone recognizes these disorders because they may show up a month or more after the vaccination, and most veterinarians dismiss anything that doesn't happen within 24 or 48 hours. However, delayed immune reactions are not uncommon.

If you know that your puppy or kitten comes from a line with vaccine-related problems, I would go for a killed vaccine on a very gentle schedule, breaking the vaccines up as much as possible. This means *never* giving something like a distemper combination booster with all seven antigens in it plus rabies and kennel cough and Lyme disease all at one time. That's a terrible idea.

If a puppy or kitten shows an adverse reaction, the schedule should be slowed way down or stopped, and I think homeopathy can help a great deal. I might use a nosode or a single remedy that matches the symptoms; it depends on the situation and the animal's reaction. *Thuja* is famous as the vaccine reaction remedy and it's often appropriate.

Whether nosodes are an effective alternative to vaccines is simply unknown at this time. A disease break is what happens when an animal is vaccinated against a disease but gets it anyway, and we've seen disease breaks in animals protected by nosodes and in animals protected by vaccinations. To me, the biggest problem with nosodes is that nobody knows what the optimum protocol is for using them. The medical literature says that nosodes don't work, but I don't believe that because I've seen them work. They may work best after exposure to the pathogen and not beforehand, but I don't know that for sure, either.

How can an owner predict how long a vaccine will last?

WYNN: There are no data whatsoever that indicate how long initial vaccines last. Ron Schultz says that the puppy vaccines last forever. He's documented dogs in which antibody titers lasted 15 years. It makes sense to think of these as lifelong vaccines because that's how some work in people. If you're vaccinated against polio as a child, you don't go in for booster shots every year.

However, because there is no published information on the time frame we're dealing with, we can't make assumptions. The way we monitor an animal's immune system status is by pulling antibody titers. Antibodies are proteins that are produced by the body in response to exposure to a pathogen. They are specific pathogen-fighting proteins, so they're easy to identify. When we measure their levels in the blood, we can get a pretty good idea of the animal's immune status. If the level is high, we can say that the animal probably still has protection against the virus being tested and can probably do without revaccination. This is all very fuzzy at the moment. Antibody titers are not a direct indication of immunity; they are an indirect measure, and from them we assume that the animal is still protected.

The important thing to remember is that even though it's an indirect measure and even though it's only an indicator, it's a much better method than shooting a virus vaccine under an animal's skin every year. You don't know anything when you've done that. You have no idea whether the animal was well enough to mount a normal immune response, and you may well be interfering with its immune system. I tend to measure only canine distemper and parvo in dogs, but there are many others as well. Where leptospirosis is a problem, I'd measure that rather than revaccinate even though it's a more expensive test. I don't think the risk of an immediate or delayed adverse reaction is outweighed by any theoretical benefits offered by a vaccine that's probably unnecessary.

It's frustrating not having data on the life of antibodies or cellular immunity measures, but statistics are being collected so that in the future we can make some educated guesses about how long immunity really lasts.

What can a pet owner do in general to help improve an animal's immune system?

WYNN: Improve the diet and avoid chemicals. If people would feed their pets a very good, fresh, natural diet and be aware of the chemicals their pets are exposed to, it would make such a difference. Animals are close to the ground so they're always exposed to stuff on the carpet and chemicals on the lawn. Well-intentioned owners put chemicals on their pets for flea control, not realizing how toxic they are and what a detrimental effect they have. When it comes to natural diet, my experience is that people don't always follow directions well, so home-prepared meals can be a problem unless there's a lot of variety and attention to detail. Most people believe that dry pet foods are good for the teeth but the published literature does not support that claim; what the literature shows is that gristly foods clean the teeth and keep the teeth and gums in good shape. The tests used oxtails, but you can feed knuckle bones and things like that.

I really dislike dry foods for cats. There is a mounting body of evidence that all the urinary tract problems so common in cats are in part due to the recent rising popularity of dry diets. I recommend that people grow wheat grass for their cats and not let them eat the pesticide-treated grass on the lawn and feed them raw meat, things like chicken gizzards, necks, stew beef and other tough, gristly meats. Gristly meats are the dental floss of dogs and cats.

While we're talking about immunity, I'd like to point out that it is a popular buzz word and much misunderstood. People want to blame the immune system for everything that goes wrong and they give it credit for preventing or curing every disease. For example, if a dog comes in with arthritis, the best way to treat it is simply to switch to a good natural diet, which will probably boost the immune system and improve the animal's mobility. A weak immune system *per se* is not always the key. Unfortunately, those who focus only on the immune system automatically want to stuff their dogs and cats full of echinacea. That's wrong, and it's even contraindicated in some autoimmune diseases. I just hate to see the word immunity overused.

Vaccination Schedules for Puppies and Kittens

The vaccination debate is an emotional issue, especially because vaccines are so widely accepted and highly regarded in our society. Keeping their animals' shots up to date is a matter of pride for many pet owners. Some volunteer activities require documentation of annual vaccinations as an assurance that only "safe" pets participate. Having an unvaccinated dog or cat is not only unusual, it's often seen as a sign of neglect, poverty, ignorance or abuse.

Holistic veterinarians spend far more time discussing vaccinations with their clients than conventional veterinarians do, although a growing number of conventional doctors are sympathetic to an owner's questions, concerns and reluctance to vaccinate. Most holistic veterinarians and many conventional veterinarians who are immunologists or researchers recommend either no vaccinations or only puppy/kitten vaccinations with no repeat vaccinations in adult dogs and cats except for rabies as required by law. All warn against vaccinating an animal that is ill, scheduled for or recovering from surgery or under stress.

If you decide to vaccinate, wait, if possible, until after four months of age to begin. The mother's immunity protects her offspring until then. Richard Pitcairn, who has a Ph.D. in immunology, says, "If you really want to play it safe, keep your new puppy isolated from contact with other dogs and just vaccinate once — at age 22 weeks or older."

Delaying vaccinations is a strategy often mentioned by critics of human immunization programs, for countries that vaccinate older children have far lower rates of adverse reactions and death than countries that give the same vaccines to infants. Is it necessary to isolate puppies and kittens? Young animals born to healthy parents and fed a fresh, natural, raw diet are less likely to contract contagious diseases than those who aren't, but it makes sense to avoid exposure to sick animals. The period between eight and sixteen weeks is so important for socialization that most trainers consider puppy play groups and interaction with older dogs an important foundation for a lifetime of good behavior. Ideally, all young puppies and kittens would be healthy enough to meet the world and everything in it without danger of infection. Until that day, owners have to decide what's best on an individual basis.

When our puppy arrived at her new home, we were warned to keep her away from other dogs and any area visited by other dogs for several weeks, but I waited only two days to introduce her to Hobbes, our Golden Retriever neighbor, who was one year old and a perfect baby sitter and companion. The two spent hours together every afternoon and I will always cherish Hobbes's patience, the games he invented to keep Samantha amused and the lessons she learned from him about getting along with other dogs. Keeping her away from areas visited by other dogs would have meant keeping her indoors, for we have a tiny backyard and many leashed dogs walk up and down our street every day. Instead of worrying about germs, we focused on diet and herbs to keep her resistance strong and hoped for the best.

Larry Bernstein, V.M.D., doesn't approve of keeping puppies and kittens in isolation. "Do you know who's at the greatest risk of picking up disease in a conventional clinic?" he asks. "It's the dog who's been hidden away in the penthouse. I tell my clients to take their pets out even when they're very young. Use common sense, of course. Don't take them to the local animal shelter to look for a little brother because shelters are a hotbed of infection, but do take them out on a limited basis. The biggest cause of problems in puppies and kittens is overhandling. The little guy has just experienced a big upheaval, moving away from mom and the rest of the litter. Now his owners are taking him everywhere and bringing company over. Mentally, the animal wants to play, play, play, but physically and emotionally, he gets exhausted. Often puppies and kittens will break with diseases three to five days after they move to their new home, and it's easy to understand why. I think the best thing to do is act the way you would with a new baby. It's nice to have company but spend some quiet time with your pup and let her rest on her own. This means protecting her from the rest of the family, too. Then take her outside. She's not going to be exposed to anything outside that you and your kids don't carry into the house. You wouldn't take your new baby to a tuberculosis ward, but you would take her for a walk on a sunny street. It's called common sense."

Holistic veterinarians recommend that their clients avoid dangerous, ineffective or unnecessary vaccines. Bob Goldstein recommends avoiding feline leukemia, FIP and Lyme disease. Susan Wynn lists FIP, feline leukemia, coronavirus, canine hepatitis and Lyme disease as vaccines to avoid and leptospirosis and kennel cough as probably unnecessary.

Beverly Cappel-King explains, "These vaccines are questionable because natural exposure to the disease is unlikely or because the vaccine causes worse symptoms than the illness itself. My least favorite vaccine is the one given to dogs for Lyme disease. I've seen it cause seizures, dementia, horrible swollen joints, paralysis and autoimmune bleeding disorders. Two Golden Retrievers who were brought to me for treatment developed kidney failure. The reaction typically shows up 10 days after vaccination. If you see one or two or a like this it could be coincidence, but not when you see 20 or 30, all with the same history of a Lyme vaccine about 10 days before the onset of symptoms. Every now and then you can get a reaction to any vaccine, a swelling at the injection site, a slight fever or lethargy, all of which are normal reactions, but symptoms like paralysis, dementia, pressing the head against a wall, kidney failure, swollen joints and autoimmune bleeding disorders are extreme."

What vaccines have a reasonably proven track record and are worth the risk?

Ron Schultz, D.V.M., Ph.D., a professor at the University of Wisconsin School of Veterinary Medicine who has documented many adverse reactions to antibiotics and vaccinations in dogs and cats, recommends only a killed distemper (feline panleukopenia) kitten series (two shots given three to four weeks apart) for indoor cats and for dogs only distemper and parvovirus. Richard Pitcairn has used no vaccines in his practice for nearly 20 years but, for those who insist, he agrees with Schultz. Pitcairn recommends giving dogs their parvo and distemper shots separately one month apart and vaccinating cats for panleukopenia only once at 16 weeks.

Most practitioners will balk at such a request, Pitcairn warns, because their suppliers would require them to buy a large quantity of each vaccine in order to treat a single patient. Instead, most veterinarians offer simpler combined vaccines, which contain only two for dogs (distemper and hepatitis) or three for cats (panleukopenia, rhinotracheitis and calici virus). Though far from perfect, he says, they are much better than the multiple combinations commonly given to dogs and cats. Combination vaccines were created for human convenience and not for scientific reasons. Immunologists warn that they are completely unnatural because dogs, cats, humans and other animals aren't exposed to more than one infection at a time. We have single diseases and so do our pets. No wonder injecting the body with five, seven, nine or more active illnesses overwhelms it.

Nosodes: Homeopathic Vaccinations

One response to the demand for safe immunizations is the creation of nosodes, or homeopathic vaccinations. In homeopathy, the products of a disease, such as the bodily secretions of a dog with distemper, are prepared in a greatly diluted solution for oral administration. Nosodes for dogs include kennel cough, leptospirosis, distemper, Lyme disease, hepatitis, parvovirus, heartworm and many others. This method of immunization was developed by a veterinarian in the 1920s and, according to Pitcairn, showed impressive results even before vaccines were developed. "When properly used," he claims, "the canine distemper nosode can protect a dog from distemper even better than the vaccine can."

Growing numbers of breeders and owners trust their dogs' lives to nosodes. In her

January 1996 *Dog World* article, Dr. Priest described Susann Everett, a Mastiff breeder, who had been using nosodes for four years while showing her dogs widely, working them as therapy dogs, using them in education programs and attending handling classes. "Her animals are rarely ill and do not experience cancer, cardiomyopathy or bloat, which are problems common in the breed," wrote Priest. She called Everett's experiences typical of breeders who have established nosode programs.

In the March/April 1994 edition of *Natural Pet* magazine, John Fudens, D.V.M., detailed his objections to orthodox vaccinations and explained why he prefers nosodes: they are given orally rather than injected, so there is no pain, discomfort, stress, shock or blood contamination; nosodes are so dilute that they contain no live or killed viruses, only energy; no drugs or chemicals enter the body; the price is a fraction of injected vaccines; the homeopathic literature documents the success of this approach in stopping epidemics and saving lives when conventional medicine could not; nosodes don't damage the body, so there is no need to spend time and money repairing it after treatment; and control remains in the hands of the client or patient, not the conventional health practitioner or government bureaucrats.

Larry Bernstein, who serves as an officer of the Academy of Veterinary Homeopathy, uses nosodes in place of vaccinations but not in all cases. "Vaccinating your animal causes problems," he told me, "but not vaccinating carries a greater obligation. If your dog lives in the backyard, eats junk food and you don't give him much attention, he's probably better off with vaccines. If you decide not to vaccinate, it is essential that you feed the animal correctly, create a healthy lifestyle for it and pay close attention to any changes or symptoms your pet may develop.

"Several years ago when I was studying homeopathy with Dr. Pitcairn, my unvaccinated Cavalier King Charles Spaniel puppy started vomiting, had diarrhea and stopped eating, all of which are typical signs of parvovirus. I tested him, and that's what it was. I was ready to intervene medically when I stood back and looked at him. He was normally gregarious, hungry, happy and cuddly and now he was cold, shivering, vomiting, uninterested in food and wanted to be left alone. Homeopathically, that just screams *Nux vomica*, so that's what I gave him. Later that night, he took a few bites of chicken and threw up. I gave him more *Nux vomica*. A little later, he ate some more chicken. The next morning he was taking things from my wife's hand and within two days he was back to normal. If I had been like most dog owners, I wouldn't have noticed or understood his symptoms until they were far more developed. This is what I mean about a higher level of owner responsibility. Raising an animal holistically pays tremendous dividends, but it involves a lot more effort."

Like other veterinarians who use nosodes instead of conventional vaccines, Bernstein reports that properly fed, healthy, nosode-treated puppies and kittens may occasionally contract a disease against which they were supposedly protected, just as animals protected by conventional vaccines do, but that unsheltered animals typically develop milder symptoms and recover faster than their vaccinated counterparts.

Preventing and Treating Reactions to Vaccination

Reactions to vaccinations can be dramatic or subtle. A mild reaction might be fatigue, loss of appetite, slight diarrhea or other symptoms lasting just a few days. Sometimes a puppy's first vaccination coincides with an ear infection. Major reactions are dramatic, obvious and sometimes fatal. As noted, rabies vaccinations are required by law and may be an annual event in your dog's life. In areas with rabies epidemics, such as the Northeast during the 1990s, cats may be required to have rabies vaccinations, too.

To help prevent an adverse vaccine reaction, be sure your pet is in excellent health. Do not vaccinate an animal that is scheduled for surgery, such as spaying or neutering, or one recovering from surgery or an accident or showing any sign of illness or parasite infestation. Don't repeat a vaccination previously given by the animal's breeder. Because stress is an important factor, avoid stressful activities that same day, such as bathing or grooming, treating fleas, visiting a stressful environment (the trip to the vet is stressful enough), training exercises or travel. Plan a quiet day for your pet.

Juliette de Bairacli Levy deals with compulsory vaccination laws encountered while traveling by neutralizing the vaccine as much as possible, which she does by immediately pressing outward around the injection site, then rubbing the area with raw lemon juice. This is followed by a day of watered milk and honey and the use of laxatives for two nights.

Homeopaths take a different approach, either following the vaccination with its corresponding nosode or treating with *Thuja* or another appropriate remedy, depending on the animal's symptoms.

Some pet owners dose their dogs and cats with extra vitamin C or other vitamins and minerals for several days before and after vaccination.

Should your pet experience an adverse reaction, you may want to telephone or visit a veterinary homeopath, for these practitioners have extensive experience with the repair of vaccine-damaged animals.

Preventing Contagious Disease

One way to make your pet a poor host to contagious diseases is to provide a natural diet. Animals in the wild have strong immune systems without any help from modern medicine. Fresh air, exercise, sunshine and raw foods are all the medicines they need. Another way is to supplement that diet with vitamins and minerals that help pets resist disease. In *How to Have a Healthier Dog*, Wendell

Belfield, D.V.M., described how vitamins and minerals enhance antibody production and immune system response in animals. "Vitamin C is a potent antivirus, antibacteria and antihistamine agent," he wrote, "and it spearheads the resistance against invading organisms." Puppies and kittens under constant stress are, he believes, incapable of producing all the vitamin C their bodies need.

B complex vitamins are important to the proper functioning of the adrenal glands. Diets deficient in pantothenic acid and vitamin B6 have been shown to produce a sharp decline in antibody production which vaccinations do not repair and diets lacking in vitamins B2, B3, folic acid and biotin result in an impaired immune response to vaccinations. Vitamin A is necessary for the production of antibodies and white blood cells; vitamin E is essential to the pituitary gland's proper functioning. Any diet deficient in vitamins, minerals, trace elements, enzymes, amino acids and other essential nutrients contributes to the "good host" status of a dog, cat, bird, rabbit, human or other animal.

Herbal Immunization

In addition to making your pet a poor host to pathogens, you can rely on herbs and vitamin C to prevent the development of infection if your animal is exposed to a contagious disease. It isn't necessary to live in an antiseptic bubble, but by counteracting some of the agents of disease, you can help your pet maintain a strong defense.

Juliette de Bairacli Levy has used no vaccines, antibiotics or other drugs for more than 50 years, and neither have adherents of her Natural Rearing philosophy. In *The Complete Herbal Handbook for the Dog and Cat,* she describes an "intensive herbal immunization" that can be used for pets exposed to active infections. The treatment is a half-day or one-day fast (water only) with a laxative that night followed by a dose of herbal antiseptic tablets, which contain garlic, rue, sage, thyme, eucalyptus, wormwood and vegetable charcoal. Alternatively, combine minced garlic with enough whole wheat flour and honey to make a dough, divide the mixture into small pills and add 1 drop of eucalyptus essential oil to each. Give 1 pill or tablet per 10 pounds of body weight once per day for several days. As a general preventive, she recommends giving antiseptic herbs to dogs just before attending shows or visiting public parks.

Using herbal immunization, de Bairacli Levy has protected unvaccinated dogs, cats, sheep, cattle and other animals exposed to epidemics. In one case, she saved 2,000 pedigree Swaledale sheep in the English Pennine mountains by dosing them heavily while the sheep in an adjacent field succumbed to a streptococcal infection that caused paralysis and blindness. None of the herbally treated sheep became ill.

Here is a review of natural immunizations that can help your pet resist or recover from contagious diseases.

Recommended Dosages for Animals Exposed to or Ill with an Infectious Disease

1. Fast the animal by withholding food for 1/2 to 1 day if exposed to an illness; if the animal has a fever, withhold food until the fever breaks.

2. Give the animal 500 mg of vitamin C per 10 pounds of body weight in divided doses throughout the day. Crush or grind tablets or use a powdered or liquid supplement for easy assimilation. For best results, use a natural vitamin C or calcium ascorbate with bioflavonoids and other C-complex substances from food-derived sources, not ascorbic acid.

3. In addition, give any of the following:

- 1 herbal antiseptic tablet or garlic-eucalyptus pill (see page 284) per 10 pounds of body weight per day as described above, or
- 1 capsule of powdered grapefruit seed extract per 10 pounds of body weight, or 1-1/2 drops of liquid grapefruit seed extract per pound, or
- 1 or 2 drops of propolis tincture per pound of body weight (10 to 20 drops for a 10-pound dog, cat or rabbit, 1 or 2 drops for a cockatoo) or 250 mg powdered propolis from capsules per 5 to 7 pounds, or
- 1 garlic extract capsule (Kyolic or a similar brand) per 10 pounds of body weight, 1/4 teaspoon garlic tincture per 10 pounds or 1/8 teaspoon finely chopped, minced or pureed garlic per 10 pounds, or
- 1 drop of echinacea tincture per pound of body weight, 1 tablespoon of medicinal strength echinacea tea per 10 pounds or 3 capsules of powdered echinacea per 10 pounds.

Adapt the label directions of any infection-fighting herb or supplement, such as olive leaf extract, noni, astragalus or colostrum, to your pet's weight. Do not feed any herb or supplement that must be taken with meals (check labels carefully) to a fasting animal.

The above are one-day dosages which should be divided into three or more servings during the day. Use any of the above alone, use any two in combination or alternate from one to another. Continue these dosages for three days as a preventive or up to 10 days to treat an active infection.

The only appropriate food for a fasting animal is raw, unpasteurized honey, which you can mix with vitamin C powder, herbal powders, crushed tablets, whole capsules, the contents of capsules, tinctures or strongly brewed herbal tea. Shape refrigerated honey into balls, feed room-temperature honey from a spoon or dilute it with just enough water or herb tea to make it liquid and gently pour it into your pet's mouth or cheek pouch. Encourage your fasting pet to drink water, and make clean water (add Willard Water extract and a pinch of unrefined sea salt) available at all times. For information about specific illnesses, see the A to Z conditions in Chapter 13.

Essential Oil Immunization

In France, where essential oils are used internally as medicines, physicians who practice aromatherapy take a culture from the infected patient and cultivate it in order to test the effect of individual essential oils on the infection. The oils that most successfully inhibit the culture's growth are combined in a prescription to be used until the infection subsides.

Some of the most widely prescribed all-purpose oils are combined in formulas that are sold over the counter to prevent infections before they spread.

In *Veterinary Aromatherapy*, Nelly Grosjean describes how to make such a blend for pets. Combine equal parts of the essential oils of thyme, cinnamon, coriander, clove, nutmeg, pine and ylang ylang, then mix this blend with an equal quantity of the essential oil of wild marjoram *(Origanum vulgare)*. Dose the exposed or infected animal three times daily with one drop of the mixture per seven pounds of body weight.

This aromatic blend helps prevent and treat bacterial, viral and other infectious diseases, and its topical use in sprays and massage oils enhances mental alertness, physical equilibrium, memory, sexual drive and cellular vitality.

In addition to giving the animal the essential oils described above, combine the following essential oils for continuous use in an aromatic diffuser: 8 parts lavandin, 4 parts eucalyptus, 2 parts each thyme, wild marjoram and rosemary and 1 part each mint and cinnamon. If you define 1 part as 1/2 teaspoon, the result will be slighty less than 4 tablespoons of the blend. If you don't have a diffuser, combine 2 tablespoons of the mixture with 4 tablespoons vodka or other 80-proof grain alcohol and add it to 1/2 cup of water in a small spray bottle. Every 15 minutes, or whenever you think of it, spray the air in the room around your pet.

The spread of airborne viruses and bacteria can be greatly reduced by spraying the air, kennel surfaces and other areas with solutions of grapefruit seed extract, tea tree oil or the essential oils of other antiseptic herbs. See Chapter 5 (Aromatherapy) for instructions.

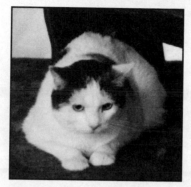

Cancer:
The Most
Feared Disease

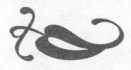

BECAUSE IT'S SO OFTEN FATAL and because its conventional treatment is so often worse than the illness itself, cancer is our most feared disease. In dogs and cats, cancer takes a terrifying toll. Breeders of pedigreed cats say the hardy stock of 30 years ago simply doesn't exist today, that it's difficult to find a line that hasn't been decimated by cancer and that the life expectancy of most breeds is only half what it used to be. Dog breeders say the same and statistics compiled by national breed clubs back them up. Animals that lived to an average age of 15 or 16 in the 1960s now die at seven or eight. The steady stream of obituary notices in therapy dog newsletters and dog club publications makes for heartbreaking, depressing reading. Here are well-loved, well-cared-for mixed-breed and purebred dogs dying at what used to be their most productive, active age.

What causes cancer? While medical researchers search for cancer genes, most physicians and veterinarians explain the epidemic in terms of heredity or exposure to known carcinogens, or they simply say no one knows. Among holistic veterinarians, the verdict is almost unanimous. Cancer, say these doctors, is most likely to develop in dogs and cats from inbred lines who are fed commercial pet foods and regularly vaccinated.

In conventional medicine there are only three approved treatments for this disease: surgery, radiation therapy and chemotherapy. In humans and other animals, these approaches have limited success, terrifying side effects and expensive price tags. Holistic and alternative therapies abound, but while these treatments have much to offer, there is no single cure for every type of cancer. What works in one animal may not in another. In cases where alternative remedies have not been shown to be effective, some holistic veterinarians recommend radiation therapy and use herbs and other support therapies to minimize its side effects. As all of the veterinarians who contributed their time and knowledge to this book repeated again and again, every case is different, and every decision depends on the patient's situation, which includes the owner's capabilities, interest and finances as well as the animal's medical condition.

Cancer is an illness for which the proverbial ounce of prevention is worth far more than a pound of cure. You can help prevent cancer by feeding a fresh, raw, natural diet, giving your animal plenty of healthy exercise and exposure to fresh air and sunlight, avoiding chemicals and pesticides, protecting your pet from environmental toxins including automobile exhaust and cigarette smoke, supplementing the diet with herbs and other nutrients, refusing unnecessary vaccinations and avoiding food additives, preservatives and coloring agents.

In all cases, Therapeutic Touch (see Chapter 7) is an appropriate support therapy that can be done at home on a daily basis. Another important factor is regular exposure to natural light (see Chapter 9). Be sure that your pet has access to natural light by spending several hours outdoors or in a screened open window or doorway every day. Color tonations are another support therapy that can be done at home; see Chapter 9.

The Holistic Treatment of Cancer
A Conversation with Allen Schoen, D.V.M.

Allen Schoen is both a pioneer of alternative veterinary medicine and a best-selling author. *His Love, Miracles and Animal Healing* has introduced thousands of pet owners to acupuncture, herbs and other therapies; he is the editor of the textbook *Veterinary Acupuncture: Ancient Art to Modern Medicine* and coeditor of *Complementary and Alternative Therapies in Veterinary Medicine: Principles and Practice*. Dr. Schoen travels extensively, teaching holistic methods to veterinarians in Australia, Scandinavia, Europe, Canada and the United States. In his clinical practice, most of Schoen's patients are dogs, cats and horses, with occasional birds, rabbits, ferrets, camels, llamas, and other exotics.

❖

Why are so many animals dying of cancer?

SCHOEN: I think the increase in cancer among animals is a reflection of the increase in cancer in people. It's a situation caused by a multitude of factors. Among animals, one is the amount of inbreeding that has been done, resulting in a limited gene pool. Certain tumors are predominant in certain breeds, like Golden Retrievers with lymphosarcoma, Boxers with mastocytomas, Ursat Danuo with ucuun mu nuues, Oermun Olimphards with human geosarcomas, and the lists go on and on.

So first you have the genetics. Second, you have the impact of diet, with all of the inferior ingredients and artificial flavors, colors and preservatives that go into the foods most people feed their pets. Third, you have the whole vaccination controversy. At veterinary conferences now, many hours are spent discussing vaccine-induced tumors in animals. The main one is fibrosarcomas in cats, but repeated vaccinations may compromise the immune systems of all animals. Fourth, you have environmental toxins and the burden they place on animals. And then there's stress. Put all these ingredients together and you get a cancer epidemic.

Then the question becomes, what are your options? In conventional medicine, you have chemotherapy, radiation therapy and surgery. In a small percentage of cases, these treatments may be beneficial in extending the length and quality of life, but it's very small. Most cancers do not respond to conventional therapies and they are expensive and have terrible side effects.

How do you treat cancer in pets?

SCHOEN: It depends on the type of tumor, the animal, the client, how far the disease has progressed and what medical treatment the patient has already been given. The true holistic approach is to look at the individual animal in its individual situation, so there isn't any single answer to your question. Some cases are so far along that I don't recommend much except enjoying the time you have left with the animal. Why get into a complicated regimen of supplements and other disruptions of the pet's life if it's already in the final stages of a terminal illness and you really don't have much time? In almost every case improved nutrition with a few basic supplements will make some difference and is worth doing. Most owners are responsive to those suggestions, but you have to consider the owners, too. Not everyone is going to follow through with a regimen of improved diet, digestive enzymes, Chinese herbs, Western herbs, homeopathy or other unfamiliar strategies even if the prognosis is excellent. I try to determine how motivated the owners are, how much time and effort they can spend, what the most realistic outcome is likely to be and what is going to work best for the animal.

My baseline recommendation for everyone is to improve the diet and give antioxidant supplements, which are vitamins A, C and E and the mineral selenium. My choice of Western or Chinese herbs depends on the circumstances, but I almost always recommend what Western herbalism calls the blood-cleansing herbs or detoxifiers. After that, it really comes down to the individual case. Sometimes I recommend supplementing the herbs and nutrition with homeopathy, acupuncture or other support therapies. I don't mean to be ambiguous, but the holistic approach depends so much on individual circumstances that it's impossible to give specific recommendations.

How do you decide on the course of treatment?

SCHOEN: Well, it's a combination of my training and experience. I graduated from Cornell Vet School and have a master's degree in neurophysiology, I'm certified in veterinary acupuncture and veterinary chiropractic, I've taken advanced training in homeopathy, Chinese herbal medicine and Western herbal medicine, and between that and 16 years of using these therapies on patients and keeping up-to-date on the literature and research conducted on animals and people, I've learned what works and what doesn't work for most situations.

How soon do you expect to see results?

SCHOEN: I give the treatment four weeks, then reevaluate. I see most cases on a weekly or monthly basis. Often the improvement is obvious — the general condition of the animal, its attitude and energy level, the color and quality of its coat, those changes are encouraging. In fact, I'd say that in nearly all cases of cancer, a holistic approach is a good adjunct for an animal and its owner. Alternative and complementary therapies can't cure every animal or every disease, but their track record is far more humane, less invasive, less expensive and more likely to result in an improved quality and in many cases length of life than the conventional therapies I recommended when I first went into veterinary practice.

In fact, that's true for not only cancer but for all of the common chronic diseases we see in animals: things like arthritis, chronic disc disease, hip dysplasia, chronic liver disease, feline leukemia, viral diseases, kidney disease and other illnesses that conventional medicine considers incurable. Some of these conditions are so easy to treat that I take their improvement for granted and I have to remind myself that not everyone knows about these therapies. Yes, many of them are unproven and untested according to scientific protocols, but is it better to let animals die while we wait for double-blind, clinically controlled, randomized trials on every single condition, which aren't likely to happen in our human lifetimes, much less our pets' lifetimes, or is it better to try procedures and methods that have been shown to produce good results in some well-documented cases and which have very little risk of adverse side effects? I believe they're worth trying.

There's a common pattern that follows the introduction of a new drug or new therapy. It happens in allopathic medicine all the time and it's true for alternatives. At first everyone's a little skeptical, but it works in a few cases and people get interested. They try it themselves and get good results. Then enthusiasm goes way up and they try it on everything hoping it will work for every case. Well, nothing does, not in allopathic medicine or in holistic medicine. After the peaks and valleys of enthusiasm and disappointment, you settle into a plateau and you realize where a particular modality fits into the whole picture. This was true for me in all of the techniques I practice, and now I appreciate that there is a place for everything, a place for conventional medicine, a place for homeopathy, a place for acupuncture, a place for Western herbs, Chinese herbs, nutrition, everything. I start every case by considering the accepted conventional treatment and whether it's reasonable for the animal and I weigh the chances of success against the risks. No one form of medicine has all the answers. If one did, we wouldn't need any others. The important thing to do is look at the best of all the different therapies and develop a new approach that incorporates all of them. I believe that this is the future of veterinary medicine.

What is the best way to find a good veterinarian?

SCHOEN: Word of mouth is probably your best reference, or check with veterinarians in the area whom you know and trust and ask for a recommendation. Conventional veterinarians are increasingly sympathetic to holistic methods. Today there are probably about a thousand veterinarians here in the U.S. who take a holistic approach, but that figure is changing fast. I think it will be a lot easier to find holistic health care for pets in the years ahead.

What single message would you most like to convey to American pet owners?

SCHOEN: In addition to learning about the different therapies in order to make informed decisions about veterinary care, nutrition and the prevention of disease, add a heaping dose of love and compassion, for that's an integral part of the healing process.

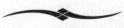

Cancer-Fighting Foods

W hile there are many holistic treatments for cancer in animals, their common denominator is improved nutrition. Packaged, processed foods containing denatured, rendered ingredients, synthetic vitamins, artificial colors or flavors and chemical preservatives are harmful to any animal fighting disease but especially so to cancer patients. The first step in every holistic cancer therapy is improving the diet.

In the treatment of human cancers, special diets abound. Do they work? Richard Walters, John M. Fink and Ralph Moss, Ph.D., are only a few of the medical journalists who have documented the effectiveness of different nutritional therapies for cancer. Not all of these approaches work, but some have enviable track records.

The foods best known as cancer fighters are fresh, raw, organically raised fruits and vegetables, such as the carrot juice that saved the life of the Dalmatian on page 78. Other juices recommended for human and canine cancer patients are combinations of beet, celery and carrot or fruits such as grape and apple.

In his book *How to Fight Cancer and Win,* William L. Fischer described the importance of sauerkraut and other lactic acid fermented foods as a support therapy in human cancer prevention and treatment. Those are fresh, raw, unpasteurized natural pickles, made without vinegar and with a minimum of salt, which are, Fischer explained, an excellent bowel tonic; they improve digestion, which in cancer patients is often compromised by a lack of hydrochloric acid and enzymes, and are themselves rich in easily assimilated nutrients. Lactic acid maintains beneficial intestinal flora while helping to eliminate harmful bacteria. According to German physician and scientist Johannes Kuhl, M.D., Ph.D., lactic acid foods are "hostile" to cancer. "No other full-value diet will do the job [of reducing cancer cases]," he wrote.

Lactic acid fermented vegetables are easy to prepare in a salad press using unrefined sea salt; see page 79. Small quantities of lactic acid fermented vegetables and freshly made yogurt or kefir, which are lactic acid milk products, are recommended for both dogs and cats.

Macrobiotic diets are sometimes successful in the treatment of human cancers, but they emphasize cooked foods, especially grains such as brown rice, which dogs and cats were not designed to consume. Although some argue that cooking improves the digestibility of foods and that any dog or cat with cancer is likely to have an impaired digestive system, cooking is a human cultural preference. Animals used to cooked foods find it more familiar and, when given a choice, may select cooked foods out of habit, but Francis Pottenger proved the deleterious effects that cooked food has on the health of animals who eat it. By gradually introducing fresh, whole, raw foods and by improving the animal's digestion, you'll supply far more nutritional support than any canned or packaged pet food or any home-prepared cooked food can provide.

One of the strongest arguments against raw meat is that it may contain parasites or harmful bacteria that the animal's impaired digestive system isn't able to deal with. While this is a valid concern, the answer is not to sterilize the food with heat but to improve the animal's digestion while reducing the risk of pathogens. See page 71 for four effective ways to disinfect raw meat. In addition, add small amounts of garlic vinegar or plain cider vinegar, lactic acid fermented vegetables, yogurt, kefir, acidophilus supplements, digestive enzymes, Willard Water and/or hydrochloric acid capsules to every meal. Juliette de Bairacli Levi credits the antiseptic herbs garlic, sage, thyme, eucalyptus, wormwood and rue, ingredients in her Natural Rearing herbal compound tablets, with preventing all types of cancer. Any or all of these herbs can be added to food in small amounts on a regular or rotating basis.

Willard Water

Catalyst Altered Water or Willard Water (see page 106) is a concentrate of microscopic particles (called a micelle) of lignite containing natural antibiotics, germicidals, amino acids and over 50 trace minerals. Since the 1960s, it has been widely used by ranchers, farmers and the owners of racing dogs and pets. John Willard, Ph.D., the chemist who discovered and patented the concentrate, collected their reports of improved nutrition and conducted his own experiments showing that it improves digestion and the assimilation of nutrients as reflected by the condition and content of the animals' droppings, their growth and weight patterns and overall health records. In addition, it reduces stress reactions, such as those experienced by livestock in transit or animals in hot weather, increases resistance to illness and reduces infection rates. In some cases the water was sprayed directly on cattle with cancer and their tumors disappeared; in others, its internal use reduced the number of cancers in livestock and poultry.

Some physicians have reported that Willard Water prevents burns in radiation therapy patients, both when sprayed on the skin and when taken internally without external application. In the May 1996 issue of *Alternative Medicine Digest*, Victor Marcial-Vega, M.D., recommended that human cancer patients drink one gallon of diluted Willard Water daily to help rid the body of toxins and heavy metals.

Some holistic pet care guides have published complicated schedules for administering Willard Water to pets, with carefully defined maximum doses and intervals between treatments. This is appropriate in the garden or greenhouse, for plants can absorb enough of the micelle to decrease its effectiveness, but daily use is safe and effective for dogs, cats, birds and rabbits. For pets under stress or during hot weather, Dr. Willard suggested adding 1 tablespoon to each quart of drinking water, which is twice the usual concentration and which is appropriate for animals undergoing treatment for cancer; otherwise, use 2 tablespoons per gallon for daily use. The only potential side effect when animals drink more than they need is mild diarrhea.

The internal and external application of Willard Water speeds the healing of cuts, burns, surgical wounds, scars, most skin conditions, poison ivy rashes, cataracts, conjunctivitis and other infections. Willard reported that when animals with infections were treated with antibiotics, veterinarians were able to reduce the drug dosage by half or more if the micelle was administered at the same time. Animals with itchy skin can be bathed in dilute solutions, or a small amount of concentrate can be added to pet shampoos. All pets, whether being treated for cancer or not, are likely to benefit from its daily use.

Vitamins and Minerals

Wendell O. Belfield, D.V.M., documents the beneficial effects of vitamin and mineral supplements on cancer patients in his books *How to Have a Healthier Dog* and *The Very Healthy Cat Book*. As he reports, researchers since 1925 have linked vitamin A deficiencies with cancer; in laboratory tests, liver and brewer's yeast, which is rich in B vitamins, protected rats fed a banned food coloring known to cause liver cancer; vitamin C protected lab animals in numerous cancer experiments; vitamins C and E plus the mineral selenium, known as antioxidants, reduced chemically induced cancers in mice to 10 percent of expected levels and enabled the mice to live longer than their unsupplemented counterparts; and many experiments have shown that diets low in zinc promote cancer in rats exposed to tumor-causing chemicals.

Where tumors are involved, Belfield is reluctant to prescribe vitamins and minerals until after surgery because most owners bring their pets to the veterinarian when growth is so advanced that time is of the essence. "I have read letters to the editor in popular nutrition magazines describing successful home treatment of pet tumors with vitamins and minerals," he wrote. "This doesn't surprise me. However, any such attempt should be conducted under the guidance or at least with the knowledge of a trained veterinarian who can monitor progress."

Belfield described a rural Missouri veterinarian, Dr. H. H. Robertson, who used vitamins C and E to treat canine tumors. His method was to inject intravenously 1 gram of sodium ascorbate per pound of body weight and give an intramuscular injection of 400 IUs of vitamin E daily for five days. Following this, the dogs were given supplemental vitamin C. According to Robertson, the average tumor took about three weeks to resolve.

Belfield also described a report of 12 canine patients treated in Ireland in the 1950s.

Dr. N. H. Lambert orally dosed the dogs with up to 300 IUs of vitamin E, which made

awkwardly positioned tumors easier to remove and in some cases eliminated the need for surgery. "The life span of otherwise doomed animals has been prolonged for as long as five years," he wrote.

At a cattery in California, an adult female purchased for breeding purposes was shown to be a carrier of feline leukemia. Belfield treated her with vitamin C, and blood tests 10 weeks later showed her to be clear of the disease. "This animal was positive two months ago and now it's negative," said the laboratory pathologist when he phoned Belfield with the news. "What are you doing?"

"There were five such cases in the past three years at this cattery," Belfield wrote in 1981. "The entire cattery is on vitamin C and, at the time of this writing, we are in the third generation of offspring without a single appearance of leukemia."

At another cattery, the feline leukemia situation was so serious that a local veterinary college had recommended the cessation of breeding in order to prevent the disease's spread. Every six months for two years, six adult cats had tested positive for leukemia. The entire cattery was placed on vitamin C and, when retested six months later, all were negative.

Therapeutic doses of vitamin C vary by individual. For best results, use a natural, food-derived vitamin C-complex rather than ascorbic acid. Many pets as well as people take Ester-C, a patented form of calcium ascorbate, which is nonacidic and is said to have a faster absorption rate than other forms. While calcium ascorbate is not a whole-food concentrate, it is superior to ascorbic acid and is often combined in capsules, powders or tablets with citrus, acerola and rose hips, all of which are natural sources of C-complex nutrients such as bioflavonoids and rutin. Start with small amounts and gradually increase the dosage to as much as several grams per day, for megadoses of vitamin C have been shown to benefit human, feline and canine cancer patients. Observe the animal carefully and dose to bowel tolerance, which occurs when the body can no longer absorb the vitamin and excretes it, causing loose stools or mild diarrhea. At that point, reduce the dosage until normal bowel movements resume.

Dogs and cats fed a raw natural diet of organically raised food (pesticide, chemical and drug residues are especially deleterious to those with cancer and other serious illnesses), including finely minced wheat grass and other greens, raw, meaty bones, fresh fruits, seaweeds from unpolluted ocean water, unrefined sea salt, fresh eggs and lactic acid fermented vegetables and dairy products, will obtain most of the nutrients they need from their food. These same guidelines are appropriate for birds, rabbits and other pets, using foods appropriate for the species. Fresh, raw, natural and organic are the key words. In addition, a trace mineral supplement and food-derived multivitamin is appropriate. Be sure that additional vitamins such as supplemental C-complex, B-complex, D, beta carotene and E come from whole food sources and are not synthetic.

Homeopathy

Homeopathy is often considered a secondary or support therapy in the treatment of cancer, but veterinary homeopath Larry Bernstein disagrees. In some cases, he claims, homeopathy does well as the primary therapy. "The disease is a reflection of the inner imbalance of the vital force," he explains. "If you work on strengthening and balancing the vital force, the disease will take care of itself. I've treated some cancer patients with homeopathy alone and they completely recovered. In other cases, where animals were brought to me as a last resort with only a week or two to live, I used homeopathy and no other therapy and they went on to live a full life happily and in comfort for anywhere from three to fifteen months. In terminal cases, the animal usually does well until the end and then goes quickly and gently. As you know, this is not what happens with patients treated with conventional methods.

"Every homeopathic remedy depends on the individual case," he continues. "You can't say all kidney cats get *Arsenicum* or all splenic hemangiomas get *Phosphorus*. Every case is different. Homeopathy works best as a cancer therapy when the illness is diagnosed early and the patient hasn't been exposed to chemotherapy or radiation. I compare cancer to a stain on a shirt. If you soak it in cold water right away, it's likely to come out but if you wash it in hot water, the stain is locked in. After that you can make it better, you can make it almost go away, but it's never going to disappear. Once you resort to chemotherapy or radiation therapy, it's just as hard to remove a cancer.

"I don't put surgery in the same category. I've dealt with cancer patients that had part but not all of a cancerous tumor removed and they did very well. I find that the hardest cancer to treat is bone cancer. Lymphosarcomas are difficult, too. I treated two cases of lymphosarcoma last summer. One of the animals is doing very well and I expect him to live a long, healthy life. That's because he was an ideal candidate and his owners were willing to go the distance with his homeopathic treatment even though it meant that some symptoms got worse before they got better. The other dog was a Cocker Spaniel who had been on cortisone. As soon as his lymph nodes increased in size, which was part of the healing process, the owner put him back on the cortisone to make the swelling go away. She had originally insisted on homeopathy, but I discovered that she really wanted him to have chemotherapy, she just couldn't afford it. Under the circumstances, her dog was unlikely to benefit from homeopathy or any other holistic therapy. She wanted something that would cause an immediate, dramatic reduction of his visible symptoms. I made some phone calls and arranged for the dog to get chemotherapy at a price she could afford. He responded well and she's delighted. I know he will have serious problems a year or two from now, because all that's been done is a massive suppression, but to me that was the holistic answer in that case."

For referrals to veterinary homeopaths experienced in the treatment of cancer, see the Resources for Chapter 6 in the Appendix.

Herbal Therapies

Some of the most impressive results in human and animal cancer treatment are obtained from herbs. Milk thistle seed (see page 157) is appropriate for all cancer patients because it supports the liver, which is probably the most overworked organ in a sick animal. All of the alterative herbs, popularly known as blood cleansers, have a place in the daily diet of cancer patients. These include burdock root, dandelion leaf and root, red clover, Oregon grape root, stinging nettle and yellow dock root, among others. Chamomile, valerian and other soothing nervines help reduce stress. Green herbs, such as wheat grass, buckwheat lettuce, rye grass, barley grass, alfalfa, spirulina and chlorella are powerful detoxifiers as well as rich sources of vitamins, minerals and other nutrients. A variety of herbs belongs in your pet's daily diet.

Aloe Vera   *(Aloe vera)*

The familiar aloe vera is a popular support remedy for those with cancer. It can be given internally with food and applied externally to growths and tumors.

In his book *Cancer Therapy: The Independent Consumer's Guide to Non-Toxic Treatment and Prevention*, Ralph Moss, Ph.D., reports that aloe, like garlic, is a member of the lily family and is primarily used as an adjuvant (helper) with other therapies. Aloe contains polysaccharides which researchers in Japan and other countries have found stimulate an immune system response. Russian scientists tested aloe juice on three types of tumors in rodents and concluded that while the juice did not affect the main tumor growth, it reduced tumor mass and the frequency of metastases at different stages of the tumors' progress. Aloe juice is often used by chemotherapy patients to help prevent the infections they are prone to as well as increase the antitumor effect of certain chemotherapy drugs. Tokyo scientists have shown that aloe provides "a significant protective effect of skin injury" caused by radiation. Its ability to protect the liver against environmental poisons makes it an important detoxifier.

For external use, apply either fresh gel from the leaf or bottled juice. If giving fresh leaf internally, peel it carefully to be sure that none of the bitter inner rind goes with the gel; the rind contains a powerful purgative laxative. As a general tonic and preventive, give 1 teaspoon of aloe vera gel or juice per 10 pounds of body weight daily; as a support therapy for cancer, give that amount twice per day. Aloe vera gel can be applied externally as often as desired, several times per day.

Carnivora

In 1980, Helmut Keller, M.D., began studying the carnivorous plant Venus fly trap *(Dionaea muscipula)* and discovered it to be not only a powerful cancer treatment but an effective therapy for ulcerative colitis, multiple sclerosis, herpes, arthritis, AIDS and most immune deficiencies. The crude extract of Venus fly trap causes troublesome side effects, but Keller created a purified extract, which he named Carnivora. Because the U.S. is unsympathetic to herbal therapies, he moved to Germany in 1981 to continue his research without government or medical establishment interference.

In cases of cancer, according to its proponents, Carnivora works therapeutically to shrink solid tumors but does not improve blood abnormalities such as leukemia. Like most alternative cancer treatments, it is most effective if the patient has not undergone chemotherapy or radiation therapy. The extract can be administered by drops, by inhalation or by injection.

Medical journalists such as Morton Walker, who reported on Carnivora in the September 1992 edition of *Natural Health,* have visited Keller's clinic, reviewed his files and interviewed patients who say they owe their lives to the extract.

A few months after reporting on Carnivora, *Natural Health* published a letter crediting the extract with saving the life of a poodle with an aggressive mouth tumor. "After removing the visible tumor and finding it was cancerous to the edges," said the writer, "our local vet referred us to a veterinary oncologist, who told us that the only way to buy time would be to remove one-third of Max's upper jaw, where the cancer had penetrated, and then use radiation or chemotherapy." The prognosis was that even with that expensive and painful treatment, the dog would die within a year. Two weeks after the first operation, a tumor as large as the original one appeared.

The dog's veterinarian had mentioned Carnivora but said it was not available in the U.S. After reading the magazine's article, the owners sent an urgent FAX to Dr. Keller, who sent the extract with instructions for the veterinarian. "Two weeks after we started giving Max injections of Carnivora, the tumor had practically disappeared," wrote the owner. "We now have what appears to be a normal, healthy dog, who continues to receive the Carnivora injections on a maintenance dose."

Allen Schoen is one of America's most experienced veterinary users of Carnivora. "I started testing it in 1990 and collected data on a small number of cases," he told me, "and I found that in certain tumor types it could be extremely beneficial but in others it didn't do anything. I found it to be most effective in the treatment of carcinomas and mast cell tumors, but I haven't found it to be very effective on sarcomas or on tumors that are so far advanced that they have metastasized and spread to other parts of the body. If it's a large but treatable tumor, I may suggest that it be surgically removed first.

"When it's effective, Carnivora works by stimulating the immune system and increasing phagocytosis of the neoplastic cells, which helps the body destroy cancer cells. Most of the time I administer it subcutaneously, injecting it beneath the skin, which I teach clients to do at home. I have them sign a release form because it's not an FDA-approved therapy; it's experimental. I have an Investigative New Animal Drug or INAD number and we're conducting clinical trials. Some of our animals with squamous cell carcinomas have been in remission for four years using only Carnivora, improved nutrition and some basic antioxidant supplements. Some animals who don't recover still experience an improved and lengthened quality of life with no adverse side effects.

"I usually suggest giving it four to eight weeks. If no improvement occurs within eight weeks, we stop the Carnivora and focus on other therapies. If the animal responds, we continue giving it. What usually happens is that an aggressive tumor stops growing, decreases its rate of growth or shrinks and disappears.

"Our present success rate is about 60 percent, which is an extremely promising statistic, but I choose my cases carefully. Altogether, I have treated about 30 animals over a five-year period with Carnivora. The dog most likely to respond well is in relatively good health, has an oral squamous cell carcinoma that has not metastasized and has not received chemotherapy or radiation. That would be a good patient for Carnivora."

Chaparral *(Larrea tridentata)*

Chaparral or creosote bush has long been used in the Pacific Southwest to fight cancer and many other diseases. In 1967, the medical establishment became interested in this bitter-tasting shrub when Ernest Farr, an 87-year-old Arizona man, went to the University of Utah Medical Center with a malignant melanoma on his right cheek. After three surgical removals of the recurring lesion, it came back again. Farr refused a fourth surgery and instead treated himself with chaparral tea. He drank two cups daily and took no other medication. When he returned a year later, the facial growth had regressed to the size of a tiny pimple and a necrotic mass on his neck had disappeared.

University of Utah doctors then tested chaparral tea on 59 patients. Of the 45 evaluated, four showed "significant tumor regression." The compound in chaparral known to have anticancer properties is nor-dihydroguaiaretic acid, or NDGA. This substance has been shown to inhibit the electron transport system of tumors, depriving them of the electrical energy they require to exist.

Chaparral received unfavorable publicity a few years ago when it was blamed by the FDA for acute toxic hepatitis, and a voluntary ban on the herb's sale was initiated by sellers. Subsequent research failed to establish any connection between chaparral and the disease, so the herb is again available.

Chaparral can be added to other tea blends and brewed as an infusion. Use 1 tablespoon per cup of boiling water and let steep until cool; chaparral tea keeps well in the refrigerator for up to a week. This is a medicinal strength tea and it tastes very bitter, so start with only small amounts in food or drinking water. Gradually increase the amount to 1 teaspoon for each 10 pounds of body weight per day. Dry or powdered chaparral can be added to food; use a pinch for small animals and 1/4 teaspoon per 25 pounds for larger dogs. Among its beneficial side effects are its vermifuge properties; chaparral repels and helps eliminate worms and other parasites. Externally, chaparral tea can be applied to wounds, itching skin or tumors to speed healing.

Essiac Tea

In the early 1920s, Rene Caisse, a Canadian nurse, questioned an elderly patient about her scarred but healed breast. She learned that several years earlier a Toronto physician had diagnosed a malignant tumor in the breast and recommended a mastectomy. Instead, the woman took an herbal tea prepared by an Indian neighbor of the Ojibwa or Chippewa tribe. Caisse asked for the formula, which she later modified and thus began her search for a cancer cure, which lasted until her death in 1978 at the age of 90.

She named her herbal remedy Essiac, which is her name spelled backward. The tea, which is said to have cured many patients of various cancers with no adverse side effects, has been at various times praised, maligned, investigated, ignored, misrepresented and widely copied. Caisse experienced mostly disappointment and frustration from her contacts with the medical establishment and adulation from patients who recovered under her care.

Caisse kept her formula secret, for she feared that if it were made public, exploiters would sell Essiac preparations that lacked the original's healing properties and she worried that the formula's simplicity would cause many to reject it out of hand.

In 1977 she was persuaded to give her Essiac formula to a Canadian corporation which had physicians on its board of directors and which planned to set up clinical trials that would prove its efficacy. Following approval from the Canadian government at a future date, the Resperin Corporation would market Essiac. Unfortunately, the corporation fell behind in its record keeping, so this goal was never reached.

Still, belief in Essiac remains alive because so many patients improve or recover, or if they die they do so with a clear mind, serene disposition and no need of painkillers.

There are many Essiac blends, recipes and products on the market today, but most follow the original formula Rene Caisse used in her Bracebridge clinic, which contained sheep sorrel *(Rumex acetosella)*, a wild perennial relative of garden sorrel and a blood tonic said to be beneficial to the heart and used to treat ulcers and kidney disorders; burdock root *(Arctium lappa)*, a well-known blood purifier and kidney cleanser; slippery elm bark *(Ulmus fulva)*, a demulcent, nutritive, tonic herb with many traditional uses; and

Turkey rhubarb root *(Rheum palmatum)*, a plant native to China and Tibet which is a liver tonic, appetite stimulant, headache reliever and digestive aid.

Essiac tea has a long history of use in people of all ages, and holistic veterinarians recommend it for use in dogs, cats and other animals. Testimonials about Essiac refer to its effectiveness in treating tumors, cancer, thyroid disorders, skin conditions and its use as a general health tonic. It is said to have alleviated and in some cases cured many chronic and degenerative conditions.

Medical herbalists suggest that Essiac not be used by those with kidney ailments or arthritis because of the oxalic acid in two of its ingredients, although it has sometimes helped dogs and cats with these disorders. Some caution against using Turkey rhubarb root during pregnancy. The formula has no documented side effects. The same precautions apply to Essiac as to any herbal blend: if disease symptoms worsen without quickly improving, or if the animal experiences an allergic reaction (rapid pulse, nausea, vomiting, diarrhea, a skin rash, violent itching or any other obvious symptoms), discontinue use.

Beverly Cappel-King recommends Essiac tea as a support therapy for cancer. "I give it to every animal I treat because it's not going to hurt and it flushes them out," she explains. "Some reports say that it kills cancer. It does not kill cancer, it just cleans the body out. You're opening up the kidneys and the liver, you're helping to purify the blood and you're soothing the gastrointestinal tract. It just flushes junk out of the body and it makes the body healthier so that it can fight cancer.

"For conditions like skin tumors, it works well on its own. I used it myself for a melanoma and it disappeared in three weeks. I went on a modified fast, took Essiac every day for three weeks and did a lot of visualization, and it was gone. We've had the same success with animals that have melanomas, suspicious looking basal cell tumors or even mast cell tumors of the skin. We put them on Essiac once or twice a day, and the tumors shrivel up within a couple of weeks."

Essiac can be purchased as a brewed tea in bottles or made at home from dry herbs. The recommended dosage is about 1 teaspoon per 10 pounds of body weight. Cats receive 1/2 to 1 teaspoon daily; dogs up to 30 pounds receive 1 tablespoon and larger dogs receive 1 tablespoon for every 30 pounds of body weight.

Hoxsey Therapy

In the 1930s and '40s, the Hoxsey Therapy was a household word. Despite founder Harry Hoxsey's lack of medical credentials, it cured thousands, whose cases are well-documented. Though far less well known today, it continues to be used successfully. There are several versions of the Hoxsey formula. Most contain red clover blossom *(Trifolium pratense)*, licorice root *(Glycyrrhiza glabra)*, buckthorn bark *(Rhamnus frangu-*

la), burdock seed *(Arctium lappa),* stillingia root *(Stillingia sylvatica),* Oregon grape root *(Berberis aquifolium),* poke root (also called red herb root, *Phytolacca americana*), prickly ash bark *(Xanthoxylum clava),* wild indigo root *(Baptisia tinctoria)* and potassium iodide. In his *Therapeutic Herb Manual,* herbal pharmacist Ed Smith wrote that the Hoxsey formula is a classic example of what medical herbalists call an alterative, depurative or blood purifier which acts through the lymph system, glands, mucous membranes and skin, enhancing the breakdown and elimination of metabolic wastes and improving the overall assimilation of nutrients.

The recommended human dose is 15 to 20 drops three times daily; this is about 1 drop per 7 to 10 pounds of body weight three times per day. Most cats would take 1 to 2 drops, dogs weighing 20 pounds would take 4 drops, dogs between 30 and 40 pounds would take 3 to 4 drops, and so forth, three times per day.

Hoxsey's famous paste for external application contained blood root *(Sanguinaria canadensis),* a North American wildflower whose root contains an alkaloid, sanguinarine, which has potent anticancer properties. Physicians and medical researchers have documented its effectiveness since 1850, when Dr. J.W. Fell, working at Middlesex Hospital in London, made a paste of bloodroot extract, zinc chloride, flour and water. Daily application to malignant growths usually destroyed tumors within two to four weeks. In the 1960s, several teams of scientists reported complete healing of carcinomas of the nose, external ear and other body parts using a paste made of bloodroot and zinc chloride. In his best-selling *Spontaneous Healing,* Dr. Andrew Weil recounted his own experiences with bloodroot, beginning with the rapid destruction of a tumor on his dog. Bloodroot also helps prevent dental plaque; it is most familiar to Americans as an ingredient in Viadent toothpaste and mouthwash and is an appropriate addition to herbal preparations for dogs with plaque.

Hsiao Chai Hu Tang

In the June 1995 edition of *Alternatives* newsletter, David G. Williams, M.D., described the Chinese herbal formula Hsiao Chai Hu Tang, also known as Xiao Chai Hu Tang in China, Sho-saiko-to in Japan and in the English-speaking world as Minor Bupleurum Formula. The remedy is sold as a tea blend or herbal tablets.

According to Williams, the formula has been prescribed for a variety of conditions including colds and flu, bronchitis, fever, chills and tuberculosis. "Where the tea really shines," he wrote, "is in the treatment of hepatitis and liver cancer. It appears to be the best medicine available (natural or synthetic) in the treatment of primary liver cancer." In laboratory tests, the formula showed no toxicity toward normal cells while inhibiting the growth of cancer cells by fragmenting cell walls and activating the body's natural defenses. At the same time, it stimulated or increased the growth of normal cells.

Additional studies have shown that the formula promotes regeneration of the liver and, at the University School of Medicine in Japan, it inhibited the development of precancerous changes in the breast.

Williams published the formula, which contains Hare's Ear Root *(Bupleuri chinense)*, Half Summer or *ban xia (Pinellia ternat)*, ginger root or *shen jiang (Zingiber officinale)*, skullcap root or *huang gin (Scutellaria baicalensis)*, jujube fruit, also called red date or *da zao (Ziziphus jujuba)*, ginseng root or *ren shen (Panax ginseng)* and licorice root or *zhi gan cao (Glycyrrhiza uralensis)*. Minor Bupleurum Formula is widely sold in Oriental markets and by traditional Chinese tea companies.

Williams instructed his patients and readers to use this tea as a preventive tonic as well as to treat all types of liver disease. When converting any human tea dosage for animal use, assume that the hypothetical human patient weighs 120 to 150 pounds and adjust accordingly. In his newsletter, Williams gave directions for brewing a strong decoction and recommended between 1 and 2 cups per day. To apply this recommendation to a 50-pound dog, give about 1/2 cup per day. A 10-pound dog or cat would receive between 1 and 2 tablespoons. For pills or tablets, convert label directions to canine or feline proportions.

The other herb known to repair liver damage is milk thistle seed (*Silybum marianum,* see page 157). Both milk thistle seed and Minor Bupleurum are appropriate support therapies in the treatment of all cancers, not just liver disease. Many herbalists suggest alternating courses of herbs, using one for several weeks, then replacing it with the other. This strategy, which prevents the body from becoming so accustomed to a remedy that its effectiveness declines, is easy to apply with these highly effective liver tonics.

Noni *(Morinda citrifolia)*

Also known as Indian mulberry, noni is a small Polynesian evergreen that grows in tropical climates. As Andrew Weil, M.D., wrote in the June 1997 edition of his *Self Healing* newsletter, the shrub produces "a little, knobby, nasty-tasting, foul-smelling fruit that has a long and respected history of use as an herbal remedy, from Southeast Asia to the Caribbean."

Biochemist Ralph Heinicke, Ph.D., who worked in Hawaii for Dole Pineapple, the Pineapple Research Institute and the University of Hawaii from 1950 to 1986, found that the active ingredient in the pineapple enzyme bromelaine is an alkaloid precursor, which he named proxeronine ("pro-" for precursor, "xeronine" for the alkaloid). Commercially grown pineapple's proxeronine content decreased with the depletion of nutrients in plantation soil and pineapple became an unreliable source of the substance, so he turned to noni, which also contains proxeronine, to continue his research. According to Heinicki, insufficient levels of xeronine may be the cause of cancer, senility, arthritis, imbalances of blood sugar, high or low blood pressure and other diseases.

Because of research in Japan showing that noni fruit inhibits the growth of cells known to be precursors of certain cancers, noni products have become popular supplements for human and animal cancer patients. Noni is reported to be an analgesic pain reliever and an antiseptic effective against harmful viruses, bacteria, including *E. coli*, fungi and internal parasites, making it an appropriate "immunization" herb. It can be applied to cuts and other wounds to help them heal without scarring.

Noni is available as a pasteurized juice diluted with other juices to improve its flavor and as a powder made by drying noni juice at low temperature. It is being used, although not always under veterinary supervision, for a variety of ailments in dogs and cats, including cancer.

Unfortunately, the multilevel marketing of any product results in the widespread publication of unverifiable anecdotal stories, wildly enthusiastic claims, high-pressure sales tactics and the denigration of competing products. It is difficult to separate fact from fiction in the early years of a supplement's widespread promotion, and these are the early years of noni's mass marketing. Because of its long history of medicinal use in tropical cultures and its lack of documented toxicity, noni is probably safe for your pet. No researchers have claimed that noni kills cancer, but it may help prevent the growth of cancer by strengthening healthy cells and cleansing the system.

To determine an appropriate dosage, adjust the label's recommendation for your pet's weight. For example, the recommended human dose for powdered noni is 1 capsule half an hour before breakfast and half an hour before lunch for five days, followed by two days off; then begin the cycle again. To administer noni to pets, open a capsule and divide its contents according to the animal's weight. Assuming that the average adult human weighs 120 to 150 pounds, use the contents of 1 capsule per day for a 60- to 75-pound animal; use a total of 1/2 capsule per day for one weighing 30 to 40 pounds; use 1/4 capsule per day for a pet weighing 15 to 20 pounds; and so on. Mix the powder with a small amount of wet food and give it with water half an hour before a regular meal, twice daily. If your pet objects to the taste, disguise it in a strong-smelling food or sprinkle small amounts in its regular breakfast or dinner.

Parasites and Cancer

One of the most unusual cancer therapies is the herbal cure offered by Hulda Regehr Clark, Ph.D., N.D. Clark has impressive credentials from the University of Saskatchewan, McGill University and the University of Minnesota, including degrees in biology and biophysics. She earned her doctorate in physiology in 1958 and worked in government research until 1979, when she began private consulting. Several years ago Clark discovered what she believes is the cause of all human cancers, an intestinal flatworm or fluke. Under normal conditions, adult para sites live only in the colon, excreted eggs hatch outside the host's body and any eggs that reach the bloodstream are destroyed by the liver.

According to Clark, exposure to toxins disrupts the liver's ability to destroy the parasite's eggs. In susceptible hosts, the eggs hatch and young parasites spread within the body, producing the growth hormone ortho-phospho-tyrosine, the presence of which is used as a common test for cancer. This growth hormone penetrates adjacent host cells, which then begin dividing and growing themselves, creating cancer.

Clark's approach is to kill parasites in every phase of their growth: egg, youth and mature adult. She does this with a simple combination of herbs and claims that within five to seven days all the flukes die with no adverse side effects to the host and the cancer dies with them.

The shortest portion of her book *The Cure for All Cancers* describes Clark's herbal cancer cure; the rest of its 503 pages are devoted to 100 case studies, instructions for building electronic devices to destroy or test for parasites and recommendations for healthy living. Clark associates all major and minor human illnesses with parasite infections, including seizures, depression, asthma, diabetes, migraine headaches and various skin conditions, linking them with roundworms, pancreatic cattle flukes, threadworms, heartworms and other parasites.

Needless to say, Clark's theories are controversial. Her diagnostic methods, like her treatments, are unconventional. But her simple protocol of using vermifuge or anthelmintic (worm-killing) herbs is inexpensive and easy to administer.

Very little has been published about Hulda Clark's cancer cure beyond its developer's books and articles, although some health magazines have printed letters from physicians who treated cancer patients with this therapy alone and whose patients made a full recovery. Clark's books give a parasite therapy for pets, though its purpose is to reduce the risk of human exposure to pet-borne parasites, not to treat cancer in animals. Clark takes an extremely dim view of dogs, cats and other animals, describing them only as a source of disease and recommending that human cancer patients avoid them. However, a growing number of pet owners, breeders and veterinarians are experimenting with her combination of black walnut hull tincture, freshly ground cloves and powdered wormwood as a support therapy for dogs and cats who have cancer. For dosage directions, see page 402 in the section on Parasites.

For information about other nutritional, herbal and alternative cancer therapies or about products mentioned here, see the Resources for this chapter in the Appendix. ◀▬

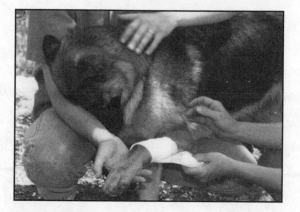

Holistic
First Aid

JUST AS YOU KEEP first-aid items on hand for yourself and your family, it makes sense to have a first-aid kit for your pets. Depending on your situation, the kit can be part of a shelf in the medicine cabinet, a collection of items in a fanny pack or enough material to fill a small suitcase.

Keep your first-aid supplies in a convenient location at home, then decide what you're most likely to need and have room for on hikes, while camping, in the car or on vacation.

The Holistic First-aid Kit

The ideal pet first-aid kit is a well-filled box or container that is easy to transport, durable, water-resistant, unlocked and easy to open. Some plastic food storage containers with press-on lids are difficult to open; test your container by having everyone in the house, including older children, open and close it. Store the container with other first-aid equipment in a duffel bag, tote bag or box. Clearly label the outside with your animal's name, DOG FIRST AID or a similar designation. Leave the kit in plain sight so it's easy to reach and everyone knows where to find it.

The following suggestions are based on the recommendations of veterinarians, herbalists and guides to emergency pet care. Start today by collecting whatever you have on hand, add new materials as you obtain them and adapt the kit so that its contents are items and products you feel comfortable using.

Tea Tree Oil. For pet use, make a 15 percent solution of tea tree oil (see page 184). This all-purpose disinfectant can be used on cuts, burns, scrapes, fungal infections, ringworm, pustules, hot spots, burns, abscesses, infected ears, tick bites, infected wounds and other conditions.

Grapefruit Seed Extract. The citrus seed extracts sold for household use (see page 152) are diluted with glycerine, but even this concentration is very strong. Apply full-strength only to pustules, ringworm and small areas when treating infection; otherwise, dilute before applying, especially around mucous membranes. Grapefruit seed extract can be used just like tea tree oil, above; it can also be taken internally as an alternative to antibiotic drugs. Keep both the bitter-tasting liquid and debittered powder capsules on hand.

Herbal Salve. A soft, all-purpose salve can help soothe and heal wounds while protecting them from bandaging materials that would otherwise adhere. Apply to burns, cuts and abrasions. Because their uses vary slightly, make or buy one salve that contains comfrey (see page 130) and one that does not, such as a salve made with plantain.

Most veterinary handbooks recommend petroleum jelly for wound protection, but a well-made herbal salve has the added benefits of disinfecting, healing ingredients.

Lavender Oil and Other Essential Oils. Lavender oil can be applied full strength to large dogs and probably to small dogs, cats and other pets because it is so well tolerated; however, to be completely safe, dilute lavender oil with an equal quantity of carrier oil. Keep the diluted oil in a glass or plastic bottle. Apply lavender oil to burns to reduce pain, swelling, redness, blistering and scarring. A natural disinfectant, lavender oil can be used on any cut, scrape or infection.

Lavender oil has dozens of medicinal uses. Other essential oils that have been helpful to pets are reviewed on pages 178-184 Select those that are most appropriate for your pet and keep them in your medicine kit.

Medicated Honey Formula. This simple product can treat just about any burn, scrape, cut or sore. Buy a plastic squeeze bottle of honey. Don't use raw honey for this purpose as it tends to crystallize, forming sharp points that are painful to burned skin; buy clear, pasteurized, filtered honey or warm raw honey until it is hot to the touch, then strain it through cheesecloth and let it cool. To 1 cup of room-temperature honey, add 1 tablespoon full-strength tea tree oil, 1 teaspoon liquid grapefruit seed extract and 1 tablespoon essential oil of lavender. Honey by itself is a highly effective burn treatment because it seals the skin, protects it from exposure to oxygen, eliminates the need for frequent bandage changes and prevents healing skin from adhering to gauze or fabric.

Most dogs dislike the bitter taste of grapefruit seed extract and the turpentine fragrance of tea tree oil, so they are less likely to lick it off. However, if they do, it won't hurt them. Tea tree oil, grapefruit seed extract and lavender oil can be added in any proportions; the measurements above are only suggestions. They add additional disinfecting, analgesic properties. Label the container "Medicated Honey for Burns and Wounds. External Use." Apply to any infected area.

Aloe Vera. Both the live plant and bottled gel can be applied topically or taken internally to treat cuts, burns, abrasions, hot spots, bites, indigestion, parasites and other conditions. When giving fresh gel from the plant, remember that the inner rind contains a strong laxative. To avoid it, slice the rind off and rinse the gel in cold water. All parts of the rind and gel are safe for external application.

Plant Identification Book. If your puppy swallows a mushroom or chews on your hedge prunings, is he in danger of poisoning himself? What if your kitten attacks a house plant and bites it? There are many well-illustrated guides that simplify the confusing world of plant identification. If you're not familiar with the plants in your yard, find someone who is and tour your backyard with an eye toward potential toxins. Get to know the trees and weeds in your neighborhood. While this information is often more important to the owners of herbivores such as horses, cows and rabbits, it can save time in diagnosing and treating the symptoms of poisoning in other animals as well.

Syrup of Ipecac, Hydrogen Peroxide. Ipecac *(Cephaelis ipecacuanha)* is a South American herb discovered in the 1600s and used in Europe ever since. Its root is famous as an emetic, a substance that induces vomiting; syrup of ipecac is sold in pharmacies.

  The 3-percent solution of hydrogen peroxide commonly sold in drug stores and supermarkets can be given to an animal to force regurgitation. Hydrogen peroxide is widely used as a topical disinfectant, but it is also a bleach and may change the color of a pet's fur.

Activated Charcoal. Available in capsules, tablets and powder, activated charcoal absorbs toxins and poisons. For emergency use, buy the powder.

Dr. Bach's Emergency Formula. Many flower essences are appropriate for first-aid kits, but this remedy (called Rescue Remedy, Calming Essence or Five Flower Formula) and yarrow essence are probably the most important. To prepare a dropper bottle for emergency use, add 4 to 10 drops of flower essence remedy to a 1-ounce dropper bottle filled approximately 1/3 with brandy as a preservative and 2/3 with distilled or pure water. Gently mix well and label. This bottle will keep without refrigeration in your first-aid kit if protected from heat and light. If you don't have a dilute solution on hand, give the remedy directly from its stock bottle.

Homeopathic Remedies. There are so many homeopathic remedies for sick and injured pets that a kit of 50 or more remedies is appropriate, but if you're new to homeopathy, consider keeping the following remedies on hand in the form of tablets or pellets:

Aconitum 30c	*Glonoine 30c*
Apis 30c	*Hypericum 30c*
Arnica montana 30c	*Ledum 30c*
Calendula 6x	*Nux vomica 30c*
Carbo vegetabilis 30c	*Phosphorus 30c*
Ferrum phosphoricum 6x	

Dried Herbs. A small metal can, plastic box or airtight plastic bag of dried plantain, echinacea or comfrey leaf belongs in your kit to pull toxins from bite wounds, infections and injuries. Because their uses vary, keep comfrey and plantain in separate containers. See instructions for applying poultices, compresses and fomentations on pages 127-129.

Some dried herbs are useful for other emergencies. For example, dried cayenne and yarrow are effective styptics which stop bleeding; dried, powdered blackberries are an astringent treatment for diarrhea; powdered slippery elm bark and psyllium husks are soothing to irritated intestinal tracts and are also effective in treating diarrhea.

Tinctures. Arnica tincture treats bruises, sprains and injured muscles. Yarrow tincture or powdered yarrow acts like a styptic pencil to stop bleeding; so does cayenne. Valerian tincture helps a stressed animal relax. Calendula tincture can be applied full-strength to burns or diluted with water to rinse or flush ears and to rinse debris from cuts and wounds. Echinacea tincture fights infection and can be used to treat snake bites. Bee propolis tincture, made from a resinous material produced by honeybees, is often called a natural antibiotic; in addition to fighting infection when taken internally, it can be applied topically to treat insect bites, scabies, mites, hot spots, ringworm fungus, cuts and other wounds.

As you become familiar with herbal preparations, you will find your own favorites. Remember that in an emergency, tinctures and essential oils are the fastest acting, most concentrated herbal preparations available.

Many first-aid kits contain rubbing alcohol, but herbal tinctures made with grain alcohol are preferred by most herbalists and many holistic veterinarians. Whenever rubbing alcohol is recommended for disinfecting purposes, substitute vodka, rum, brandy or an herbal tincture.

Insect/Tick Repellent. This item should be part of your daily grooming routine for outdoor animals, but indoor pets can be exposed to mosquitoes, fleas, flies and other insects, too. For suggested formulas, see pages 171-172.

Clay. Clay is widely revered for its medicinal properties and in some emergencies, it's essential. Clay water can pull toxins from the body, disinfect the intestinal tract and stop a diarrhea attack; a clay poultice helps disperse toxins pulled from the skin by herbs like comfrey, wheat grass or plantain; a thick clay paste can be wrapped around a broken bone with gauze to create a temporary cast. Look for green or bentonite clay at your health food store or herb shop. See also Herbal Melange, page 326.

MISCELLANEOUS SUPPLIES

Gauze Bandages, Cotton, Tape, Q-Tips. A box of 3x3-inch gauze bandages or pads, two rolls of 3-inch gauze, a half-pound roll of cotton and a roll of white porous adhesive tape will absorb blood, protect and cushion wounds, act as a temporary splint, tape a dog's mouth shut as an emergency muzzle and hold bandaging material in place. Nonstick adhesive tape and elastic bandages are often recommended. Long Q-tip sticks can be used — very, very cautiously — to clean ear canals.

Tweezers, Scissors and Other Tools. Use good-quality, all-purpose tweezers for removing ticks and splinters. In addition, keep a pair of sharply pointed tweezers for removing small splinters or thorns. A small magnifying glass can help with all tweezer tasks.

If you live in porcupine territory, keep needle-nose pliers or heavy forceps on hand for quill removal.

Good-quality nail trimmers can be used for routine nail or claw care and to repair broken or torn nails in the field.

Your kit should contain a pair of scissors sharp enough to cut tape quickly and small enough to trim hair away from cuts and other wounds.

It should also contain an empty eye dropper bottle or a small rubber ear syringe for administering liquids by mouth.

Towels and Blankets. A thick beach or bath towel and a warm, thick, strong blanket will help prevent shock and the loss of body heat while cushioning the animal.

Old bath towels can be used to restrain an injured animal. Bath or dish towels can be torn into cloth strips for bandage materials. Keep a roll of paper towels handy for cleaning up.

Thermometer. Buy the short, heavy type appropriate for rectal use, not the long oral human type. Ear thermometers work well in animals that hold still long enough to produce an accurate reading. Practice using the thermometer so you can perform this task in an emergency and, while practicing, write down your pet's normal temperature (take three readings a few days apart) so you have a baseline for comparison.

Salt, Salt Water. A saline solution of pure water (distilled or boiled filtered water is best for this purpose) is an effective wash for cuts, scrapes and other wounds. Add just a pinch of salt, so the solution is about as salty as human tears. For convenience, keep a bottle of pure or distilled water in your kit with a small amount of salt in a plastic bag and add the salt just before using.

Eyewash. In an emergency, use plain water or a slightly saline solution of water and salt to rinse your pet's eyes if they contain foreign matter. When there's time to prepare an eyewash, brew chamomile tea and, as it cools, add a pinch of unrefined sea salt. Filter through cheesecloth, fabric or a coffee filter before rinsing your pet's eyes. Alternatively, add a tiny amount of sea salt to a dilute solution of Willard Water and keep it on hand for emergency use.

Pet Stain and Odor Remover. Enzyme products are essential whenever you're housebreaking a puppy, when an older animal becomes incontinent or sprays in the house or when your pet gets sprayed by a skunk. Keep a quart on hand for emergencies.

Willard Water. A spray bottle of dilute Willard Water solution belongs in your pet's first-aid kit. If desired, add a pinch of unrefined sea salt. Apply to burns, cuts, abrasions or infections before applying salve. This solution can be sprayed or dropped into an animal's eyes as an eyewash or applied by gently pressing a well-soaked cotton ball against the eye.

Plastic Bottles. Plastic pint- or liter-sized soda or water bottles are convenient ice packs and hot water bottles.

For ice packs, fill plastic bottles to within an inch of the top, leaving room for ice expansion, cap tightly and leave in the freezer until needed. Other ice pack material is appropriate for pet use, too, such as sports gel packs and traditional ice bags filled with ice cubes.

When a hot water bottle is needed, fill an empty plastic bottle of the appropriate size with warm (not scalding) water and wrap a towel around it.

Simple Soap. Keep a small plastic bottle of liquid unscented olive oil, castille or vegetable oil soap, not a detergent, dish washing liquid or disinfectant hand soap. Your health food store probably carries at least one brand of vegetable oil soap, such as Dr. Bronner's. Add tea tree oil (see page 186) for disinfectant soap.

Emergency Veterinary Care

Pet emergencies are stressful for everyone: the owner, the animal, friends, family, witnesses and those you call on for help. Don't wait until your dog is hit by a car or your cat is unconscious from exposure to a toxic chemical to find out whether your veterinarian offers 24-hour emergency care. If he or she does not, ask for referrals to clinics that do or look for veterinarians who can accommodate you. Check with local trainers, groomers, humane societies and breed clubs for advice. Some veterinarians make house calls and so do some veterinary ambulance services. Find out what emergency services your community offers and write everything down in one place. It is not unusual for holistically oriented pet owners to have two or even three veterinarians, one for routine matters such as parasite exams, heartworm tests, minor injuries or required rabies vaccinations, another for nutritional support or the treatment of serious conditions and a third for emergencies.

While some emergency clinics are willing to work closely with an animal's regular doctor even if that veterinarian has an entirely different philosophy of healthcare, such as homeopathy or holistic medicine, unfortunately sometimes there is a conflict between what the staff of an emergency hospital wants to do and what the owner or the animal's primary veterinarian prefers. It is difficult to think clearly and assert yourself when people with impressive credentials wearing white lab coats scowl at you and announce in authoritative voices a course of action. Always try to reach your primary veterinarian or a consultant for information and support. If you can't reach anyone, trust yourself. You are the one who's responsible for your pet's life and welfare. You may agree wholeheartedly with an emergency doctor's recommendations, but if you don't, assert yourself.

Keep emergency phone numbers in an obvious place, such as on your refrigerator and in your purse or wallet. Update this information on a regular basis. Anxiety often interferes with one's ability to remember the obvious, so remind yourself from time to time where to look for this information and whatever emergency equipment and reference books you have on hand.

If you travel without your pet, be sure your pet sitter or boarding kennel understands your treatment preferences and is provided with appropriate phone numbers, clear instructions and authorizations.

If you travel with your pet, spend at least some time considering what you would do in different emergencies. If you're going to be in one place for some time, ask holistic veterinary referral services whether they have members in the area or ask your pet's veterinarian for suggestions. Always take at least some first-aid equipment with you. Fortunately, the odds of anything happening are very small; most people hike, hunt, fish, swim, sail and engage in all kinds of outdoor activities with their dogs without mishap. Still, whenever I spend an afternoon reading gory stories in dog magazines or discuss pet injuries, accidents, poisonings and other mishaps with veterinarians, hunters, breeders, trainers and hikers, I think Samantha shouldn't go anywhere without a MediVac helicopter.

It is some consolation to know that a pet born to healthy parents, fed a well-balanced raw diet and treated with holistic medical care is more likely to survive an accident, poisoning or other injury than its conventionally fed, conventionally treated counterpart. Celeste Yarnall practices natural rearing and so do the people who adopt her kittens. When one of her raw-diet, unvaccinated kitties fell from a rooftop, he was rushed to an emergency clinic where the veterinary staff marveled over his strong bones and excellent health; in fact, an attending vet tech realized she had never seen a truly healthy cat before and the following day she called Yarnall to make an appointment to look at her kittens.

The most obvious ways to protect your pet's health are to strengthen the animal with natural care and nutrition, provide a safe, wholesome living environment and prevent accidents before they happen by exercising common sense.

Disaster Plans

I f you live in an area prone to floods, earthquakes, hurricanes, forest fires or similar disasters, you have probably prepared an emergency evacuation plan for your family. Here's how to make one for your pet.

Boarding strategy. Look to the north, south, east and west to friends, relatives, pet-friendly motels, hotels, bed and breakfast inns and boarding facilities that might take your pets in an emergency. Boarding kennels for dogs and cats usually require up-to-date vaccinations. In most cases, unvaccinated animals are either refused, vaccinated by kennel staff or, if space is available, quarantined at additional expense. While holistic boarding kennels are the exception, facilities sympathetic to natural pet care do exist and are worth seeking. There is nothing more stressful to an animal than losing its home and its people at the same time. It is worth making every effort to find a place where you can stay with your pets. By making arrangements or cultivating relationships ahead of time, you are more likely to be welcomed in an emergency.

Identification. Your pet should have more than one form of identification. An ID collar is a must because that's the most visible, familiar and obvious. Pets found without ID tags are assumed to be strays even though they might carry a tattoo or microchip. In addition to collar ID tags, a permanent identification (tattoo or microchip) is a sensible backup.

Carrier, cage or kennel. A sturdy airline-quality plastic, wire or luggage-style carrier should be part of your pet's evacuation plan. Cardboard boxes and pillow cases don't provide adequate protection. Train your cat, rabbit, dog or bird to come when called and enter the carrier; do this by making it a daily game and a pleasant experience. Cats and rabbits can be leash-trained. If there isn't time to transfer your small pet to its carrier, carry it from house to car in a pillow case that's tied closed, but place it in a sturdy carrier as soon as possible.

Evacuation kit. In addition to your regular first-aid kit, prepare a disaster kit for your pet. Keep these supplies in a box, suitcase or tote bag in a convenient place (such as the animal's carrier) where it can be reached quickly. Review the kit periodically to replace stale supplies and revise the contents. Emergency kits are more likely to be remembered and used when they're regularly inspected. The kit should contain the following.

1. First-aid supplies as described above.

2. A week's supply of food for your pet. If you're feeding a natural diet, you won't keep fresh food in the kit, but have a small or medium size cooler on hand for whatever fresh or frozen food you can take with you. Keep a week's supply of nutritional supplements in a tightly sealed plastic bag in the cooler and replace it with fresh supplements on a regular basis. Also, this being an emergency kit, buy a high-quality canned pet food or jars of meat baby foods for your dog or cat in case there isn't anything in the freezer or fridge when disaster strikes. Canned foods are an appropriate emergency ration (keep a hand-operated can opener in the kit as well), especially with added enzymes and other supplements; after the crisis, you can return to a natural diet.

3. Bottled water. Water supplies are often reduced or contaminated during disasters. Keep on hand clear plastic quarts or gallons of the water your pet normally drinks as part of your emergency supplies.

4. Lightweight dishes for food and water. Plastic is not generally recommended, but

in an emergency, lightweight, unbreakable plastic is more reliable and convenient than glass or ceramic.

5. Sanitary supplies. For cats, this means a litter pan and cat litter; for dogs, plastic cleanup bags; for rabbits, whatever the rabbit is used to; for birds, newspaper for lining the cage. Keep a roll of paper towels, a bottle of pet stain remover, a package of wet wipes and some kitchen-sized garbage bags in the kit as well.

6. Medication. If your pet is taking any prescription drugs, keep a supply in a waterproof plastic bag. Be sure your pet's first-aid kit contains Dr. Bach's emergency formula (Rescue Remedy/Calming Essence/Five Flower Formula) and/or herbal tinctures of relaxing nervines such as valerian, skullcap, passionflower, hops, lobelia, chamomile or a blend of nervines. A few drops on the tongue will help your pet sleep well, relax and deal with stress.

7. Copies of important papers including dog license, rabies vaccination, health records, prescriptions, etc., stored in a waterproof plastic bag.

8. Phone numbers. Keep in the kit a current list of numbers for your veterinarian, humane society, animal control office, dog club, friends, pet-friendly motels and anyone who might be able to help you find temporary housing for you and/or your pet.

9. Mylar thermal blanket. This metallic, lightweight blanket, available at sporting supply stores, protects against cold, hypothermia and shock; it takes up much less space than conventional blankets and works well when wet.

10. Extra collar, leash or harness and ID tags.

11. A favorite toy or two.

12. A familiar soft towel or small blanket to help the animal relax and sleep.

Keep all of these items in sturdy tote bags that are easy to carry, stored in or next to your pet's emergency crate or carrier or in an equally obvious location. In an evacuation, take your pet with you if at all possible; don't assume that rescue workers will be able to find or provide for pets left behind. Unfortunately, Red Cross shelters do not admit pets; only service dogs are admitted to these facilities. This is why it's important to plan ahead. Don't wait until a disaster strikes to consider what you might need or where you might go.

Hazards at Home

Accidents can happen any time, but with pets they are most likely to happen when puppies, kittens, dogs or cats are left unsupervised. Young puppies will chew on anything. When my dog was eight weeks old, she was either in her crate or beside us on her leash or at our feet. The day after she arrived, I took her downstairs to my sewing room and left her playing with a rope toy for 30 seconds while I ran around the corner to pull clothes from the washer and toss them in the dryer. By the time I raced back, she was contentedly chewing on a box of black fabric dye. Fortunately, she hadn't broken the package, but that experience sharpened my eye for puppy hazards, and they were everywhere.

Small items like cat toys are not appropriate for teething puppies. Neither are electric cords, phone cords, knives, sharp objects, drapes, carpets, shoes or boots. Puppies swallow amazing things, like rubber gloves, steel wool soap pads, books, door mats, coins, rocks and tubes of toothpaste. One living legend ate a neighbor's chain saw.

Bitter Apple, which is sold in pet supply stores, and other nasty tasting substances, including hot pepper sauce and tea tree oil, can be applied to items you don't want a puppy to chew, but no deterrent will work for every dog. The easiest way to prevent problems is to provide a crate, kennel or cage that is the puppy's private retreat and supply healthy chew toys and raw bones to keep her busy and happy.

Kittens aren't likely to chew your drapes, but they may try to climb them. They'll squeeze behind furniture, jump into open ovens, curl up in clothes dryers, walk across stoves, leap into open windows, hide in file cabinets and otherwise give you a heart attack. Always check and double-check appliances before you turn them on. Kittens love to pounce, but if they swallow or become tangled in dental floss, rubber bands, twine or yarn, their play drive can be fatal.

Keep a close eye on your kitten and when you can't, be sure he or she is in a safe place where accidents aren't waiting to happen. The best toys for kitties are soft and sturdy. Fishing wand toys with long lines should be put away after use because cats playing on their own can become entangled and panic, causing serious injury or even strangulation. Christmas tree ornaments or tinsel, small decorations at any time of year and lit candles are other health hazards.

Don't let your kitten or puppy play with or chew on leather toys from countries where tanning chemicals may leave harmful residues and, when feeding your pet, avoid the use of colorful imported ceramic dishes that might contain lead glaze. Good-quality bottled water is a safeguard against lead in water pipes and other contaminants. Pesticide residues are a concern in catnip as in all foods and herbs; look for organically grown catnip or grow the herb yourself.

Always check pet toys for good construction. Try to pull or pry the toy apart. Look for reinforced stitching, nontoxic materials and a sensible size. Birds are inordinately fond of mirrors, bells, shiny objects and novelties, but the sharp beak of a cockatoo or macaw can demolish anything that isn't built to withstand wire cutters. Look at every prospective purchase while asking yourself, "What's the worst that could happen?" Cat tunnels should be smooth inside, with no sharp edges that could scratch. Cat trees and scratching posts should have a solid, heavy, stable base to prevent tipping. Jingle bells are a questionable addition to cat toys; if your cat tends to rip toys apart, a tiny jingle bell is a health hazard. If your dog tears soft toys to shreds, give her rope chews and other toys that are built to last.

The most important feature of any pet's toy is its owner's good sense. No toy is 100 percent safe in all circumstances, but an observant caretaker can prevent most accidents before they happen.

Every day pets are taken to emergency rooms for the treatment of preventable tragedies. Dogs tied to truck or car bumpers are badly scraped when people drive away without untying them; cats seeking warmth in winter climb into automobile engine compartments and are badly hurt when someone starts the car; dogs traveling in cars or pickup trucks go through windshields and are thrown out of storage compartments; pets fall out of open windows; dogs and cats drink water in toilet bowls containing continual-release cleaning products; declawed cats are allowed to jump on balcony ledges by people who forget that without claws they can't hold on the way they used to; birds fly out of open doors and windows; dogs wearing choke chains are strangled on all kinds of things; pets can be suffocated by plastic bags, even by the plastic liners of empty cereal boxes; rabbits have died from loud noises, such as music from stereo headphones held to their ears; pets of every description are left in hot cars in the hot sun; dogs have died from eating the fragrant garden mulch made from cocoa hulls; the list is endless.

Pets riding in cars should be fitted with seatbelt harnesses or carriers that attach to seatbelts. If your car has a passenger-side air bag, don't let your dog sit up front; just as children have been decapitated in minor accidents when these safety features inflate, dogs can be fatally injured. A dog riding in the back of a pickup truck should be in an attached kennel that prevents him from jumping out and protects him, at least to some extent, if the truck is in an accident. At home, window screens should be checked and repaired. Hazards such as broken glass, antifreeze, rat poison, garden chemicals, prescription drugs, sharp objects, bleaches, cleansers and electrical cords should be removed, locked away or placed where they are less likely to shorten the life of your companion animal.

Think of your puppy, kitten or bird as a mischief-making two-year-old and do everything you can to child-proof and pet-proof your home, car, truck, boat, camper and garden shed.

Poisons, Pesticides and Other Chemical Hazards

Commercial pesticides and pets are *not* compatible. Chemical flea dips, flea collars, tick collars and insecticide sprays place a serious burden on the animals they treat. Every veterinarian I spoke with mentioned these "safe" chemicals as contributing to the health problems of America's dogs, cats and other pets. In addition, accidental exposure to toxic chemicals is a leading cause of death.

Even the recommended use of a lawn or garden pesticide can be harmful. Pets often display symptoms of poisoning after their owners' lawns are planted with chemically treated grass seed or sprayed with herbicides or other chemicals.

A few years ago our townhouse was sprayed by a tree service whose driver went to the wrong address. We filed a complaint with the New York State Department of Environmental Protection and when the inspector visited, he told us one horror story after another, most involving legally applied pesticides that killed dogs, cats, horses and birds. His work has convinced him to avoid all pesticides, even "benign" chemicals made from plant sources, and he had nothing good to say about Integrated Pest Management, the latest buzz word in agricultural circles. It's one thing to read dry statistics and official reassurances; they make chemical problems sound remote and unlikely. It's entirely different to hear a state official describe his hands-on experiences with dead and dying animals, ecological disruption and other chaos caused by the lawful application of lawn and garden chemicals.

Dogs are frequent victims of accidental poisoning because of their mobility and curiosity, but all pets are at risk. Sweet-tasting automobile antifreeze, ant or roach bait, rat poison, chips of lead-based paint and household products like toilet bowl cleaner, dishwasher detergent, paint remover, garden chemicals, prescription drugs and recreational drugs are only a few of the hazards that have shortened the lives of America's companion animals.

Agricultural chemicals pose such a threat that many farms, commercial orchards, ranches and large greenhouse operations keep emergency medical equipment, including intravenous drips, oxygen and antidote drugs, on hand for animals exposed to organophosphates, defoliants and other commonly used chemicals.

Help! What Should I Do?

The most important first step in treating a poisoned pet is accurate identification. What did the animal drink, breathe, touch or walk on? All hazardous products sold in the U.S. carry warning labels with instructions for emergency care, some saying to induce vomiting at once, others warning not to induce vomiting but to flush the body with large quantities of milk or water or to administer mineral or vegetable oil orally.

Some products carry their own emergency phone numbers for 24-hour assistance.

Always read the label of a product before using it. Keep the original container or copy the emergency treatment information before disposing of the container.

If your product's emergency information is confusing or if you can't find it, phone the ASPCA National Animal Poison Control Center (see Resources for this chapter, page 503) or call your veterinarian and authorize him or her to do so on your behalf.

Observe the animal carefully so that you can describe his or her symptoms. Typical symptoms of poisoning are:

• Muscle twitches, tremors and convulsions

• Loss of bodily fluids through vomiting, drooling,
diarrhea, tearing, involuntary urination and nasal discharge

• Abdominal cramping and diarrhea or vomiting

The animal's breathing may be labored or shallow; the pulse may be rapid or slow; the eyes may be dilated and unfocused; or there may be other symptoms. Note the symptoms your animal is displaying, their severity and how long they have lasted.

In cases of poisoning, time is of the essence. So is knowing the correct protocol. If the ingested substance is an acid, alkali, petroleum distillate or an irritating plant such as fresh nettle, do not induce vomiting. These substances are easily breathed into the lungs or may cause other damage if regurgitated. Acids include household cleaning agents and bleaches; alkalis include lye, drain cleaner, laundry detergents, ammonia and paint removers. Petroleum distillates include gasoline, kerosene, paint thinners and charcoal lighting fluid. Nettles include not only the beneficial herb with its irritating, burning sting, but the bull nettle and nettle spurge as well. *Do not* induce vomiting if your pet swallows one of these substances. Instead, rinse the mouth and any parts of the body that came in contact with the substance and give 1 to 2 tablespoons of vegetable oil, cooking oil or mineral oil. To speed the removal of toxins from the body, feed small amounts of substances that will absorb or bind with toxins, such as wheat grass juice or clay water. Juliette de Bairacli Levy often recommended castor oil and in France and other European countries, magnesium chloride (Epsom salts) is the preferred purgative laxative.

If the substance is not caustic and you know your pet has ingested the material, don't wait for symptoms to develop. Induce vomiting immediately. If symptoms are already obvious, your quick action is even more important. Most veterinary experts agree that removing the toxic substance from the animal's digestive tract is a crucial first step in emergency treatment. Chemical bird repellents, rat poisons, herbicides, insecticides, fertilizers, soil-sterilizing chemicals, fungicides, heartworm-preventive medicines, pharmaceutical drugs, chocolate, antifreeze, automobile brake fluid, transmission fluid, lead paint, wood preservatives, tobacco, poisonous mushrooms, bufo frogs, poisonous California salamanders, toxic house or garden plants and illegal drugs are potentially fatal to small animals. Note that many of these toxins have complicated treatment protocols. While the first-aid steps outlined here are the only treatment an animal needs for some exposures, they are merely an essential first step in helping animals recover from others.

Emetics and Activated Charcoal

To induce vomiting, give your pet any one of the following emetics with the aid of a spoon, eyedropper or small syringe:

- 1 heaping teaspoon salt dissolved in 1 cup warm water, 1 teaspoon (small animal) to 1 tablespoon (large animal) every 15 minutes, three doses maximum; or

- 1 to 2 teaspoons of 3-percent hydrogen peroxide plain or mixed with milk every 10 minutes, three doses maximum; or

- 2 to 3 teaspoons of syrup of ipecac, given once; or

- small amounts of soapy water (use a simple soap, not dishwashing liquid).

Do not induce vomiting if the animal is unconscious or in a stupor.

Not all animals will respond to these treatments. If yours has the undisturbable digestion of a goat, veterinary treatment may be necessary. Always keep your veterinarian's phone number and the phone numbers of the Animal Poison Control Center with you so you can obtain the information and assistance you need in an emergency.

If you have Dr. Bach's emergency formula (Rescue Remedy, Five Flower Formula or Calming Essence), rub it into your pet's gums, spray the animal lightly or both. Take some yourself. This flower essence helps calm the stress and anxiety felt by all involved.

While waiting for the emetic to work, mix activated charcoal with enough water to form a liquid consistency and give 1 teaspoon to animals weighing less than 25 pounds or 2 teaspoons for dogs weighing more. Place the slurry in the animal's cheek if he or she doesn't want to swallow it. Repeat this treatment after the animal regurgitates.

If the poison is caustic and you should not induce vomiting, give activated charcoal immediately. In either case, give up to 1/8 cup of the slurry to a small animal and up to 1 cup to a large one.

In all cases of poisoning, wrap your pet in a blanket to prevent shock. Keep the animal warm and as quiet as possible.

Homeopathy: Give 2 pellets of *Nux vomica 30c* whole or crushed on the tongue every 15 minutes for a total of three doses. If symptoms worsen, do not continue this treatment.

Follow-up Treatment

Depending on the poison involved, your animal may require extensive medical care. No matter how simple or complicated the protocol, you can support the follow-up therapy with herbs and nutritional supplements.

Herbal Therapy: Wheat grass and wheat grass juice help prevent toxic reactions and rid the body of toxic metals, harmful inorganic chemicals and other poisons. Wheat grass juice or other green juices or powders given in small, frequent doses can supplement whatever medical treatment your pet requires, and they can be given at any time, including while you are waiting for an emetic to work or while you are treating an animal that should not be forced to regurgitate.

I have used the Austrian product Herbal Melange for years and would definitely feed it to a pet exposed to anything toxic. Herbal Melange is a dark mud-like beverage concentrate from peat moors. Extensive European research has shown that Herbal Melange stimulates digestion and the absorption of nutrients, absorbs gas, binds acid, lowers alcohol levels, reduces cholesterol, helps repel parasites and harmful bacteria and detoxifies the entire gastrointestinal system.

Any animal recovering from exposure to a poison has an overworked liver, for the liver is the body's primary filter of toxins. Milk thistle seed powders, teas and tinctures help repair liver damage and are appropriate additions to the diet for weeks or months after toxic exposure.

Poison Prevention

Chemical exposure doesn't have to come from the great outdoors. Mothballs destroy liver cells and a cat locked in a moth-treated closet can be seriously harmed. Furniture polish, air fresheners and other household products hold similar dangers. So do outgassing carpets, solvents, paints, tobacco smoke and construction materials.

"Sick building syndrome" affects pets as well as people. Insufficient air circulation, electromagnetic hazards, toxic construction materials, paints, glues and contaminated water are all potential hazards. Wherever possible, use nontoxic building materials, paints, natural carpet and carpet mats, etc. Keep doors and windows open as much as possible. Install air filters and a jungle of house plants in hanging baskets and other locations that are not accessible to your pet. Let your pet spend as much time breathing fresh air and exposed to natural light as possible, either outdoors or in an open window.

Read pet products labels carefully. Never use a dog product on a cat and always follow directions to the letter. Even products labeled natural, organic or holistic can pose
hazards. Unfortunately, some of the most potentially toxic products have the most confusing label instructions. A feline friend of mine was poisoned by his well-intentioned
family when they couldn't make sense of the directions on a supermarket flea dip and
used too strong a concentration.

In addition to the environmental hazards they face, pets may be exposed to pesticides and other chemicals in the food they eat. Most farm animals raised for human consumption in the U.S. are fed grain or fodder treated with pesticides, antibiotics and hormones, residues of which remain in their organs and muscles. Remember that animals
in the 4-D category (dead, diseased, dying or disabled), which are rejected for human
use, are denatured before being sent to rendering plants. Denaturing is any process that
makes a substance so unpalatable that no one will consume it. Grain alcohol is denatured before being sold at low cost for external application; the result smells and tastes
so terrible that no one is tempted to drink it, thus protecting state and federal government alcohol tax revenues. The denaturing of diseased and contaminated meat is a similar process, this one designed to protect human health. If 4-D carcasses were left undisturbed, they would probably find their way to market, but denatured meat is so
obviously tainted that no one tries to sell it as food for people. As Wendell O.
Belfield reported in "A Gruesome Account of Food Not Fit for a Pet" in the May
1992 edition of *Let's Live,* the denaturing materials approved by federal meat
inspection regulations are fuel oil, kerosene, crude carbolic acid and citronella.
Belfield was a veterinary meat inspector for the U.S. Department of Agriculture and
the State of California for seven years, and he saw first-hand the chemical treatment
of condemned carcasses sent to rendering plants that turned them into ingredients
for pet food.

In addition to residues of denaturing chemicals and the antibiotics and hormones fed to farm animals raised as meat, there are traces of other drugs in pet
foods. On February 19, 1990, the *San Francisco Chronicle* printed the second of two
articles by investigative reporter John Eckhouse documenting questionable ingredients in pet foods. The articles raised a storm of controversy and indignant denials
by pet food industry executives, but the facts are as Eckhouse stated. Federal and
state agencies, including the Food and Drug Administration, the American
Veterinary Medical Association and state veterinary organizations all confirm that
dogs, cats and other pets are routinely rendered after they die in animal shelters or
are disposed of by health authorities, and the end product, labeled tallow, meat
meal or bone meal, serves as raw material for pet foods. According to veterinary
researchers quoted by Eckhouse, many of these dead pets were given the euthaniz-
ing drug sodium pentobarbital, which is not removed or altered by the rendering

process. In addition to containing trace amounts of sodium pentobarbital, rendered products are preserved with chemicals such as BHA (butylated hydroxyanisole) and BHT (butylated hydroxytoluene), both known to cause kidney and liver dysfunction. Their use is prohibited in several European countries. Ethoxyquin, another fat stabilizer in common use, has been the subject of many articles in holistic pet magazines, for it is a suspected carcinogen and has been linked with a number of possible health problems in animals. Propylene glycol, an ingredient in semimoist pet foods, is chemically similar to the antifreeze ethylene glycol and it destroys red blood cells.

While the trace amounts of toxic chemicals, lead and other contaminants in commercial pet foods won't cause the dramatic symptoms of acute poisoning, their cumulative effects can be detrimental to any animal. Pets being weaned from commercial pet foods in favor of a raw, natural diet usually benefit from the daily use of wheat grass and other green foods, antioxidant vitamins and minerals, herbs that support the liver, other detoxifying herbs or supplements and occasional doses of activated charcoal to help rid the body of accumulated toxins.

Poisonous Plants

Any plant, even the most beneficial herb, can cause digestive distress or other symptoms if consumed in large quantities, but some plants are more toxic than others. Few adult cats or dogs are attracted to dangerous plants, but a playful kitten or chewing puppy might ingest anything. An adult retriever might play with garden prunings, and any pet that touches plant secretions may ingest them while grooming. Toxic plants include Barbados (kukui) nut, castor bean, dumb cane (dieffenbachia), English holly, purple foxglove, poison hemlock, water hemlock, horse chestnut, hydrangea, English ivy, great or mountain laurel, lily of the valley bulb, amanita and other mushrooms, deadly nightshade, oleander, pokeweed, privet, black walnut hulls, English walnuts and yew.

Some of these, like black walnut hulls, are beneficial in small amounts added to food but in larger quantities can produce vomiting, diarrhea and convulsions. Apple seeds contain cyanide, and a small animal that consumes several apple cores might display the symptoms of cyanide poisoning, which include red gums, involuntary elimination, convulsions, labored breathing and coma. Cyanide poisoning can also be caused by various cherries, hydrangeas and apricots. Laurels cause vomiting, excessive salivation, abdominal pain, weakness and staggering. Some toxic mushrooms kill by destroying the liver; symptoms of amanita mushroom poisoning include vomiting, bloody diarrhea, trembling and weakness. Pruning your garden's landscaping plants may expose your pet to privet, yew or oleander trimmings that cause vomiting, abdominal pain, diarrhea and other symptoms.

the holiday poinsettia contains an irritant sap that can cause skin inflammation, vomiting or diarrhea, but it is not fatally poisonous the way castor beans and foxglove leaves are.

If you know your house and garden plants and the symptoms they cause, you will be able to make intelligent decisions about an exposed animal's treatment. For more detailed information about specific plants and their adverse side effects, see the recommended reading list for this chapter. As with all health hazards, common sense is your best guide. Don't let your puppy play with the daffodil bulbs you plant in autumn, don't toss potentially toxic shrub prunings for your retriever to fetch, don't drag a kitty string up the sides of your dieffenbachia and keep toxic vegetation out of bird and rabbit cages.

Treating an Injured Animal

Injured animals are unpredictable. The most gentle dog or cat may snarl or bite in pain or fear. If your pet will enter his carrier or if your dog will enter your car, it may be possible to drive to an animal hospital without mishap. If not, it may be necessary to restrain your pet, not only to protect yourself from a bite or scratch but to protect him from additional injury.

Calming Your Pet

Spray the area around your injured animal with Dr. Bach's emergency formula. Speak gently, softly and reassuringly; say your animal's name. Approach from behind or from the side.

If your pet will allow you to do so, place several drops of Dr. Bach's emergency formula in his mouth or place them on your finger and massage his gums; place two pellets of homeopathic *Arnica 30c* on the tongue every 15 minutes for a total of three treatments; or calm the animal with several drops of valerian, chamomile or lobelia tincture. If your pet is extremely upset and likely to bite, dissolve any of these remedies in a small amount of milk or water and squirt or drip it into his mouth from a safe distance using a rubber ear syringe or rubber eye dropper.

If your animal seems reassured by your presence and does not struggle to get away, center yourself by relaxing and breathing slowly and deeply. Position your hands just above his fur or feathers and gently stroke from head to tail as described in the section on Therapeutic Touch, page 227.

Massage his ears, assuming they haven't been injured. The tips of the ears are especially sensitive and responsive. Run his ears through your fingers by pressing each ear between your thumb and forefinger and slide your hand from base to tip.

By lightly stroking and massaging your pet, by giving him flower essences or calming herbs, by speaking calmly and by focusing your own thoughts, you can interrupt the panic, hysteria and fear that might cause further injury and which interfere with your pet's self-healing mechanisms.

If Your Pet Is Unconscious

Is your animal breathing? This is the first vital sign to check in cases of drowning, lightning strike or electric shock and whenever an animal is unconscious. Gently turn her on her side and watch her lungs, place your hand over her chest and check for any rise and fall, place a mirror under her nose and watch for the condensation that accompanies exhalation or place your ear next to her nostrils and listen for sounds of breathing.

Is her heart beating? Place your ear on her chest and listen or place your hand on her chest from the side, just under the armpit, and feel for a pulse.

If your pet is breathing, *do not* give her artificial respiration or cardiopulmonary resuscitation (CPR). If she is in a dangerous location, such as on a road, move her to safety; if possible, slide her onto a board or a tautly held blanket without bending her spine or changing her body's position. Check her for injuries, try to stop any bleeding, massage Dr. Bach's emergency formula onto her gums, give her a dose of homeopathic *Arnica 30c*, wrap her in a blanket to keep her warm and get her to a veterinarian as quickly as possible.

If she has been pulled from the water, hold her upside down by her hind legs to allow water and fluid to drain from her airway; gently pound on her lungs to accelerate the removal of fluid.

You are probably familiar with the Heimlich maneuver, which has saved many choking victims. The maneuver has helped drowning victims as well, for it clears obstructions from the trachea and sometimes triggers breathing on its own. To perform the Heimlich maneuver on a dog or cat, lift the animal to a four-legged standing position and, if possible, elevate the front of the body slightly. Form a fist with one hand and place it in the animal's solar plexus, which is a network of sympathetic nerves and ganglia high in the back of the abdomen; position your hand in the center of the upper abdomen just below the rib cage. In people, this position is directly above the navel. For small animals, use your bent thumb or a fingertip. Cover your fist or finger with your other hand and with both hands abruptly thrust upward into the abdomen, aiming toward the head. This action forces air out of the lungs and clears the breathing passageway. You will of course need far more force on a Rottweiler than a kitten, so practice on yourself to try to gauge the impact you will need for your pet. Performed too forcefully this procedure can cause injury, so err on the side of caution when you first try it. If nothing happens, repeat the maneuver using additional force if necessary. If the animal does not respond by breathing on her own, give her artificial respiration. Open her mouth, pull her tongue out and check the back of her throat to be sure there are no obstructions. Clear away any mucus, blood or debris that's in the way and replace her tongue.

If your homeopathy kit is handy, place two pellets of *Carbo vegetabilis 30c* on her tongue. Hold her mouth closed and place your mouth over her nostrils. Exhale and breathe into her nose, filling her lungs, then release your mouth and let her exhale. Breathe in six times per minute (every 10 seconds) for a dog and 12 times per minute (every five seconds) for a cat.

No Breathing, No Pulse

If your pet's heartbeat has stopped, use a needle, pin, your fingernail or a sharp object to press or jab the emergency acupressure point under her nose (see page 217).

If she does not respond, alternate mouth-to-mouth resuscitation with external heart massage or CPR. Place your animal on her side on a firm surface. For a cat or small dog, use one hand; for a larger animal, use two. Press firmly over the lower chest directly behind the elbow and release quickly. Do this once per second, 60 times per minute. Don't press too hard, for too much pressure can cause additional injuries. Use a firm but gentle percussive touch.

Check her gums as well as her pulse. When the heart stops beating, the gums become pale from lack of blood; when it resumes, they become pink again. As soon as her heartbeat resumes, discontinue the CPR. As soon as her breathing resumes, discontinue the artificial respiration.

After five minutes of mouth-to-nose resuscitation and/or CPR, place two pellets of *Arnica 30c* on her tongue.

Beginning five minutes later and repeating the treatment every five minutes until breathing resumes, place several drops of Dr. Bach's emergency formula in her mouth, on her nose, behind her ears, on her abdomen and on her paw pads. If you're working alone, place the drops in her mouth and don't worry about applying it elsewhere. After her breathing is restored, give the flower essence every 30 minutes until you reach help.

If conditions permit, perform a color tonation by shining lemon yellow light on the animal's face and front side. Follow with magenta over the heart.

If Your Pet Is Bleeding

If the animal is bleeding, your first priority should be to stop the flow of blood. To protect yourself from a possible bite or scratch, especially if the animal seems agitated, badly frightened or about to panic, slowly approach from behind or from the side and place a towel or blanket over him, then gather the animal and blanket together to complete the restraint. Don't try to move him if you suspect a fracture of the neck or back. If appropriate, fashion a temporary muzzle for a dog that might bite by looping a long gauze or fabric strip over the nose and mouth; tie it once under the chin, then tie the ends over the top of the neck. Tie the muzzle with a single loop that is easy to untie quickly. Do not muzzle a dog that is vomiting, has trouble breathing or has a flat face or small nostrils.

To stop the bleeding of a wound, first locate the source of bleeding. Flush the wound with salt water or plain water to remove any debris that might cause further injury. If the animal has long hair, cut hair away from the wound so you can see what you're doing.

If you don't have any supplies with you, do the best you can with a scarf, handkerchief, T-shirt, your belt or the dog's leash, whatever you can use to create a pressure bandage.

If the wound has been bleeding severely, don't try to clean or treat it when bleeding stops. Disturbing the dressing or bandage might cause bleeding to resume. Get the animal to an emergency clinic as soon as possible.

When the application of pressure is successful, bleeding usually stops within five to ten minutes. If you cannot stop bleeding from a leg or the tail, apply a tourniquet just above the bleeding area by wrapping a strip of clean fabric or a heavy rubber band just tightly enough to stop the bleeding. As soon as it stops, clean the wound with warm salt water and pack the wound with styptic herbs (see below) to prevent bleeding from resuming when you release the tourniquet. After five minutes, slowly loosen the tourniquet. Retighten it if bleeding resumes. Try to estimate how much blood your animal has lost so that you can report it to your veterinarian.

Herbal Therapy: Pack the wound with powdered cayenne pepper or powdered yarrow, both of which have styptic properties, or dilute yarrow tincture or calendula tincture with a small amount of water and apply it to the wound. Using a clean towel or gauze pads (dry, coated with a soft, healing salve or saturated with diluted tincture), press down on the wound for five to ten minutes. If this does not stop the bleeding, press a nonstick bandage to the wound (use nonstick bandage material or coat a gauze pad or fabric with salve or honey as described on page 334) and secure it by wrapping gauze around the leg or body. The wrap should be snug enough to hold the pressure bandage in place but not so tight that it restricts the animal's breathing or circulation. Hold the gauze wrap in place with adhesive tape. Watch the animal carefully; if swelling occurs or the animal has trouble breathing, remove the wrap at once. Use a tourniquet only to slow uncontrollable bleeding.

Alternatively, apply a comfrey or plantain poultice (see page 127) or cover the wound with a thick layer of honey or a soft herbal salve. Hold the poultice in place or protect the wound with gauze bandages. Fresh comfrey or plantain leaf can be mashed, chewed or simply applied whole and held in place with a pressure bandage; dried comfrey or plantain can be applied as a dry powder, softened with water and applied as a poultice or brewed as a strong tea with cool water and applied as a compress. Of these two herbs, both of which are highly regarded by American herbalists, comfrey seals wounds faster because it contains the cell growth stimulant allantoin. I know people who have treated deep cuts in their own hands or legs with fresh comfrey by tying the herb in place with bandages and leaving it undisturbed for several hours. By the time the poultice was removed, the skin had healed over the cut, embedding pieces of the herb. Comfrey was their only treatment and their deep cuts healed rapidly without infection, complications or scarring.

Homeopathy: Give three doses of *Arnica 30c* 15 minutes apart. If the animal doesn't improve, give three doses of *Phosphorus 30c* 15 minutes apart.

To protect against shock, keep the animal warm by filling a plastic soda bottle with warm water, wrapping it in a small towel and placing it against him. The animal should be lying on and covered by a towel or blanket.

Internal Bleeding. Because internal bleeding is not visible, check for it by inspecting your pet's gums. Blood loss is usually reflected by a color change from reddish pink to pale pink, white or grey. This is very serious and requires prompt veterinary treatment. On your way to the hospital, do what you can to keep the animal calm and warm. Use blankets and warm water bottles to help prevent shock.

Homeopathy: To treat internal bleeding, give three doses of *Arnica 30c*, one every 15 minutes. If that is not sufficient, give one tablet of *Ferrum phos. 6x* every hour for four treatments.

Herbal Therapy: Cayenne pepper and yarrow are natural styptics. If your pet is bleeding internally, mix powdered cayenne, hot pepper sauce, yarrow tincture or powdered yarrow with a small amount of milk or water and give it by mouth. Any combination of these ingredients may be helpful, in just about any quantity. Another herb that helps stop bleeding is shepherd's purse. If the animal is unconscious, place a small amount of any liquid styptic in the side of the mouth and wait for her to swallow before giving more.

Burns and Scalds

The first step in treating any burn or scald is to cool the skin. Immerse the burned body part in cold water, pour cold water over it or hold ice to it. Another burn-cooling treatment is the application of a grain alcohol tincture. A badly burned man was treated with calendula tincture at an herb farm when he carelessly ignited the brush he was clearing. He was treated with calendula tincture before being taken to the hospital emergency room and, by the time he arrived, his skin was already healing. The tincture had stopped the burn, removed the heat, disinfected the injury and stimulated rapid repair.

Herbal Therapy: After removing heat from the burn and covering the skin with calendula, chamomile, St. John's wort or comfrey tincture or full strength aloe vera juice or gel or lavender essential oil or a dilute solution of tea tree oil, cover the burn with a generous coating of plain honey or the honey salve described on page 312. As beekeeper Ross Conrad reported in a 1993 edition of the *Northeast Herbal Association Journal,* when honey is the only dressing, burns heal quickly and dressing changes are painless and require no scraping. Coating a burn with honey retards oxygenation by sealing the wound, which alleviates pain within seconds. Honey is hydroscopic, absorbing moisture from its surroundings, so it doesn't dry out and its pH is too acid for bacterial growth.

Ever since a chemist burned his hand and impulsively plunged it into a vat of pure lavender oil, this essential oil has been recognized as an effective burn treatment. If applied immediately, lavender oil by itself can prevent pain, blistering and further tissue damage. Similar claims are made for tea tree oil. When treating animals, do not apply tea tree oil full-strength; dilute it first with an equal quantity of carrier oil.

If you don't have honey or a honey salve, apply an appropriate tincture or essential oil and cover the area with a thick layer of soft salve containing skin-healing herbs such as calendula, St. John's wort and comfrey (see page 130).

Alternatively, dilute an alcohol tincture such as calendula or chamomile tincture with twice as much water, soak a thick gauze pad and place it over the burn. Hold it in place with a bandage. Don't let the gauze dry out; apply more solution as needed.

Vitamin E is well known as a wound healer. Its application to any burn, abrasion or cut will help prevent infection and scarring. Empty the contents of a natural vitamin E-complex capsule by pricking one end with a pin or scissor and squeezing the oil out.

To help your pet relax and rest, administer valerian or chamomile tincture by mouth using about 1/8 teaspoon per 5 to 7 pounds of body weight; give a 10-pound dog or cat 1/4 teaspoon and a 60-pound dog 1 teaspoon. If your valerian or chamomile tincture is extra-strength, made according to the directions on page 127, use half that amount.

Homeopathy: Administer *Arnica 30c* every 15 minutes for up to three doses. If available, follow with *Cantharis 30c* every 15 minutes for up to six doses.

Flower Essences: Give several drops of Dr. Bach's emergency formula and/or yarrow essence or yarrow special formula every 15 to 20 minutes.

Color Therapy: Shine blue and indigo on the affected area until the pain subsides; an extended tonation may be useful. Follow this with turquoise and green systemics that includes the affected areas. If kidney function is affected, treat with scarlet over the kidney area as well.

Heat Stress, Heat Stroke, Heat Prostration

Pets left in hot rooms or closed cars develop heat stroke in summer; so do dogs working in fields or on long hikes. Dogs and cats cannot dissipate heat by sweating. Their only way to cool down is by panting.

To prevent or reduce heat stress, which is not life-threatening, let your pet become accustomed to climate changes naturally and gradually, the way animals adapt in the wild. Schedule long walks for earlier or later in the day but spend some time outdoors during warmer hours, too. Unless your climate is dangerously hot, your pet can be comfortable for short periods. Stay in the shade, have ample water on hand for drinking and to spray on your pet, pour water on his coat or let him cool down in a creek, pond or pool. Indoors, keep air circulating with a fan and have a cool surface for your pet to lie on, such as a tile floor or the cool metal floor of a wire kennel. Keep your bird's cage in the shade. Outdoors, use a well-ventilated dog house in a shady location with a cool sleeping surface.

If your dog is panting from the heat, fill empty plastic bottles with water, freeze them and let him lie on them. Young puppies, especially those from breeds that thrive in cold climates, love frozen-water-bottle pillows. Any of the adaptogen herbs, such as ginseng or fo-ti, can help an animal adjust to climate changes.

Never leave your pet in a car during hot summer months. The temperature in a closed car can increase several degrees a minute and quickly reach 150° F.

Brain damage occurs when the body's temperature reaches 106° to 107°F. The symptoms of heat stroke or heat prostration include a warm nose and foot pads, glazed eyes, heavy panting, rapid pulse, a dark red tongue, fever, dizziness, vomiting or diarrhea.

To treat heat stroke, work fast. Move the animal to a shaded area. If you can't lift the animal yourself, find someone to help you. Two or three people may be needed to lift a large dog. Have someone call the police and a local veterinarian. If there's a stream, pond, fountain, horse trough or bath tub nearby, gently immerse the animal in cool water. Otherwise, wet the animal thoroughly, beginning with the head and extremities. Pour a continuous stream of water from a hose, watering can, bottle or pan, or saturate towels and wrap them around your pet's legs, abdomen, neck and chest. If you have ice, place ice packs or frozen water bottles around the head, body and feet; rub ice on the gums.

Place a pinch of unrefined sea salt on your pet's tongue or dissolve 1/4 teaspoon salt in 1 cup water and give the animal half a dropperful every 10 minutes.

Homeopathy: The homeopathic remedies recommended for heat exhaustion are *Glonoine 30c* and *Bryonia 30c.* Use *Glonoine* unless the animal is nauseated, in which case *Bryonia* is the preferred treatment. Place 2 pellets on the tongue.

Flower Essences: Administer Dr. Bach's emergency formula every 10 minutes until you reach the animal hospital.

Color Therapy: Scarlet systemic front and back. This color is appropriate because although red shades tend to be warming rather than cooling, heat prostration usually brings a drop in blood temperature and circulatory failure.

Acupressure : Stimulate point SP6.

Hypothermia, Frostbite

Hypothermia and frostbite are serious disorders. While dogs and cats can survive exposure to very cold weather, doing so requires acclimation. Indoor pets shouldn't be left outdoors in cold weather unless they can make the transition gradually.

Hypothermia is a thorough chilling that causes the body's core temperature to drop below normal, to as little as 94 to 96 degrees F. An animal suffering from hypothermia shivers excessively, breathes shallowly and appears uncoordinated and disoriented. Frostbite is the freezing of small blood vessels in the skin, causing blood to clot, and unless treated promptly, tissue fed by affected blood vessels dies. Ear tips, tails and foot pads are common frostbite locations. Pale or reddened skin, especially in the extremities, and white or whitish hair are the main symptoms. Seek emergency veterinary care at once if your pet is in severe pain or is aggressively biting or licking the area. Frostbite causes permanent damage, especially if the skin is injured or mutilated. To treat frostbite at home, wrap your pet in a blanket, have the animal stand in ankle- or knee-deep warm (not hot) water or wrap him in towels heated in a clothes dryer.

Herbal Therapy: Soak a towel in warm oatstraw, comfrey, chamomile or calendula tea and place it over white or frozen body parts. Thawing the skin this way helps prevent gangrene and tissue damage, but you must act immediately to be successful. Brew the tea with hot tap water if necessary; cool it to lukewarm with ice and apply as a warm compress. Because comfrey contains allantoin, a powerful cell growth stimulant, keep powdered comfrey root or dried comfrey leaves are ideal for this purpose. If you don't have comfrey, oatstraw, chamomile or calendula on hand, pour hot water over oatmeal and use the milky white liquid.

Give the animal vitamin E, 400 IU for cats and dogs weighing up to 50 pounds and 800 IU for large and giant dogs. In addition, puncture a vitamin E capsule and spread the liquid on affected skin after treating it with a warm herb tea compress.

Apply aloe vera juice or gel as a final treatment. Continue applying comfrey, vitamin E and aloe vera until the area heals. If skin breaks open and falls away, see your veterinarian.

Flower Essences: Give Dr. Bach's emergency formula or a yarrow formula at once. Administer every 10 to 15 minutes.

Puncture Wounds

Teeth, claws, thorns, porcupine quills and other sharp objects puncture the skin and often trap infection.

Wash the wound with plain soap and water and/or flush it with salt water, calendula or echinacea tincture diluted in 2 to 3 parts water, grapefruit seed extract diluted in 4 to 5 parts water, a 15-percent tea tree oil solution, a similar wash made with lavender oil or a medicinal-strength herbal tea made with plantain, echinacea, sage, thyme or other antiseptic, disinfecting herbs.

Use tweezers, your fingernails or whatever tool you have to pull embedded hair from the puncture and rinse the wound again.

Herbal Therapy: Mash a fresh plantain leaf, mix dried plantain with water to make a thick paste, mash or grind fresh wheat grass to a pulp or mix powdered wheat grass or a similar green grass powder with water and apply the herb as a poultice. Alternatively, cover the wound with a thick layer of plantain salve. Note that comfrey is not usually recommended for puncture wounds because it heals the skin so quickly that infection may be trapped inside. Plantain and wheat grass are "drawing" herbs; they help pull embedded splinters, thorns, hair, debris and infection from wounds. Keep the poultice or salve in place with a gauze bandage.

Homeopathy: Give the animal *Ledum 30c,* 2 pellets every two hours for a total of four doses.

Flower Essences: Give Dr. Bach's emergency formula and/or yarrow flower essence or yarrow special formula. Give either or both of these emergency flower essences every

15 to 30 minutes for the first hour or two, then give the essence two or three times a day as the animal recovers or whenever you think it would be helpful.

Color Therapy: Indigo on the affected area until bleeding stops, then turquoise systemic to include the effected area and green and magenta on the area.

Snake Bite

Few injuries are so alarming and terrifying as a snake bite. If you live in an area where poisonous snakes are common, become familiar with their appearance, behavior and habitat.

If you can recognize the snake, you'll be able to tell whether the bite is venomous or not. If it isn't, treat it as a puncture wound, above. If it is venomous, pour echinacea tincture over the bite, apply an echinacea leaf poultice and/or give your pet echinacea tincture by mouth, up to 1 or 2 teaspoons for a small pet and 1 or 2 tablespoons for a large dog. Today's echinacea therapy for snakebites is based on the Plains Indians' treatment of rattlesnake bites, for which they chewed one leaf and applied it externally, then chewed and swallowed another.

In *The Complete Book of Essential Oils & Aromatherapy*, Valerie Ann Worwood, Ph.D., mentioned that lavender has long been used effectively against the venom produced by adders in the mountainous regions of Europe. "It is about the best essential oil to use from the travel kit until you can get help," she wrote. Apply 10 drops of full-strength lavender essential oil every 30 seconds until you reach medical help.

The more calm and relaxed your animal is, the better. A pulse made rapid by panic only accelerates the distribution of venom through the body. Dr. Bach's emergency formula, Therapeutic Touch and other calming techniques will help both you and your pet survive this crisis.

Snake-bite kits that employ suction devices work only on bare skin; even the hair on human arms and legs interferes with their use, which is why these kits include razor blades for shaving affected areas. There is practically no hairless area on a dog or cat and even if you were able to shave one, the animal's anatomy might prevent the use of a suction device. If the bite is on a wide part of a dog's nose or his relatively hairless abdomen, this device could probably help. I haven't been bit by a snake, but I did use a snakebite kit when a bumblebee stung my arm and I was surprised at how powerful the suction was and how quickly it worked; the pain stopped immediately and a large drop of venom emerged within a second or two.

Today's first-aid experts do not recommend cutting the bite area with a knife to increase bleeding, an old-fashioned way of releasing venom, or, if the animal is bitten in the lower leg, tying the limb with a tourniquet. A snug bandage a few inches above the bite on a leg or tail may help slow the spread of venom, but don't make it tight enough to cut off circulation.

Because ice slows the spread of venom, wrap ice in a cloth and place it against the bite for 10 minutes, remove it for five minutes and reapply for 10 minutes. At the same time, keep the animal warm with warm water bottles and blankets to help prevent shock. Seek veterinary care immediately.

As mentioned on page 204, homeopathic *Aconite 30c* given every 15 minutes for three or four doses is appropriate for snake bites. Although this remedy does not neutralize venom, it helps calm both animal and caretaker.

Insect, Tick and Spider Bites and Stings

The following work as well on people as they do on pets, so consider using these effective remedies for the entire family.

For a sting by a honey bee, which leaves its stinger behind, gently remove the stinger with tweezers or flick it away with your fingernail. Don't squeeze or press the stinger, as that may release more venom.

Remove ticks with tweezers as described on page 393.

Herbal Therapy: Place mashed or puréed fresh wheat grass, plantain, comfrey or just about any green herb on the bite. If the area is swollen with infection, tie or hold the poultice in place for as long as possible; replace it with a fresh poultice every hour until swelling subsides. If fresh plants aren't available, mix powdered wheat grass juice with water to make a thick paste or combine dried herbs with warm water and let them soak for a few minutes before using.

Aromatherapy: Apply diluted tea tree oil or, for medium to large dogs, a single drop of full-strength tea tree oil. Tea tree oil relieves itching and disinfects bites.

Aromatherapist Valerie Ann Worwood recommends the following essential oil first-aid treatments. For bee stings, apply full-strength chamomile oil three times a day for two days. Rinse wasp stings with cider or wine vinegar and apply a blend of equal parts lavender and chamomile oil three times daily. For spider bites, mix 3 drops lavender and 2 drops chamomile oil with 1 teaspoon of vodka or other alcohol and apply to the area three times per day. A single day of treatment is usually sufficient. For a venomous spider bite such as the black widow, apply 10 drops of full-strength lavender oil every two or three minutes until you reach medical help.

Broken Bones

If your pet breaks a leg, you will want to reach a veterinarian as soon as possible. If you're in a remote location, that may not be for hours or days, so do what you can to make your animal comfortable until you can reach professional help. Treat his most serious symptoms first, such as bleeding, and prevent shock by keeping him warm. Give the animal and yourself Dr. Bach's emergency formula and/or calming nervine herbs such as valerian or skullcap to help both of you relax. Before moving or treating your pet, tie a temporary muzzle as described on page 332.

To lift your pet without disturbing the break, ease him onto a board or a tautly held towel or blanket. Move him to a safe location as necessary. Protect the break from further damage by preparing a temporary splint. Depending on your animal's size, this may consist of cotton and gauze wrapped around the leg and held in place with tape, a combination of cotton, gauze and a small piece of wood taped in place or an initial wrapping of gauze followed by a thick layer of clay (mix powdered clay with enough water to make a paste) applied to gauze or fabric strips, wrapped into place and allowed to dry.

Be sure that the temporary cast is not so tightly wrapped that it interferes with circulation.

If *You* Are Bitten or Scratched

Serious, life-threatening dog bites should be treated by a physician, but even minor bites and scratches can pose health risks.

Cat scratch fever is a mystery. No one knows what causes it or who is likely to succumb. Symptoms, which can include fever, exhaustion and swollen lymph nodes, typically develop one to two weeks after a feline scratch or bite. To prevent cat scratch fever, keep your own resistance high with whole foods and supplements and keep your cats healthy. If you are injured, soak the scratch or bite in a solution of 1/4 cup sea salt or Epsom salts dissolved in 2 cups hot water to encourge bleeding, then treat it with a 15-percent solution of tea tree oil, full-strength tea tree oil, the antiseptic concentrate described on page 186, undiluted grapefruit seed extract, 3-percent hydrogen peroxide, full-strength lavender oil or a blend of the essential oils of thyme, lavender, eucalyptus and chamomile. Repeat the application every six hours for one to two days. In addition, if the scratch or bite is deep, place a plantain leaf or wheat grass poultice over the wound to pull toxins out. Take grapefruit seed extract, other infection-fighting herbs and large quantities of vitamin C internally for a few days to reduce the risk of infection.

The greatest danger from animal bites is the risk of rabies. Identifying biting dogs and documenting their vaccination history is a public health requirement. Any contact with an infected animal can be hazardous, including wild animals such as raccoons. Never approach an unfamiliar animal that looks dazed, uncoordinated or unwell.

Before leaving this topic, do you know what animal gives the most serious bite containing the largest variety of bacteria and producing the most serious infections? If you guessed human beings, you're right.

Other Conditions
Additional conditions requiring first-aid treatment appear in the following A to Z section.

Chapter

A to Z
Ailments
in Dogs, Cats, Birds
and Rabbits

T HE FOLLOWING SECTION describes conditions commonly found in dogs, cats, birds, rabbits and other small animals, many of which also occur in horses, cattle, goats, sheep, domestic fowl, wild birds and other animals.

In all cases, the key to preventing an illness or condition is a natural, healthful lifestyle: raw food based on whatever the species consumes in the wild, daily exposure to natural light, pure water, clean air, regular exercise and a peaceful environment.

Some of the illnesses described here are acute. That is, they develop quickly, display their symptoms quickly and subside quickly, often on their own. Others are chronic, developing slowly, over a period of weeks, months or years; their symptoms usually increase in number and severity and seldom resolve or disappear on their own or with conventional drugs.

When a course of treatment is effective in an acute condition, whether it's a homeopathic medication, herb, essential oil, acupuncture, acupressure, massage, flower essence or color tonation, the animal's improvement is usually obvious within a few minutes or hours. Chronic conditions, which take much longer to develop, take longer to resolve; improvement may not be obvious for weeks or even months, depending on the condition's history and severity. If the patient experiences a healing crisis, which is a temporary worsening of one or more symptoms, those symptoms usually begin to improve within a few hours or one day in acute conditions and within several days or a week in chronic conditions. Just as the right diet, exercise and living conditions help prevent disease, they help an animal recover from whatever illnesses do occur. A well-nourished, healthy pet with a strong immune system can recover from most acute infections on his own, but an animal depleted by internal and external parasites, malnutrition and a compromised immune system could die from just about any infection. This is why the most important step in combatting harmful bacteria, viruses, parasites, fungi and other pathogens is a lifetime of good nutrition, just as it is the easiest way to prevent the chronic conditions we consider "normal" in pets, like arthritis, cataracts, skin and coat problems and illnesses such as diabetes.

As the veterinarians quoted throughout this book remind their clients, no single cure works for every patient, patient responses to the same treatment differ and not all patients treated with holistic methods recover. However, most pets experience an improved quality of life and an overall improvement of health as a result of the therapies described here.

The basic methods for preparing and administering the recommended treatments are described in the preceding chapters. Before giving your pet an herbal tea, dried herbs in capsules or an herbal tincture, see the recommended dosage chart on page 136. For the internal use of essential oils and hydrosols, see the recommended dosage charts on page 174. For homeopathy guidelines, see Chapter 6. For the administration of flower essences, see page 248. For acupressure and other hands-on therapy instructions, see Chapter 7. Please take the time to read these sections before treating your pet for a specific condition.

Space limitations make it impossible to list all the illnesses and conditions experienced by dogs, cats, birds, rabbits and other domestic animals. The following section emphasizes the most common illnesses, and you will find others in the preceding chapters. To locate the information you need, check both the A to Z listings and the index at the back. In addition, refer to any of the pet health guides recommended throughout this book.

Abscesses and Pustules

Abscesses are local infections that form when a puncture wound heals on the surface while trapping bacteria or infected debris beneath the skin. The cause might be a cat scratch or bite, a porcupine quill, splinter, thorn or other material. Pustules are small pus-containing blisters that sometimes develop between an animal's toes for no apparent reason.

Abscess Prevention

Abscesses can be prevented if injuries are treated promptly, which involves removing embedded material, disinfecting the wound and supporting the animal with oral doses of herbs and vitamins.

Use any or all of the following treatments to prevent the development of an abscess.

Herbal Therapy: Apply a 15-percent solution of tea tree oil or diluted grapefruit seed extract, calendula tincture diluted in 2 to 3 parts water, plain salt water or soap and water. Flush and rinse the wound well. Apply full-strength aloe vera juice or gel or essential oil of lavender mixed with an equal part of aloe vera or water.

If a splinter, thorn, embedded hair or other object is visible, remove it with tweezers. If embedded material remains, apply a poultice of fresh or dried plantain or wheat grass to pull it from the wound or substitute a compress of wheat grass juice or plantain tea. If the wound site or the animal's disposition makes it difficult to hold a poultice or compress in place, apply a thick layer of a drawing salve made with plantain and other herbs.

Internally, dose the animal with grapefruit seed extract, using 1 capsule per 10 pounds of body weight once per day if the injury is minor, such as a thorn or splinter you were able to remove promptly, or twice per day if the animal was bitten or scratched in a fight or still has part of a porcupine quill or splinter embedded in the skin. In the case of a minor injury, two days of grapefruit seed extract should be sufficient; for more serious injuries, treat for five to seven days.

In addition to or instead of the grapefruit seed extract, dose the animal orally with echinacea tea or tincture.

Nutritional Therapy: Vitamin C is the premier infection fighter. If the injury is minor, increase the animal's daily intake of vitamin C by about 250 mg per 10 pounds of body weight per day for two or three days. For more serious injuries, give vitamin C to bowel tolerance as described on page 101 for several days, or until the wound heals.

Echinacea, garlic and bee propolis can also be given with food to help prevent infection. See the natural immunizations described on pages 285-286.

Any liquid trace mineral supplement can be applied topically to a wound, abscess or pustule, or use a seawater-strength solution of unrefined sea salt and water. Repeat either application three or four times daily.

Homeopathy: If given immediately after the injury, *Lachesis muta 30c* may prevent an abscess from forming. Give 1 pellet or tablet every four hours for a total of three treatments.

Abscess Treatment

If an abscess has already formed, it will be tender, swollen, filled with pus and hot and painful when touched. The animal may develop a fever, which is one of the body's methods of fighting infection. To treat an established abscess or pustule, use all of the above herbal and nutritional therapies plus any of the following.

Herbal Therapy: Apply a fomentation (hot compress) of strong oatstraw or plantain tea to the inflamed area, including the skin several inches above it. Place a drop of essential lavender oil on the abscess before applying the fomentation. If the foot or lower leg is involved, prepare a jar or bowl of comfortably hot tea and immerse the leg. Keep the fomentation or the submerged limb in place for several minutes and repeat several times. This will help the abscess come to a head and drain, removing the embedded splinter or infection.

Apply 1 drop of full-strength grapefruit seed extract to any abscess or pustule, being careful to keep it away from the eyes, nose, mouth, ears and mucous membranes. Full-strength grapefruit seed extract is especially effective for pustules between the toes.

Homeopathy: For extremely painful abscesses, give *Hepar sulph 30c* every 4 hours for a total of three treatments. If the abscess has already burst or is about to, substitute *Silica 6x* and give 1 tablet or pellet every 4 hours for 24 hours.

Note that if a thorn, quill, splinter or other material is so deeply embedded that these treatments don't remove it, surgery may be necessary. To prepare for surgery, give the animal extra nutritional support as described on page 437.

Color Therapy: If the abscess has not yet come to a head, give a green systemic front followed by indigo on the affected area. A few orange and yellow tonations may help drain the abscess. Give magenta or purple over the chest area and a blue systemic front in case of fever.

If the abscess is already draining, stimulate healing with a turquoise systemic front over the affected area followed by indigo on the abscess.

Allergies

Every allergy that inconveniences humans has its counterpart in dogs, cats and other pets, including allergic reactions to drugs and chemicals, food sensitivities and contact dermatitis. Both people and their pets can have adverse reactions to insect bites; in dogs and cats, flea allergies are common.

Most allergies in pets are caused by poor nutrition. Well-nourished animals don't get allergies and animals that have them often get rid of them if they eat a well-balanced, natural, raw diet. This is not to say that the cure works quickly, for just as diet-related allergies are slow to develop, they are slow to reverse. Many of us are impatient and want instant results, but if you think of the life you want your animal to be living a year from now, the benefits of this gradual approach are obvious. Cortisone and other drugs may mask or suppress allergic symptoms, but they don't reverse them, and, over time, the condition of drug-treated animals usually deteriorates.

To determine whether your pet is allergic to a specific food, see the instructions for diagnosing food allergies on pages 92-94.

Even if your pet's allergies seem unrelated to food, they are probably connected. Hot spots, skin eruptions, inflamed toes, anal itching, inflamed ears, lick granulomas, most digestive problems and several immune system disorders have their roots in diet. Because nutrition is such an important factor in treating allergies of all types, changing to a raw, natural diet is the single most important step you can take to improve your pet's health. Once your pet is eating whole, natural foods, taking nutritional supplements and herbs that improve digestion and the activity of beneficial intestinal bacteria, drinking pure, uncontaminated water, dining from glass, ceramic or stainless steel dishes, getting the right kind of exercise, spending several hours per day exposed to natural light and enjoying a life of reduced stress, his or her allergic conditions should improve and gradually disappear. The other strategy most recommended by holistic veterinarians is the elimination of annual revaccinations.

In addition, treat your pet's allergic symptoms by using appropriate herbs, nutritional supplements, homeopathy, massage and essential oils; see *Respiratory Illnesses* and *Skin and Coat Conditions* as appropriate.

Color Therapy: Support any treatment for allergies with a lemon systemic on both sides of the body followed by a yellow systemic front for two weeks, then an orange systemic front for two weeks. In addition, tonate specific symptoms, such as respiratory congestion or skin problems, as they occur.

Hands-on Therapies: Any of the physical therapies described in Chapter 7 are effective support treatments for allergies.

Anal Scent Glands

The anal glands of dogs are much like the scent glands of skunks, and, if you've ever been with a dog who was frightened enough to blow his anal glands or if you've ever manually expressed them or been with your dog when a veterinarian did, you've had a malodorous experience.

Healthy anal glands secrete a strong-smelling fluid. Impacted anal glands are obstructed — often because of constipation, poor diet or inadequate exercise — and anal glands sometimes develop abscesses. To relieve the discomfort of these conditions, dogs often scoot across the ground, the floor or any rough surface.

Nutritional Therapy: Improve the diet; see Chapter 2. The fiber in bran, psyllium husks, carrots and other grated raw vegetables will help keep the glands exercised. Eliminating foods to which the animal is sensitive is also important.

Herbal Therapy: Apply fomentations of hot chamomile, lavender, calendula or red clover tea. Test the temperature on your bare arm before applying the saturated cloth to be sure it isn't too hot; hold the fomentation in place for three to five minutes and repeat. This treatment by itself will loosen, soften and stimulate impacted anal glands, helping them flow on their own. For anal gland abscesses, add several drops of grapefruit seed extract or tea tree oil and apply the fomentation twice a day for three days or longer, if necessary.

If the glands are severely impacted, you can manually empty them with a gentle "milking" pressure on either side; hold gauze pads in both hands to cushion the pressure and collect the glands' contents.

Homeopathy: For anal gland abscesses, give *Belladonna 6c*, 1 pellet or tablet every 4 hours for three treatments. The following day, give the tissue salt *Silica 6x* every 4 hours all day. For impacted anal glands, give *Silica 6x* once per day for 10 or more days or until the condition improves.

Color Therapy: Follow the schedule for abscesses.

Anemia

White or pale gums, physical weakness and a fast pulse are common symptoms of blood loss in dogs and cats, which may be caused by wounds, parasites such as fleas or intestinal worms, toxic chemical exposure or a serious disease such as feline leukemia.

The more serious conditions require veterinary attention, but mild anemia caused by blood loss can be treated at home.

If the blood loss is caused by intestinal worms or fleas, remember that even the most benign chemicals can be fatal to puppies and kittens drained of blood by parasites. Use the most gentle treatments possible, such as removing fleas with a flea comb, improving the diet and making the animal a less hospitable host.

Nutritional Therapy: Feed a natural diet with additional blood-building nutrients such as liver, nutritional yeast, leafy green vegetables, seaweed such as kelp and vitamin C, which increases the absorption of iron during digestion. Make these nutrients easy for your pet to digest by puréeing them before adding them to regular foods.

Herbal Therapy: Feed herbs that support the liver, such as yellow dock root and milk thistle seed.

Homeopathy: To treat weakness and loss of strength caused by blood loss, give *China officinalis 6c* once per day for four weeks.

Color Therapy: Give red and lemon systemic fronts that include the feet.

Antibiotic Side Effects

When penicillin appeared on the medical scene, it ushered in a new age and was revered around the world as a miracle-working wonder drug. Now, half a century later, public sentiment about penicillin and other antibiotics is beginning to change. Thanks to the overuse and misuse of these drugs in medicine and agriculture, antibiotics are often ineffective against the infections they were designed to treat. As a result, drug-resistant bacteria have become a public health menace. Allergic reactions and other adverse side effects are common not only in people but in their pets, for veterinarians routinely prescribe over a dozen of these powerful drugs to treat common infections. Antibiotics can treat many conditions caused by bacteria, fungi or protozoa, but they are often prescribed when no infection is present or when the problem's cause is clearly a virus, against which antibiotics have no effect. "People are so used to giving their kids antibiotics, taking antibiotics themselves and giving their dogs and cats antibiotics that no one gives them a second thought," says veterinarian Beverly Cappel-King. "Most physicians and veterinarians hand them out like candy. Sometimes people act disappointed when I don't prescribe an antibiotic, they're so conditioned to expect one. People in our culture have a difficult time understanding how powerful and potentially damaging these drugs really are."

Although not always apparent, the side effects of antibiotics can be severe. Pets as well as people die from allergic reactions. As veterinary homeopath Christopher Day reports, guinea pigs are allergic to penicillin, streptomycin and erythromycin, hamsters to penicillin and streptomycin and birds to streptomycin and procaine penicillin. Antibiotics have been blamed for birth defects in kittens, puppies and other animals conceived while either parent was taking the drug or born to mothers who were treated while pregnant. Because they disrupt an animal's intestinal flora by destroying beneficial as well as harmful bacteria, antibiotic treatment is often followed by bouts of indigestion, *Candida* yeast infections, thrush, ear infections and other problems caused by the opportunistic growth of bacteria no longer held in check by natural defenses.

Another inconvenient side effect is the disruption of scent detection in hunting, tracking and search and rescue dogs. Some experts theorize that by destroying the beneficial bacteria in a dog's nose, antibiotics confuse the animal's ability to detect and process the minute information that makes his or her sense of smell 300 million times more acute than our own. This temporary disability is often apparent during the second week of antibiotic treatment and up to two weeks after treatment stops. If you are engaged in activities that depend on your dog's good nose, a visit to a holistic veterinarian for natural infection fighters will avert this side effect.

No one says that antibiotics should never be used for any patient under any circumstances, for antibiotics can and do save lives, but veterinarians like Cappel-King criticize their casual use, especially when their side effects outweigh the benefits and when natural therapies are equally or more effective.

Your pet is most likely to benefit from antibiotics when taking them for a short course (typically seven to fourteen days) for a serious condition such as a paralyzing attack of Lyme disease, a dental abscess that is poisoning the entire body or a life-threatening bladder infection. Your pet is far less likely to benefit from the long-term use of antibiotics for chronic or recurring infections.

Alternatives to antibiotic therapy include the herbal immunizations described on pages 285-286, which can be used to prevent or treat most infections caused by bacteria, viruses, protozoa, fungi and other pathogens, and homeopathic remedies appropriate to the patient and his or her symptoms.

The following support therapies are appropriate for patients taking antibiotics.

Nutritional Therapy: Holistic veterinarians who prescribe antibiotics often give large amounts of vitamin C at the same time, such as double or triple the animal's normal daily dose or dosing to bowel tolerance.

Because antibiotics kill beneficial as well as harmful bacteria, your pet's intestinal balance will be disrupted. There is no point in trying to correct this imbalance until the course of treatment ends because any beneficial bacteria you introduce will be killed as well.

The day antibiotic treatment ends, begin dosing your pet with large quantities of acidophilus supplements, freshly prepared yogurt or kefir, lactic acid-fermented vegetables and other foods that contain or feed beneficial bacteria. Review Chapter 3 for specific instructions.

Homeopathy: Veterinary homeopaths rarely recommend antibiotics for they have an effective arsenal of remedies to use for every type of infection. Consult an expert before treating any serious condition to be sure you're using the correct preparation. If your pet has taken antibiotics in the past or has to take them in the future, consult a veterinary homeopath for posttreatment guidelines.

Herbal Therapy: Garlic taken the week after therapy ends helps cleanse the intestinal tract and makes it more hospitable to the friendly bacteria introduced by acidophilus and other supplements. In addition, fresh cleavers and dandelion act as tonics for the spleen and lymph, helping restore normal function to the entire system. Add either or both to your pet's food as available.

Appetite, Loss of

An animal might lose its appetite for several reasons. Remember that in the wild, dogs and cats have a sporadic food supply, feasting one day and fasting the next. If your pet is otherwise in good health, she may not be hungry because she overate the day before, the weather is unusually hot, she's unusually tired from hard work or she dislikes a new food. These are all temporary self-correcting conditions. If she has just lost a favorite companion or if she's miserable in a boarding kennel or unhappy about a family relocation, her appetite will probably return as she adjusts. Flower essences, hands-on therapy and patience are most helpful in those cases.

It is not uncommon for kittens, puppies, dogs and cats to go without food for several days after receiving a vaccination. If this is the only side effect, appetite should return quickly. You can help prevent adverse reactions to required vaccinations with the help of a veterinary homeopath.

The other major reason for appetite loss is infection. By letting its digestive system rest, the body frees energy for the more efficient operation of other glands, organs and systems that combat bacteria, viruses and other pathogens.

Never force an otherwise healthy animal to eat if the loss of appetite lasts only a day or two. Take your pet's vital signs and compare them to her normal resting temperature, pulse and respiration rates. Practice Therapeutic Touch while checking her for unusual symptoms. Provide ample drinking water. If she doesn't regain her appetite the second day, call your vet with an accurate description.

If the appetite loss results from a serious condition such as liver disease, weight loss and malnutrition can interfere with healing. Your holistic veterinarian can help you plan nutritionally dense meals and a feeding schedule your pet will respond to. In that situation, several small meals may replace one large one, digestive enzymes or hydrochloric acid supplements may help the animal absorb nutrients and freshly prepared carrot juice can accompany or replace solid foods as necessary.

Hands-on Therapies: Acupuncture stimulates the appetite in some cases, and the acupressure massage of point ST36 does as well. Massage and therapeutic touch are appropriate in all illnesses.

Color Therapy: In humans, anorexia nervosa is treated with green and magenta systemic front tonations and yellow across the abdomen. This same treatment would be appropriate for underweight animals with little interest in food.

Arthritis, Hip Dysplasia, Elbow Dysplasia and Other Joint Problems

Arthritis is so common in dogs, people think of it as inevitable and natural. It isn't. Arthritis is a cooked food disease, as researchers all over the world have demonstrated repeatedly. Whenever identical animals have been fed the same diet, with one group eating the food raw and the other cooked, the group fed raw food experiences improved health or maintains good health while the health of the group fed cooked food deteriorates.

Hip dysplasia, elbow dysplasia and other joint problems are now common in the most popular breeds. There is much debate in veterinary circles about whether these conditions are hereditary and whether they can be treated. Many dogs with only minor symptoms have been euthanized after being diagnosed with hip dysplasia. The following information about arthritis applies to hip and elbow dysplasia as well.

The orthodox treatment for arthritis is the use of cortisone and anti-inflammatory drugs, neither of which addresses the problem's cause. These treatments may suppress symptoms but they don't interrupt joint deterioration. When the drugs stop working or are discontinued, symptoms are usually worse than before because the disease itself is worse.

Nutritional Therapy: Put your pet on an appropriate, well-balanced, freshly prepared raw food diet.

If raw food is impossible to provide on a daily basis, digestive enzymes will help prevent arthritis. Nineteen years of field use, research and clinical tests demonstrate that ProZyme, a plant-derived enzyme supplement described in Chapter 3, increases the absorption of essential nutrients and fatty acids from cooked food. A ProZyme videotape for veterinarians shows, among other things, a ten-year-old Golden Retriever with well-documented hip dysplasia jumping over hurdles and acting like a puppy. Enzyme supplements have become so popular that there are now several brands to choose from. Of course, even the best enzymes can't create nutrients that aren't in the food to begin with, so a home-prepared diet is almost always preferable to commercial pet foods.

Shark cartilage has become popular in the treatment of arthritic dogs and horses, as have collagen products derived from chicken and cattle. All kinds of conflicting claims are being made for and against these products, which can be expensive, take several weeks or months before showing improvement and cause digestive disturbances. Each manufacturer claims that its brand is superior to everything else on the market, and it is difficult to separate fact from exaggeration.

In humans, at least one conventional study has verified the use of cartilage powders. In 1993, Harvard Medical School and the Boston Veterans' Administration Hospital studied 29 arthritis patients scheduled for joint replacement surgery. The volunteers were given a heaping teaspoon of ground, dried chicken cartilage in orange juice every morning for three months. Within 10 days, their pain and inflammation had disappeared. In 30 days, the subjects could open pickle jars that had never been opened and at 90 days, all had maximum return of function. Although no similar trial has been conducted with dogs, veterinarians and owners report encouraging results from their use of shark, bovine and poultry cartilage powders and extracts.

The easiest way to give your dog or cat cartilage is by feeding raw bones as described in Chapter 2. Chicken drumsticks and wings, lamb neck bones, beef spareribs and other gristly bones are rich sources. Veterinarian Wendell Belfield uses vitamin C to treat and prevent arthritis and hip dysplasia, explaining that it nourishes the body's collagen. The combination of vitamin C and raw bones can be your version of the Harvard Medical School treatment.

Another sea creature that has helped arthritic dogs and other animals is a starfish cousin, the sea cucumber found on Australia's Great Barrier Reef. Dried, powdered sea cucumber is combined with processed sea vegetables as a food supplement, and researchers who have tested human patients report that the supplement both reduces arthritis pain and slows or reverses the disease itself. Most sea cucumber supplements have a pronounced fishy odor that appeals to dogs and cats.

Other supplements said to help human, canine, feline and equine arthritis patients include chondroitin sulfate (derived from cartilage), glucosamine sulfate, cetyl myristoleate, superoxide dismutase (SOD), fish oils and antioxidant vitamins and enzymes.

Food sensitivities often manifest as arthritis, so in addition to upgrading your pet's diet, test for his or her reaction to individual foods. Pasteurized milk is a common culprit.

Herbal Therapies: The herbs boswellia, feverfew, devil's claw root and yucca root are only a few of the herbs considered specifics for joint pain. The external application of arnica tincture is another. Bupleurum, burdock root, dandelion, horsetail and nettle are important support herbs. See pages 145 to 159 for descriptions of these important plants. Wheat grass and other green grasses are recommended as well.

In recent years celery seed has become a popular supplement for those with arthritis. Your pet may respond well to a celery seed extract, tincture or powder added to food.

Cayenne pepper increases circulation and relieves pain when taken internally and applied externally. Although some human arthritics are sensitive to plants in the nightshade family (potatoes, tomatoes, eggplant, peppers and tobacco), this response is not commonly reported in dogs, cats, horses and other animals, although it is certainly possible. Infuse whole fresh, dried or powdered cayenne in any appropriate carrier oil or brew a cayenne pepper tea to use as a massage lotion. Give cayenne pepper in capsules with dinner or, if your pet enjoys the spice, simply add it to food.

Aromatherapy: Any essential oil that increases circulation through the joints can be applied in a massage oil. Basil, cinnamon, coriander, nutmeg, rosemary, lavender and pine are often used for this purpose.

Homeopathy: George Macleod's book *Dogs: Homeopathic Remedies* lists nine remedies for canine arthritis due to infection, nine for simple or rheumatoid arthritis, five for ankylosing spondylitis, seven for osteoarthritis and six for bursitis. In homeopathy, individual diagnosis is essential for effective treatment, especially in chronic conditions. For best results, consult a veterinary homeopath or study the books recommended in Chapter 6.

Light and Color: As John Ott discovered, exposure to unfiltered natural light can be an arthritis cure in itself.

In addition, Darius Dinshah suggests the following color tonations. For bursitis, give a green systemic that includes the affected area followed by blue or indigo on the affected parts. If the bursitis is chronic, start with a lemon systemic front and then use orange and, if the area is still painful, add blue. For acute attacks of osteo or rheumatoid arthritis, begin with green and magenta systemics that include the affected areas and follow with blue or indigo. For chronic osteo or rheumatoid arthritis, begin with lemon and magenta systemics over the affected areas and follow with turquoise and/or indigo for painful joints and orange on areas of bone atrophy.

Hands-on Therapies: Acupuncture, acupressure, massage, Tellington TTouch, Therapeutic Touch, myotherapy and chiropractic are all recommended for arthritis, rheumatism, hip or elbow dysplasia, bursitis and related conditions.

Other Treatments: Hydrotherapy, the simple application of water from a garden or grooming hose, can be helpful to arthritic dogs. The pressure does not have to be strong; in fact, the massage provided by a gentle flow is more effective. Follow with a brisk but gentle toweling and the application of arnica tincture or warming herbs.

Because hard surfaces jar and irritate arthritic joints, orthopedic pet beds containing foam rubber shaped in an egg crate design have become popular. Any bed that cushions the animal and insulates the body from cold floors will be appreciated. Check pet supply catalogs for bean-bag bed sacks, large cushions filled with fluffy material, cedar chip bedding and other designs.

Asthma: See *Respiratory Illnesses*

Autoimmune Disorders

Although increasingly common in animals fed commercial pet foods, given long-term treatments of steroids, antibiotic or other drugs, vaccinated annually or exposed to toxic substances, immune system disorders are unusual in pets fed a natural diet, given pure water, vaccinated seldom or never, exercised daily, exposed to unfiltered natural light and provided a safe, comfortable, healthful lifestyle.

Because autoimmune disorders can be difficult to diagnose and treat, consult a holistic veterinarian. He or she will probably recommend a change in diet, nutritional supplements, Chinese or Western herbs, a homeopathic remedy, acupuncture and/or other therapies described in this book.

Behavioral Problems

Veterinarians are often asked for advice about behavioral problems, but unless they have spent considerable time living with or training the same type of dog, bird, rabbit, cat or other animal, their suggestions may be limited. Before agreeing to put your pet on chemical tranquilizers or a psychoactive drug like Prozac, examine the situation from a different perspective.

Nearly all of America's pet problems are caused by some combination of the owner's ignorance (lack of knowledge about the animal's needs or basic nature, an inability to read body language or a misunderstanding of appropriate training methods) and poor nutrition.

To better understand your pet's behavior, study Chapter 1 and some of the books it recommends. Talk with breeders, owners, trainers and others whose animals you admire. The solution to your problem may be a simple change in your own behavior.

Take your pet to a holistic veterinarian in order to screen out medical reasons for unwanted actions. Sometimes heavy metals or environmental toxins cause behavior changes that disappear when these substances are eliminated from the body. In some cases, behavior changes are caused by prescription drugs or other medical treatments. The hormone cycles of intact dogs and cats can create problems, in which case spaying or neutering makes a substantial difference. Or an illness might be the cause, such as a urinary tract infection that interferes with your cat's use of his litter pan.

Nutrition: Improve your pet's diet. The simple step of replacing chemical preservatives, artificial colors, artificial flavors, synthetic vitamins and inferior foods with a natural diet eliminates a host of behavioral problems by itself. Many otherwise well-behaved dogs and cats begin ripping into trash bags, stealing food and scrounging under dumpsters after being switched to "lite" or low-calorie dry foods. No wonder they act as though they're starving — they are! Lick granulomas, often considered an obsessive-compulsive disorder, are rare in dogs fed raw foods.

Light and Exercise: Insufficient exposure to unfiltered natural light causes people and animals to manifest all kinds of personality disorders. Let your pet spend as much time as possible outdoors, on a screened porch or near a screened, open door or window.

Increase or improve your pet's exercise. This is especially important if you have a young dog from a sporting or working breed or if your pet has abundant nervous energy. A tired puppy is a good puppy. Don't assume that if you have a large backyard, your dog gets sufficient exercise. She can be as much a couch potato on five acres as she is on the living room sofa. Dogs are pack animals; they need companionship and group play. Go for walks with your dog, play fetch, invite other dogs to visit and romp, take up agility training, scent tracking or another canine sport or take her swimming.

Play with your cat every day using a fishing wand string toy, crinkly balls of aluminum foil, empty paper bags, cardboard boxes and whatever he most enjoys. If your rabbit doesn't have the run of the house or a safely fenced yard, take him outdoors on a leash. Bunnies are wonderful companions and enjoy petting and handling if you start when they're young. Provide a large cage for your bird and bring her out for regular bathing, cuddling and play. Large, intelligent birds like cockatoos have an almost inexhaustible play drive, and their human companions have a real challenge keeping them entertained. Some birds' favorite games are making the bed (this involves two people and a trampoline-like blanket toss) and dancing (any music will do, with much swooping and turning while the bird perches on a hand or arm). Nothing alleviates depression in an African grey or other smart, curious bird like a bag of shiny new toys, the brighter and noisier, the better. Whatever your animal, holistic pet care involves keeping her busy and happy with appropriate exercise.

Flower Essences: Nearly every behavior problem that doesn't have a physical cause can be helped with flower essences, for their strength is the treatment of underlying emotional issues. See pages 249-256.

Herbal Therapies: If the animal is anxious and hyperactive, a blend of relaxing nervine herbs such as chamomile, passionflower, hops, oat grass, blue vervain, valerian, lobelia or skullcap will probably help.

Hands-on Therapies: Acupuncture, Therapeutic Touch, Tellington TTouch and massage therapy can also make a difference. Even aggressive behavior can be interrupted, as Linda Tellington Jones has repeatedly demonstrated with TTouch and as Suzanne Clothier explains in her booklet *Body Postures & Emotions: Shifting Shapes, Shifting*

Minds. See the Resources list for Chapter 7 for recommended books and videos.

Just as we train ourselves and our children to relax, sit down, breathe deeply and take a time out when feeling angry, upset, scared or unable to function, we can teach our dogs to do the same. Sitting is a neutral position, standing is assertive and lying down is submissive. By elevating a dog from flat-on-the-floor submissive to neutral by placing her in a sit, you can change a frightened animal's behavior. A similar strategy shifts an aroused, potentially aggressive standing-on-all-fours-with-fur-straight-up dog into neutral. With either animal in the neutral sit, it is possible to create new responses by reshaping posture, facial expression, ear position and tight muscles. Food treats are not always appropriate, and timing is everything; see Clothier's handbook for detailed instructions. Gentle stroking, massage, Therapeutic Touch, Tellington TTouch and the application of flower essences or essential oils can interrupt old habit patterns and make your dog far more receptive to new ideas.

Acupuncture, acupressure, chiropractic and myotherapy have similar results. Before his acupuncture and chiropractic treatments, Java, the snarling Doberman, was tearing after every dog in the waiting room. After, he floated past them in a state of bliss. Don't underestimate the power of hands-on therapies to transform problem behavior.

In some cases, special equipment or products help, such as the puppy crates and odor-control products that simplify housebreaking, battery-operated collars that release a harmless spray of citronella under the nose of a dog that barks excessively, battery-operated leashes that whistle or beep whenever the dog pulls, electric fences that keep off-lead dogs in the yard, head halters that prevent pulling, harnesses that prevent jumping, seat belt harnesses that keep pets from moving around inside a moving car, scat mats that startle pets when they jump on forbidden furniture and well-built scratching posts that keep cats happy and out of trouble. Check pet supply catalogs, magazines and trainer recommendations for the right equipment.

Bird Care

For optimum health, your bird needs a well-balanced diet of fresh, raw foods including sprouting grains, grasses, fresh herbs, greens, fruits, vegetables, nuts and seeds. Add small amounts of a liquid trace mineral supplement or Willard Water extract to your bird's drinking water. Birds in the wild eat all kinds of things, including insects and worms; free-range chickens devour slugs, snails and mice; even tropical birds known for their love of fruits and seeds occasionally eat meat. Your bird may enjoy occasional raw meat trimmings or a suet cake embedded with insects such as those designed for backyard bird feeders. Study descriptions of your bird's life in the wild to determine what's appropriate and provide similar foods as much as possible. See Chapter 2 for nutritional guidelines.

In addition, give your bird access to unfiltered natural light. Whenever possible, place her cage in the shade outdoors, leave her perch near an open door or window or take her with you into the garden. Although full-spectrum lighting is not the same as natural light, install full-spectrum tubes where your bird spends the most time when she can't be outdoors or near an open window. The best combination may be standard fluorescent (not pink or orange "soft light" or energy efficient) tubes with a single ultraviolet black-light tube or a combination of standard incandescent (not "full spectrum" incandescent) bulbs with a Vita Lite fluorescent tube. The worst light for your bird's room is from standard fluorescent tubes with a pink or orange glow or energy-efficient tubes that make familiar colors look strange. Malillumination will cause problems far more serious than unhealthy looking feathers.

Fresh air is important, too. When your bird has to stay in a closed room, keep a fan running to keep air moving. Use house plants and an air filter to improve the quality of the air. Because out-gassing carpets pose a serious health hazard to birds, consider keeping your bird in a room with a wood floor or avoid synthetic fibers when installing new carpet. Also note that fungal spores can proliferate in carpeting, causing respiratory problems in birds.

A good supply of fresh, clean water and an opportunity to bathe often is another factor in feather health. Birds in the wild swallow sand, gravel, dirt and dust, but indoor birds are deprived of these natural sources of grit. Depending on your bird's size, fill a large or small ceramic pet bowl with fresh water and add a handful of sterile compost, grated cuttlebone, oyster shell and limestone and leave it where your bird can rummage to her heart's content.

Spray your bird with a mister several times a day using plain water, chamomile tea, lavender hydrosol or a favorite herbal infusion. In addition, let her bathe in the sink, bathtub or shower. The owners of tropical birds are often reluctant to bathe their pets in winter, fearing the stress of chills, but as Donna Hefton wrote in the April 1997 *Bird Talk*, winter is when parrots most appreciate frequent bathing. The tropical rain forests in which they evolved receive six to eight feet of rainfall a year, far more than most captive birds receive in their very long lifetimes. Bathing is a fundamental part of parrot grooming, and it does far more than relieve dry, itchy skin. Bathing is an exciting, fun, wing-spreading, splashing good time. Some birds love the shower (cool water, please — anything close to body temperature is unnaturally warm); others prefer to dip in partly filled sinks, bathtubs or pans of water. The feathered area at the base of the neck covering the crop is literally a hot spot; its contents are warmer than the rest of the body, and most birds love to soak this area. One theory is that if bacteria are not flushed from the skin near the crop, they proliferate and cause itching that may lead to feather pulling.

If your bird isn't used to bathing, she may love it at once or resist strenuously. If she really dislikes it, be gentle and patient; provide the opportunity but don't force her, and mist her frequently with dilute solutions of Dr. Bach's emergency formula or other flower essences.

But isn't the water too cold in winter for bathing? Hefton's answer is "If the house is warm enough for me, it is warm enough for my birds." Nighttime temperatures in the world's rainiest jungles can drop to 50° F. and birds survive there very well. Unless your house is colder than that, which would be remarkable, continue to bathe your bird even in the most frigid weather.

What if your bird shakes? That reaction, says Hefton, has nothing to do with chilly weather; wet birds shake even when the temperature is 95° F. They quickly expand their down feathers and warm themselves just as they would in the rain forest. Warnings about the dangers of drafts have sent bird owners through their houses with lighted candles looking for anyplace the flame might flicker, but that isn't necessary. Healthy, well-nourished parrots in excellent plumage do not die from exposure to mild drafts.

Bathing is the highlight of the day for many birds, so continue and even increase this activity during winter months. Let common sense be your guide. Have your bird dry off in a warm room and don't expose a bird with health problems to extreme temperatures. Protect your bird from soap, shampoo and other chemicals in your shower, tub or sink; even residues are dangerous because they can interfere with your bird's natural waterproofing. Some birds enjoy being dried off with a blow drier set on gentle heat and used at a safe distance; others prefer to air dry near a sunny window or radiator. If you use a heat lamp or other device designed for bird use, be sure it's mounted securely at a distance, for birds have been burned after falling on such equipment or having it fall on them. Also, be sure your bird can move far away from the heat source, as she can overheat quickly, even when wet.

Crop Statis or Sour Crop

The proventricula just below the crop is like the gizzard in chickens; both are muscular organs that move swallowed food toward the stomach. If the proventricula is weak, food stays in the crop too long and sours.

Crop statis usually responds quickly to a raw, natural diet and the increased fiber it provides. Be sure your bird's water dish contains gritty material as described above.

Egg Binding

If your bird becomes lethargic, quiet, huddles at the bottom of her cage and has a distended lower abdomen, she may be egg-bound.

According to Fred Bauer, egg binding is usually caused by nutritional deficiencies including an imbalance of calcium and other minerals. To prevent egg binding, feed your bird a well-balanced, raw natural diet that emphasizes sprouting grains and a variety of fresh fruits, vegetables, insects, worms and other foods as appropriate.

To treat egg binding, Bauer recommends warming the bird by placing her in a cardboard box with a thermometer and raising the temperature to 110° F. with a portable heater or other heat source. "Twenty to thirty minutes of carefully controlled warm heat will often solve the problem," he says. "People should avoid using a steam generator or vaporizer because the noise it makes can cause further trauma, and dosing the bird with oil at either end does more harm than good. We use heat and homeopathy with excellent results."

Homeopathy: Christopher Day recommends *Caulophyllum,* homeopathic blue cohosh, which is a specific for the female genital system during labor or egg laying. *Sepia* has similar uses. Give 1 dose of either remedy every four hours for a total of three treatments. If there is no improvement, switch to the other remedy and use the same schedule.

Additional Therapies: Therapeutic Touch is always an appropriate support therapy, and so is Dr. Bach's emergency formula or yarrow flower essence.

Feather Plucking

Nesting birds pluck some of their own feathers to line the nest, but feather plucking in pet birds is entirely different. Often called a behavioral or emotional problem, plucking is a preening habit that won't stop. It leaves feathers broken, damaged, crushed, twisted or pulled out completely. The bare spots it leaves behind depend on the type of bird and the amount of time it devotes to plucking. The chest, abdomen, wings and upper legs are common plucking sites, but some birds remove every feather they can reach, leaving them naked except for the top of the head.

Feather plucking is not a disease, it's a symptom. The underlying cause is most often a combination of poor nutrition, malillumination, owner neglect and the bird's own stress levels. A medical diagnosis might point to bacteria, parasites, fungi, hormone imbalances or liver disease, but these conditions are easy to prevent with a natural diet, herbs and holistic therapies. Most cases of chronic feather plucking are called "nonmedical" because they have no obvious cause.

Birds are highly sensitive animals who need attention, affection, play, interaction and companionship. In addition to improving the quality of your bird's life and diet, consult a holistic veterinarian for appropriate homeopathic remedies, Chinese herbs or acupuncture treatments, all of which have helped birds break this destructive habit, and read the descriptions of flower essences in Chapter 8 to determine the most appropriate remedy.

Herbal Therapy: Any of the relaxing nervines may be appropriate. Fred Bauer reports that birds that continue to pluck their feathers after changing to a raw natural diet may respond well to the Polynesian herb kava kava, which he has found to be effective in the in birds as well. Passionflower, which Boyer recommends for nervous disorders in baby birds, may help a bird relax and stop pulling its feathers. Valerian, skullcap, chamomile and California poppy have similar properties. No herb can compensate for a deficient diet and a lack of exposure to natural light, but the relaxing nervines are appropriate in the holistic treatment of feather plucking and other nervous conditions.

Aromatherapy: The essential oil of neroli is a stress reducer for birds; it can be given in food in tiny doses (1/4 drop twice daily for parrots and canaries) or dispersed in the air for five minutes at a time near the bird's cage four to five times daily. Either of these treatments can be given for three to five days at a time. Another soothing blend for birds is 10 parts lavender, 4 parts marjoram and 1 part neroli essential oil.

Infectious Diseases

To prevent infection or to combat an active illness caused by bacteria or a virus, see the natural immunization described on pages 285-286 as well as respiratory infections on page 421 and viral infections on page 451.

Bladder Stones or Infections: See *Urinary Tract Problems*

Bloat: See *Digestion*

Breeding: See *Reproduction*

Bronchitis: See *Respiratory Illnesses*

Burns: See Chapter 12, *First Aid*

Cancer: See Chapter 11, *Cancer*

Cardiac Problems: See *Heart Disease*

Cataracts: See *Eyes, Vision*

Chewing, Excessive

Tail chewing, self-chewing and foot chewing are common symptoms in dogs and cats with allergies, fleas or nervous disorders. Similar behavior is seen in birds.

To treat allergic reactions, change the diet and remove obvious allergens from the environment. If the chewing is sudden and out of character, look for a physical cause, such as exposure to fiberglass insulation or a similar irritant. If the animal has fleas, use an appropriate treatment and build your pet's resistance with improved nutrition. If the cause is emotional or nervous, be sure your pet gets sufficient exercise and use an appropriate flower essence, herbal blend or hands-on therapy.

If the animal is a teething puppy, adolescent dog, rabbit of any age or bird with a sharp beak, his need to chew may result in damaged furniture, shoes or other items. This is not a behavior problem; it's a reflection of the owner's poor planning. Raw bones and a cage of his own can keep a puppy busy and his surroundings tidy for hours. Refill the hollow center of marrow bones with cheese or peanut butter for an encore. Pet stores are full of chew toys designed for dogs of all ages and sizes for between-meal gnawing.

Supply clean hardwood blocks, thick dowel rods or appropriate chew toys for rabbits and birds. Hard-shelled nuts are good for cockatoos, macaws and other large birds.

Boredom contributes to nervous chewing, so be sure your pet has interesting toys and spends time every day in meaningful play with you, the other people in your house or other animals.

See also: *Behavioral Problems, Bird Care* and *Lick Granulomas.*

Cold Weather

Cold weather takes a toll on pets just as it does on their owners. New seasons bring climate changes that affect us all, indoors and out. Wild animals and pets that spend most or all of their time outdoors prepare for cold weather by growing thick, protective coats of heavy fur. Shorter hours of sunlight and dropping temperatures trigger this transformation. Even indoor pets respond to the cycle of seasons, though less dramatically.

Hot forced-air heating systems circulate dust and dry indoor air, stressing our furred and feathered companions. Sunlight streaming through windows can quickly heat a room, and because the sun's angle is lower now, its path has changed. Be sure your dog's crate and your bird's cage are in comfortable locations, far from heat registers and direct sun.

When humidity drops, everything dries out. Static electricity generates static sparks and makes fur and feathers unruly. Dehydration increases your pet's need for water. Keep your animals comfortable with a humidifier and refill water bowls frequently.

If your dog sleeps outdoors or in a garage, provide shelter to keep him warm and dry. A dog sleeping on a cold surface, such as a cement floor, can experience cold-weather lameness from lying on one side through the night. Guard against this by installing a thick layer of blankets or an insulated dog bed.

Animals younger than six months, elderly animals and those in poor health are more adversely affected by cold weather than those in their prime. Be cautious in scheduling outdoor activities and err on the side of caution.

Protect rabbits from sudden changes of temperature. Rabbits are very susceptible to hypothermia, especially when ill.

Never leave your pet outdoors and unattended in a snow storm; blizzards are very disorienting. If your dog needs to go out, put him on a long leash and hold the other end.

Herbal Therapies: Dogs' and cats' paw pads can be irritated by ice, snow, road salt and chemical de-icers, especially between the toes. If your pet is exposed to road salt or sidewalk chemicals, soak his feet in chamomile, yarrow, oatstraw or black tea, or mix 2 cups warm water with 1/4 cup oatmeal for foot soaking. If sores develop between his toes, apply comfrey tincture or grapefruit seed extract diluted with an equal quantity of water, full-strength aloe vera gel or a 15-percent tea tree oil solution. Prevent this type of damage with one of the natural wax or balsam products sold in pet supply stores to protect dogs' paw pads from road salt, melting chemicals and ice in winter and from hot sidewalks in summer.

If your pet is sensitive to cold temperatures, feed warming herbs like ginger root and cayenne pepper and stimulate acupressure point ST36.

Nutritional Therapies: Be sure your pets' winter diet is rich in essential fatty acids. Natural cold-pressed olive, sesame and avocado oils are often recommended for winter use. In cold weather your dog's calorie needs increase, so if her exercise routine remains the same, increase her rations. Tom Holcomb, D.V.M., who writes the Veterinary Clinic column for *Gun Dog* magazine, recommends a modest weight gain for working dogs at the beginning of cold weather so that energy reserves are available when needed. "Going into hunting season," he writes, "I like to see dogs carry a light to moderate covering of fat over the rib cage. Also, diets high in fat should be used during extended hunting periods to maintain condition."

Antifreeze Warning: As the seasons change, be careful with antifreeze. Many pet lovers are switching to dog-friendly antifreeze, but most antifreeze is still sweet and deadly, thanks to its ethylene glycol. As little as four tablespoons can kill an adult dog and 1 teaspoon can kill a cat. Two-thirds of the veterinarians polled in a recent survey report that they treat at least one case of antifreeze poisoning every year. Clean up spills promptly and dispose of drained antifreeze and empty containers so no animals can reach them.

See also: *Bird Care* **(winter bathing) in this chapter and** *Hypothermia* **and** *Frostbite* **in Chapter 12,** *First Aid.*

Circulatory Problems: See *Heart Disease*

Cirrhosis: See *Liver Disease*
Colitis: See *Digestion*

Conjunctivitis: See *Eyes, Vision*

Constipation

Constipation is common in inadequately exercised pets fed a commercial diet and rare in well-exercised pets fed a natural diet.

The easiest way to prevent this condition is to provide a nutritious raw diet with ample drinking water, fresh air and exercise, frequent opportunities to eliminate and, for cats, a clean litter box.

The one factor in a raw-food diet that may cause problems for dogs and cats is raw bones. If your pet isn't used to this essential food, he may experience temporary constipation or diarrhea while his system adjusts. Feed raw meaty bones every few days rather than every day; give the bones immediately after the largest meal of the day; start with single servings and boost digestion with enzymes, hydrochloric acid supplements, cider vinegar or bitter herbs such as fresh minced dandelion.

If your pet is constipated, follow the above strategy and use any or all of the following.

Nutritional Therapy: In addition to the well-balanced, variety-filled raw diet recommended throughout this book, provide additional grated carrots, apples and other minced or puréed fruits and vegetables. If stools are dry, increase fluid consumption by adding fresh carrot juice, apple juice or water and a pinch of unrefined sea salt to each meal. In addition, add 1/2 to 1 teaspoon of olive, sesame, avocado or fish oil to food twice daily. Soak bran, powdered psyllium husks, pectin or a combination of these fibers using 1/4 teaspoon per 10 pounds of body weight in a small amount of juice or water until soft and fully hydrated and add it to food, giving half in the morning and half at night. Most dogs and some cats enjoy fresh figs and dates as well as dried figs and prunes that have been soaked overnight. Feed directly or purée and add to food in small amounts. Juliette de Bairacli Levy recommends adding freshly grated coconut and sesame tahini to food for dogs and cats.

Be sure to provide ample drinking water and encourage your pet to consume extra fluids to avoid any possibility of intestinal obstruction.

Homeopathy: Give 1 tablet of *Nux vomica 6c* every 12 hours for three days to pets that strain to produce small amounts without relief, especially if the animal avoids petting, withdraws and acts irritable. Use *Silica 6c* when weak rectal muscles do not expel fecal matter and it slips back in; give 1 tablet every 12 hours for three days. A single dose of *Sepia 30c* is recommended for severe chronic constipation in cats.

Herbal Therapy: Add finely minced wheat grass and garlic to food.

If constipation continues, add a small pinch of powdered senna leaf or cascara sagrada, both of which are mild laxatives, to juice or water in the morning and at night for one or two days. If normal bowel movements do not resume, increase the dosage for two additional days.

Color Therapy: Lemon systemic front, yellow over the lower back and, if the condition does not respond, orange over the lower back.

Exercise: This is so important, it deserves special mention. Take your dog for long walks, let her run and jump, take her swimming, keep her out in the fresh air and natural light and give her every opportunity to relieve herself. Follow the same advice as much as possible for cats, rabbits, birds and other pets.

Acupressure: Stimulate points LU7 and SP6. In cases of dry constipation, use ST36 as well.

Other: Richard Pitcairn warns that aluminum toxicity can cause constipation by weakening rectal muscles. Sources of aluminum include cookware, dishes, pet food sold in aluminum cans, processed cheeses, refined table salt, white flour and some tap water. If you suspect this problem, remove all sources of aluminum and consult a holistic veterinarian. Pitcairn recommends high levels of vitamin C (500 mg to 3 g daily) with a chelated zinc supplement (5 mg for cats and small dogs, 10 mg for medium dogs and 20 mg for large dogs) to help remove aluminum from the body.

Cuts, Wounds: See Chapter 12, *First Aid*

Dandruff: See *Skin and Coat*

Dental Problems: See *Teeth and Gums*

Diabetes

Once rare, diabetes is now common in pets in North America. Who are its victims? Animals, primarily dogs and cats, fed cooked and processed foods, especially a monotonous lifetime of commercial grain-based pet food. Semimoist treats and foods containing sugar and other refined carbohydrates are major contributors, but all canned and packaged foods contribute to the disorder. In pets given a well-balanced raw diet and healthful lifestyle (adequate exercise, exposure to natural light, etc.), diabetes simply doesn't exist.

The insulin deficiencies that define diabetes cause blood sugar to be excreted through the urine, resulting in a chronic state of semistarvation, weakness, abnormal thirst and excessive urination. Although insulin injections control these symptoms, they do not cure diabetes. As the illness progresses in dogs and cats, diabetes often causes weight loss, pancreatic inflammation, cataracts in the eyes and urinary tract infections.

If your pet is already being treated for diabetes, work with a holistic veterinarian to reduce or discontinue insulin injections, a process that should be carefully monitored.

Nutritional Therapy: A natural, raw diet is a must for diabetic dogs and cats. Feed two or three small meals rather than a single meal to help reduce stress on the pancreas. Many veterinarians recommend a low-fat diet to further help the pancreas because its secretions are necessary to digest fat. While this is more important on a cooked-food diet, and while a very low-fat diet is unhealthy in its own way, trimming some of the fat from raw meats is probably a good idea.

Brewer's yeast, which is rich in chromium, is often recommended for diabetic pets. Give 1 teaspoon to 1 tablespoon with each meal, depending on the animal's size.

Vitamin E reduces the need for insulin. Give 25 to 200 IU of a food-based vitamin E-complex daily. Vitamin C is another important nutrient; if your pet isn't already taking vitamin C, use a good quality supplement (not ascorbic acid) and give up to 500 grams per 20 pounds of body weight, starting with smaller doses, for as long as the disease remains active.

Juliette de Bairacli Levy notes that although carrots are often forbidden to diabetic patients, they contain a natural insulin and are really beneficial, as are Jerusalem artichokes. Use either vegetable raw, grated, pressed with unrefined sea salt, juiced or puréed. Jerusalem artichoke flour is sold as a probiotic food supplement. Although a steady diet of sweet fruits is not recommended and dried fruits are a concentrated source of sugars, a daily apple, banana or other fresh raw fruit can be part of your diabetic pet's diet.

If you have a source of raw milk, especially goat's milk, feed it often. If the sale of raw milk is illegal in your state, make your own yogurt or kefir with the best quality milk you can buy (whole, organically raised, not homogenized) and feed it to your pet as soon as it's ready. Don't rely on supermarket yogurts because these foods are most therapeutic when only a few hours old.

Herbal Therapy: The leaf of the olive tree *(Olea europaea)* is a traditional European remedy for diabetes, and modern research indicates that it reduces a diabetic's need for supplemental insulin. In her *Complete Herbal Handbook for the Dog* and Cat, de Bairacli Levy recommended 1 teaspoon of olive leaf tea daily for diabetic pets. If you have access to an olive tree, you can brew your own decoction (the olive's leathery leaves require simmering) or make a concentrated tincture. Because the leaf can cause gastric symptoms, these preparations should be taken after meals and not on an empty stomach. Recent innovations in the manufacture of olive leaf extracts have produced powders with no adverse side effects for which a variety of claims are made. See page 493.

The Chinese herb fo-ti *(Polygonum multiflorum)* is a specific for diabetes and hypoglycemia. An adaptogen, it helps restore balance and corrects deficiencies througout the body. Fo-ti can be given as a tonic for long periods.

Devil's club *(Fatsia horrida, Panax horridum* or *Echinopanax horridum)* is a ginseng cousin that grows in the Pacific Northwest and has a long history of use among Native Americans for adult-onset diabetes. Devil's club root tincture is popular with human diabetics who use it to replace or reduce their daily insulin, and a growing number of pet owners give it to their diabetic dogs and cats.

Bean pod tea is another blood sugar balancer. The pods of green beans contain an insulin-like hormone that helps control diabetes. Add raw green beans (string beans, not lima beans) to your pet's diet, put them in the juicer with carrots and other vegetables or brew bean pod tea with fresh green beans or with dried bean pods from an herb shop or health food store.

Garlic is helpful to diabetics and so are the blood cleansing herbs dandelion and burdock.

Homeopathy: One of the most dramatic adverse reactions to homeopathy Larry Bernstein has ever seen followed his treatment of a diabetic cat. Dr. Bernstein prescribed a single homeopathic remedy and instructed the owners to wean the cat off his daily insulin while improving his diet. They gave the remedy correctly but neglected to monitor his glucose as directed; less than a week later, the cat went into insulin shock. "That was a dramatic demonstration," says Bernstein. "The reaction occurred because the cat no longer needed the level of insulin he was receiving. The patient is fine, by the way. He recovered as soon as his owners gave him sugar and he's been well, and completely off of insulin, ever since."

There is no single homeopathic remedy for diabetes. "That's because its symptoms are so common," explains Bernstein. "There are over 100 remedies listed in the homeopathic literature for sugar in the urine, over 250 for increased thirst and over 100 for excessive urination. When you look at a case of diabetes, you always see the same symptoms, so it is important to prescribe homeopathically according to other symptoms that are more specific to the case or symptoms the pet may have shown prior to the onset of the disease.

"For example, in the literature there are less than 20 remedies each for desiring to hide and desiring warmth, and only one of them belongs to both categories. That's

Arsenicum. In this example, *Arsenicum* might be appropriate for a dog or cat manifesting these two symptoms, depending on the animal's other behaviors. Characteristic symptoms like these provide a much better clue to the best remedy for a specific animal than any general guidelines can, and this is why homeopathy is such a complex system of medicine. It's science mixed with art, and everything depends on the practitioner's education and level of experience. This is why I suggest that your readers consult a veterinarian with advanced training in homeopathy before attempting to treat an animal for this or any other serious illness."

Hands-on Therapies: Therapeutic Touch, acupuncture and acupressure are all appropriate in cases of diabetes. Massage acupressure point SP6.

Aromatherapy: Nelly Grosjean recommends a blend of the essential oils of eucalyptus, juniper and lemon.

Color Therapy: Lemon systemic front followed by yellow on the upper and lower abdomen and a magenta systemic front.

Flower Essences: Because stress contributes to diabetes, consider the flower remedies most likely to help your pet. See page 249.

Diarrhea

The frequent or uncontrollable evacuation of loose, watery stools can result from chemical poisoning, a bacterial or viral infection, food sensitivities, prescription drugs, internal parasites, swallowing a foreign object or the acute stage of a progressive disease such as liver failure. There is no single right treatment for diarrhea because it is not an illness in itself; it is merely a symptom reflecting the body's need to remove something from the digestive system as quickly as possible.

If you suspect poisoning, if your pet has a serious illness, if the animal is bleeding internally (dark or bright red blood in the stool) or if the animal is acutely ill, call your veterinarian immediately.

In most cases, diarrhea is the result of a viral infection, eating spoiled food, overeating or intestinal worms, and the symptom is sufficiently mild to treat at home. If your dog develops diarrhea after taking an herb, nutritional supplement or prescription drug or after eating certain foods, such as dairy products, discontinue and see if the symptom goes away. Most cases of diarrhea in dogs and cats are self-correcting and last only a few hours.

Regardless of its cause, diarrhea's most dangerous side effects are dehydration and the loss of essential minerals. Young and small animals are always at risk and so are adult dogs with copious diarrhea. Conventional veterinarians recommend electrolyte replacement products sold for human infants, but their labels show refined salt, preservatives, artificial flavors and other questionable ingredients. You're better off making your own with 2 cups water, 1 tablespoon unrefined sea salt, 1/4 teaspoon liquid colloidal trace minerals and 1/2 cup raw honey. In case the problem's source is water contamination, use bottled water or boil filtered tap water before using it. Give this solution from a bowl, spoon or eyedropper, 1 tablespoon solution per five pounds of body weight every two to three hours. If the animal is fighting an infection or illness, add any of the natural immunization herbs or supplements described on pages 285-286. If the animal is severely dehydrated and vomits frequently or refuses water, administer the fluid rectally with a bulb syringe or infant enema, raising the hindquarters for several minutes to improve absorption and assimilation. Repeat the rectal application of small amounts of fluid every three to four hours until the animal no longer retains the liquid.

Fasting is an important treatment for diarrhea because it allows the digestive tract to rest. Don't feed solid foods but offer fresh, raw carrot or apple juice or honey mixed with water if your pet is hungry.

Any sudden change in diet can produce diarrhea in rabbits; so can shock, cold chills or eating milk products. Rabbits are fond of milk but, as veterinary homeopath Christopher Day wrote, "It is a wholly unsuitable food." Owners can inadvertently cause diarrhea in their rabbits by keeping their cages scrupulously clean. Rabbits produce two types of fecal pellet: pale green droppings that have been through the digestive system once and dark shiny droppings that are the final product. If not given access to their first-stage droppings, they develop digestive disorders and vitamin deficiencies.

Nutritional Therapies: There are two schools of thought about diarrhea. One says that diarrhea is an essential part of cleansing whatever toxins are causing problems and that diarrhea should be allowed to run its course until the animal is clear of infection. The other says that diarrhea should be slowed or stopped because there are other ways to clear infection without diarrhea's side effects, which include dehydration and the loss of essential nutrients.

One of the most effective ways to slow diarrhea is with clay, which absorbs toxins and removes them from the body while "gluing" fecal matter together. Use green bentonite or montmorillonite clay powder sold for cosmetic purposes, liquid bentonite clay sold for intestinal cleansing or Kaopectate, which contains clay and pectin. If you are using clay powder or a very thick liquid, mix it with enough water to make it easy to pour and let it stand for 10 minutes to be sure it's fully hydrated. Give about 1/2 teaspoon of liquid clay or 1 teaspoon Kaopectate per 10 pounds of body weight and repeat the dose every four hours for one to two days. Give plenty of water and other fluids at the same time.

We associate powdered psyllium husks with accelerated bowel function because it's usually recommended for those with sluggish elimination, but when the problem is diarrhea, psyllium has the opposite effect: it slows things down by absorbing fluid and by helping create well-formed stools. Pectin has a similar effect. Clay, psyllium and/or pectin can be used together in juice or water. Avoid breathing psyllium husk powder; it can be allergenic. Add psyllium husk powder by itself or with pectin and/or clay to enough water or juice to make a slurry that's gelatinous but thin enough to pour (let it stand 10 minutes before using to be sure you've added enough liquid) and follow the dosage schedule for clay, above. Large, frequent doses of clay and fiber are a nutritional concern because they may leach minerals from the body. Trace mineral supplements help prevent deficiencies, especially if given between (not with) these treatments. In addition, the Austrian peat liquid Herbal Melange (see page 326) is appropriate.

Activated charcoal is always appropriate because it quickly absorbs toxins. If the diarrhea was caused by spoiled food or any type of poisoning, this is an effective first-aid treatment. See the instructions on page 325 for administering.

One of the most flavorful diarrhea cures is the ripe blackberry. Some herbalists keep dried blackberry powder on hand to treat diarrhea and, in a pinch, even blackberry jam has stopped an attack.

Another diarrhea cure is colostrum, the "premilk" secretions of nursing mothers, human and animal. Containing concentrated nutrients and immunity factors, colostrum prevents most bacteria, viruses and parasites from surviving in a newborn's digestive tract. For years, dried bovine colostrum has been a popular subject of veterinary research, for it prevents intestinal infections in livestock. More recently, bovine colostrum has become available as a human food supplement headlined for its beneficial effects on the immune system and for, among other things, its ability to cure and prevent diarrhea.

Acidophilus supplements are important in restoring intestinal health and they help prevent and control diarrhea. Use high-quality acidophilus supplements in amber glass jars from your health food store's refrigerator or make fresh yogurt or kefir for your pet.

Herbal Therapies: If the diarrhea is caused by a viral or bacterial infection or by internal parasites or protozoa, dose the animal with any of the natural immunizations described on pages 285-286.

After letting your pet fast for a day or until his fever subsides or other symptoms improve, soothe his digestive tract with demulcent herbs such as powdered slippery elm bark, comfrey, fenugreek seed or carob. Any of these can be mixed with water as a soothing gruel, as can oatmeal or Jerusalem artichoke flour. Aloe vera is another intestinal soother and it has antibacterial properties as well (see notes on laxative rind, page 143 and 313).

Aromatherapy: According to Grosjean's *Veterinary Aromatherapy*, cinnamon is the best essential oil to give for diarrhea.

Homeopathy: As with any widely experienced symptom, there are many factors to consider before prescribing a homeopathic remedy for diarrhea. Does the animal strain before, during or after bowel movements? Does the stomach churn and gurgle? What color is the diarrhea? Is there gas or flatulence, abdominal pain or pain during defecation? Is the anus sore or tender? Is the evacuation forceful, involuntary or effortless? How is the animal's behavior or personality different?

Dogs and Cats

The following homeopathic remedies work in most cases, according to Richard Pitcairn's *Natural Health for Dogs & Cats.*

- For diarrhea that gushes forcefully and smells terrible, *Podophyllum 6c,* a homeopathic preparation of mayapple, may be effective. Give 1 tablet every 4 hours for a total of three treatments.

- Dysentery's frequent bloody stools produced by painful straining, which results from eating a toxic substance or from a viral infection, often responds to *Mercurius corrosivus 6c* given as above.

- For diarrhea resulting from eating spoiled meat and accompanied by chills, weakness, thirst and frequent bowel movements that produce small quantities, give *Arsenicum album 6c* as above.

- For long-lasting, dark, offensive-smelling diarrhea in cats that act uncomfortable after eating, give *Natrum muriaticum 6c* as above.

- Overeating or eating food that is too rich or fatty can produce diarrhea as well as an upset stomach. Unlike most cases of diarrhea, thirst is not usually a symptom. For this condition, give *Pulsatilla 6c* as above.

Birds

In *Homeopathic Treatment for Birds,* Beryl M. Chapman wrote that diarrhea caused by starvation in birds is often bright green and liquid; it responds well to *Arsenicum 30c* given for 3 or 4 doses over two days. For dark or light brown diarrhea that continues for more than two days, give *Alum 30* on the same schedule. If the bird has a chill and diarrhea in wet weather, give *Dulcamara 30.*

Hands-on Therapies: Stimulate acupressure points L11 and SP6. If the diarrhea is watery and contains undigested food, use point ST36. In all cases, Therapeutic Touch will soothe your pet and help stimulate the healing process.

Flower Essences: Diarrhea doesn't always result from a pathogen, toxin or infection; its cause is sometimes emotional. Even if the cause isn't directly connected to your pet's state of mind, her response to it is. Flower essences such as Dr. Bach's emergency formula, yarrow formulas and other essences are appropriate support therapies.

Color Therapy: Give a yellow tonation over the entire abdomen once, then a turquoise systemic front. If the condition does not improve within 24 hours, give an indigo systemic front.

Digestion

Indigestion in various forms is discussed throughout this book. There are many types of indigestion, and although the conditions are not identical in pets and people, many of the same terms apply. For example, colic causes spasmodic abdominal pains, flatulence and other symptoms of indigestion; colitis is an inflammation of the colon that causes alternating bouts of diarrhea and constipation; gastritis is an inflammation of the stomach's lining that causes short-term discomfort or chronic pain; irritable bowel syndrome (IBS) is a chronic disorder in which the muscle of the lower colon produces exaggerated contractions causing pain, gas, bloating and alternating constipation and diarrhea; "leaky gut" syndrome results when incompletely digested food accumulates in the stool and small particles are absorbed into the body causing allergic reactions and other problems.

Bloat or gastric dilation is a serious condition in dogs, especially large breeds. Two to six hours after eating (the problem is most common in dogs fed large meals and almost always involves commercially prepared dry food) the stomach swells with liquid and gas; typically, the dog drools, attempts to vomit, forages desperately for grass and eventually becomes weak and collapses.

Remember that animals fed a fresh, raw, well-balanced diet with a healthful lifestyle don't have indigestion, colitis, irritable bowel syndrome, chronic bloating, flatulence and similar complaints. The following give temporary relief from the symptoms of indigestion and in some cases help strengthen the system, but they are no substitute for feeding the right foods in the first place.

Nutritional Therapy: Any of the above conditions may be caused or exacerbated by ingredients in commercial pet foods. Prevent bloat by feeding large dogs two or three small meals rather than one large one and never feed foods that will absorb fluid and swell in the stomach. Check for food sensitivities while improving the animal's diet. Give digestive enzymes with meals. If stools contain undigested food, the animal may have a deficiency of hydrochloric acid; try adding apple cider vinegar or a hydrochloric acid supplement when feeding meat.

apple, carrot or other fruit or vegetable juice for a day or two every week (use half-day fasts for very young or small animals) and whenever indigestion is severe.

If your rabbit suffers from diarrhea or indigestion, see the note on page 371.

A dog that has suffered one bloat attack is likely to suffer a worse one next time, and this condition is life-threatening. If possible, get the animal to a veterinarian at once. As an emergency treatment, prepare fresh cabbage juice and give 4 tablespoons to a giant breed and half that amount to a spaniel-sized dog every 15 minutes, or until symptoms subside. If you don't have cabbage on hand, dose with Herbal Melange (see page 326) or give the animal strongly brewed chamomile tea, several drops of chamomile essential oil or a teaspoon of licorice root tincture mixed with water.

Herbal Therapy: To relieve intestinal irritation and soothe a growling stomach, use demulcent, mucilaginous herbs like comfrey root, slippery elm bark, oats or arrow root. Add water-soluble fiber to the diet such as psyllium husk powder or pectin.

To prevent or relieve gas or flatulence, add any of the following to food as a tea, powdered herb, tincture or essential oil or give with a small amount of water: angelica root, aniseed, caraway seed, cardamon seed, catnip, cayenne pepper, celery seed, chamomile, cinnamon, cloves, fennel seed, ginger, lemon balm, licorice root or peppermint. In severe cases, give 1 or 2 capsules containing activated charcoal with water every 20 minutes until symptoms subside.

Ginger is an all-purpose digestive aid for dogs, cats, birds and other animals. Add fresh grated or dried powdered ginger or ginger tea or tincture to food; add fresh ginger to your juicer when making carrot juice for your pet. Chamomile is another specific for most canine and feline digestive disorders. It can be used in any form as often as desired.

Aromatherapy: The essential oils most recommended for indigestion or flatulence are caraway, nutmeg, coriander, cumin, mint and chamomile.

Color Therapy: For indigestion or flatulence, tonate with orange over the entire abdominal area. Darius Dinshah notes, "If tonated for a full hour too soon after eating, vomiting may result, which is usually beneficial."

For colitis, give a green systemic front followed by one or two yellow tonations over the entire abdomen and indigo on the same areas.

For acute indigestion (gastritis), tonate once with orange over the stomach and upper abdomen, then give a turquoise systemic front followed by indigo over the stomach and upper abdomen.

For chronic indigestion (gastritis), give a lemon systemic front followed by orange over the upper abdomen/stomach area.

Homeopathy: As veterinarian Larry Bernstein explained in the description of diabetes, there is no single homeopathic treatment for any disease with common symptoms. Accurate prescribing depends on symptoms other than those most associated with the disorder. For best results, keep a homeopathy handbook and basic remedy kit on hand. Dr. Pitcairn's *Natural Health for Dogs & Cats* gives several treatments for indigestion and bloating. For example, as described in Chapter 6, he recommends *Carbo. veg. 30c*, 1 dose of 3 crushed capsules every 15 minutes for a total of 3 treatments for a dog with bloat, especially if the animal is greatly distended with gas, looks very ill, has cold legs and ears and has a bluish color in the tongue and gums. A dog that has had at least one serious episode from which it has not fully recovered can be treated with a single treatment.

Flower Essences: Many digestive problems have emotional foundations. Experiment with essences that seem to fit your pet or consult a flower essence practitioner.

Hands-on Therapies: Any massage or therapeutic touch can be helpful. Stimulate acupressure point ST36.

You may notice symptoms of indigestion as your pet's diet changes to include more raw, whole foods. If that happens, treat the symptoms as they appear and make the transition slowly. Flower essences may help your pet adjust to a new diet.

Distemper, Canine Distemper/Chorea/ Feline Panleukopenia: See *Viral Infections*

Dysplasia: See *Arthritis*

Ear Problems

Every pet's daily or weekly health check should include a quick inspection of the ears. How do they look? How do they smell? If you wipe them gently with a cotton ball, ear wipe or tissue, is there a dark or greasy-looking residue? Does your dog or cat shake her head, paw at her ears and pull away from hands petting her ears or does she groan and lean hard against petting hands for a really deep, satisfying scratch?

If the ears look inflamed, have a yeasty or cheesy smell and leave a residue on your cotton ball, your pet may have an ear infection caused by bacteria, fungi or yeast or she may be allergic to pollen in the air or a food she's been eating. Dogs with allergies often chew their front feet and scoot on their rear ends across the floor so if you see these behaviors, be sure to check the ears.

Conventional veterinarians are quick to prescribe antibiotic ointments and pills. These may help clear the infection but do nothing to prevent its recurrence; in fact, by destroying beneficial bacteria in the body, antibiotics contribute to reinfection. Surgically installed drainage tubes don't solve the problem, either.

Minor ear infections and ear mite infestations are easy to treat at home, but get your pet to a veterinarian if he is shaking his head continually. It is not uncommon for dogs and even some cats to burst a blood vessel this way, and the resulting hematoma requires medical attention. Obviously, blood or pus coming from the ear is a serious symptom that should be examined by a veterinarian.

Ear wax and bacteria are normal inhabitants of an animal's ears. In fact, ear wax is a product of elimination, as are sweat and urine. Toxins, and the wax and oils that carry them, collect in the ear canal where resident bacteria break them down into a liquid that flows out naturally. However, when the animal's resistance is low or when beneficial bacteria have been destroyed by antibiotics, other bacteria proliferate and create infection.

How to Clean Your Pet's Ears

Prepare or purchase an ear wash or oil (see *Herbal Therapies,* below) and put it in an eye dropper or squeeze bottle. Heat the bottle in warm water to body temperature. Gently squirt or drop the liquid into your pet's ear and hold the ear flap shut before your pet can shake it out. Massage the skin and fur over the ear canal while holding the ear erect for half a minute or so. Release the ear and let your pet shake his ears, which will remove some of the wax and debris. Use a cotton ball or an ear wipe to clean the inside of the ear flap; deeper cleaning with a cotton swab is unnecessary and potentially harmful. Wipe the animal's head and neck.

Owners who are zealous about keeping their dogs' ears squeaky clean can create ear problems where none existed. If your floppy-eared dog loves to swim, it isn't necessary to flush her ears with drying chemicals every time she comes out of the water; just wipe them gently with a piece of cotton wadding or a soft cloth. If you notice a dark discharge, don't assume it's a bacterial or fungal infection; it may be nothing but wax. Take her to the vet if an infection becomes serious or causes obvious discomfort.

If the discharge in your pet's ears looks gritty, like dried coffee grounds, if the ear looks inflamed and your cat scratches her ears when you rub them or your dog shakes his head and scratches his ears frequently, ear mites are the likely culprit. Prepare an ear oil as described below in *Herbal Therapies* and apply it every other day for a week, let the ears rest for three days, then apply the oil every three days for an additional month. The oil will smother the tiny mites, and its repeated application will treat new generations, preventing a recurrence.

Wipe away any oil that spills on your pet's fur and, if necessary, clean the area with a mild soap or pet shampoo. At the end of this course of treatment, rinse your pet's ears well with the herbal ear wash described below. If desired, wash him with a mild liquid soap or pet shampoo first, rinsing the ears well.

Nutritional Therapies: Keep your pet on a natural raw diet and check for food sensitivities. Chronic ear infections often disappear when an animal stops eating dog biscuits, sugary treats and other processed foods. Give large doses of acidophilus and, if your pet tolerates it well, fresh yogurt or kefir. Some owners and veterinarians report good results in desensitizing the animal to airborne allergens by adding small amounts of bee pollen to food for several weeks in early spring. If you decide to try this strategy, use pollen from a local beekeeper. Another bee product is propolis, which helps prevent and clear infections. Give animals weighing up to 35 pounds 250 mg twice daily (divide a 500 mg tablet or capsule in half); animals up to 85 pounds can take 500 mg twice daily and giant breeds 1,000 mg twice daily. Follow this schedule for 10 days, then give the propolis once daily for two weeks.

In addition, increase the dosage of vitamin C to bowel tolerance until the infection clears.

Herbal Therapies: If your pet's ear problems worsen in spring and summer pollen seasons, add stinging nettle or mullein leaf to food. If you suspect a yeast or bacterial infection, add grapefruit seed extract, echinacea tincture and/or other infection-fighting herbs for short periods, such as five to seven days at a time. If the ears improve, repeat this therapy as needed, supplementing with acidophilus and probiotic foods at the same time.

Prepare an ear wash by making a 15-percent tea tree oil solution as described on page 185. To 1 cup of strongly brewed chamomile, comfrey, plantain or calendula tea add 1/2 cup of the tea tree oil solution and 10 drops of liquid grapefruit seed extract. Apply as directed above. Alternatively, add 1/8 teaspoon essential oil of lavender to 1 tablespoon calendula tincture, black walnut hull tincture, echinacea tincture or a blend of all three. Add this mixture to 1 cup aloe vera juice or gel and mix well. Or combine 1/8 teaspoon lavender essential oil with 3/4 cup witch hazel extract (the liquid sold in drug stores), 1 tablespoon powdered boric acid (another drug store item) and 1/4 cup aloe vera juice or gel. This preparation will help keep the ears dry, dissolve wax, remove debris and soothe the ears. Shake well before using.

Prepare an ear oil by making an olive oil infusion of fresh or dried mullein blossoms or garlic or both. Both are traditional ear "cures." If desired, add several drops of tea tree oil, vitamin E oil, grapefruit seed extract or essential oil of lavender. To treat ear mites, the oil can contain garlic, rue or other vermifuge herbs.

Acupressure: Massage point LI4. For chronic wax buildup, chronic moist problems or acute ear infections, stimulate point LI11. If the ears are red or inflamed, use point LU7.

Eczema: *See Skin and Coat*

Epilepsy, Seizures

Epilepsy has become common in dogs and is sometimes seen in cats. Holistic veterinarians have long associated the condition with incorrect feeding and vaccinations. Before deciding when and how to vaccinate your dog or cat, review the pros and cons with your holistic veterinarian or veterinary homeopath. This is especially important if your pet has ever had seizure symptoms or if any of its siblings are epileptic. Because epilepsy or a susceptibility to having seizures can be inherited, pets with this disorder should be neutered or spayed and not allowed to reproduce.

Nutritional Therapy: A natural diet is a must, for just about everything in commercial pet foods can worsen the animal's health. Extra zinc, B vitamins, vitamin C, trace minerals and other nutrients in whole foods help strengthen the nerve sheaths and prevent attacks.

Veterinarian Wendell Belfield notes that vitamin B6 deficiencies have long been associated with seizures in all mammalian species. In his experience, animals on a good vitamin and mineral program don't have epilepsy. "Whenever an animal is brought to my office suffering from seizures," he wrote in *How to Have a Healthier Dog,* "I ask the owner if the dog has been on supplements of any kind and invariably the answer is no." Belfield recommends 50 mg vitamin B6 daily for an average size dog and 100 mg for larger breeds; use B6-Niacinamide from Standard Process, Inc., or another brand made from whole-food sources for best results.

Belfield gives dogs suffering grand mal seizures a central nervous depressant such as Dilantin for one month in combination with vitamin-mineral therapy. The drug has no curative powers but sharply reduces the intensity of seizures while the vitamins build up the animals' system. Then he gradually withdraws the drug and continues the supplements. In most cases, he reports, the animals stay seizure-free. The use of an herbal nervine, as described below, may be equally effective in giving the animal relief from seizures while vitamins and other nutrients strengthen the body.

Belfield explains that worm infestations can cause seizures because internal parasites such as roundworms release toxins that have an adverse effect on the nervous system. Before treating an animal suffering from seizures, he runs a fecal exam and checks for eggs. If there is a parasite infection, he deworms the animal after injecting .5 gram of sodium ascorbate (vitamin C) per pound of body weight. "The worming procedure is toxic," he explains, "and I want the animal protected as much as possible." Vitamins and minerals don't prevent infestation but they buffer the host animal against toxins from both the parasites and worming medication. High doses of vitamin C for two weeks after worming protect against residual toxins.

Martin Schulman, V.M.D., reported in the *Journal of the American Holistic Veterinary Medical Association* (May 1996) that mineral deficiencies often contribute to the development of seizures. In his clinic, a review of the medical histories of patients diagnosed with epilepsy revealed that an "astonishingly high percentage" showed significant manifestations of pica, an eating disorder caused by malnutrition. In one case, a female German Shepherd had a history of licking wrought iron and eating Christmas tree lights and glass. Treating the patient for pica with an improved diet supplemented with plant-derived colloidal minerals, digestive enzymes and probiotic foods cured the pica within 21 days and the dog had no additional seizures.

Food sensitivities and allergies are important triggers. Placebo-controlled double-blind trials have shown complete recovery from epilepsy in human patients when offending foods were removed from the diet, and there is evidence that certain chemicals, such as industrial air pollutants, pesticide sprays, smoke, solvents, volatile compounds and food additives can cause human seizures. The same factors are blamed by holistic veterinarians for seizures in pets. In fact, switching a seizure-free dog from a high-quality diet to a commercial dry food can trigger a relapse, as a friend of mine recently demonstrated.

Herbal Therapy: If your dog has been taking a prescription drug to control seizures, work with a holistic veterinarian when using alternative therapies. Give extra support to the liver with herbs like milk thistle seed to any pet taking pharmaceutical drugs, especially over a long period of time and especially when those drugs are reduced or discontinued.

American herbalist John Christopher was famous for his successful treatment of epileptics. He discovered that even the most severe, untreatable cases responded to what he named B&B tincture, made of equal parts blue cohosh, black cohosh, blue vervain, lobelia and skullcap. Instead of taking the tincture orally, his patients placed the tincture in each ear before bed, holding it in place overnight with cotton. Dr. Christopher considered blue cohosh, black cohosh and blue vervain specifics for the medulla oblongata, the base of the brain stem, which forms the major pathway for nerve impulses leaving and entering the skull and which contains centers that regulate circulation, respiration, salivation and swallowing. Lobelia is an excellent catalyst, especially for nerves, and skullcap is a well-known nerve healer. In his long years of medical practice, Christopher treated all types of nerve damage with B&B tincture, and it repaired even long-standing disorders.

I know people who have tried this remedy on their epileptic dogs with immediate results. My sample is tiny, but all of these dogs have been seizure-free without prescription medication and with no adverse side effects since their first use of the tincture. According to David Christopher, Dr. Christopher's son and the director of the School of Natural Healing, the protocol for treating humans with epilepsy is 4 drops of B&B tincture in each ear twice a day, 1 dropperful massaged into the skin at the base of the skull every hour during the day and 2 dropperfuls taken orally three times a day. An animal who has been taking seizure-prevention drugs can use the same dosages adjusted for his or her weight. For example, a dog weighing 60 pounds would take half these amounts. David Christopher recommends that pet owners begin with small doses and increase to the recommended quantities within a week. Continue at the maximum dosages for three weeks and, if the animal remains free of seizures, gradually taper to a maintenance dose of 5 to 10 drops orally per day. Several dogs have made the transition to a drug-free, seizure-free life on 2 oral dropperfuls daily. The above protocol, with its frequent external applications, may be most appropriate in severe casses.

Physical and emotional exhaustion can trigger attacks. Either skullcap tincture or B&B tincture is an appropriate preventive in times of stress, upheaval or exhaustion.

Homeopathy: If seizures are caused by vaccines, *Thuja 30c*, homeopathy's vaccine-clearing remedy, may be helpful. Give the remedy at least an hour after food or water, then wait at least an hour before letting your pet eat or drink. Richard Pitcairn recommends a single dose of *Thuja 30c* followed one month later by a single dose of *Silicea 30c* for epilepsy in dogs and cats.

If seizures are the result of a head injury, give *Arnica 30c* once every 12 hours for three treatments.

If either of these remedies is ineffective, consult a veterinary homeopath. When epilepsy responds to a homeopathic remedy, it does so at once and there is no need for further treatment.

Hands-on Therapies: Acupuncture can be very effective in the treatment of epilepsy. Therapeutic Touch, TTouch and other massage techniques help soothe a stressed animal and heal neural pathways.

Color Therapy: Give a purple systemic front, then treat the head and upper body, front and back, with lemon and yellow for two weeks followed by lemon and orange for four weeks.

Eyes, Vision

Keep your pet on a well-balanced raw diet with ample exposure to natural light and she'll see well into her old age.

In cases of injury or serious infection, see your veterinarian. Any of the following drops and washes can be used to help heal a scratched or injured eye or to rinse debris from the area.

Cataracts

Cataracts usually develop because of nutritional deficiencies or an injury to the eye. Cloudiness in the eyes of older pets does not necessarily interfere with their vision; they can often see well despite the scar tissue that thickens the lens.

Nutritional Therapy: A natural diet with vitamin supplements derived from whole foods is essential to any animal with vision problems. Dogs respond well to the carotenes in freshly made carrot juice; cats derive more benefit from animal sources of vitamin A such as liver. In *How to Have a Healthier Dog* Wendell Belfield described veterinarians who used vitamins A and E and the mineral selenium to prevent, reverse and eliminate cataracts in dogs. In addition to supplementing the diet with these antioxidants, provide a good quality vitamin C with bioflavonoids and trace minerals. The eyes use more zinc than any other organs in the body, so be sure your supplement provides this essential mineral.

As cat owners discovered when commercial pet foods did not include taurine, a deficiency of this amino acid can cause blindness in cats. Dogs and cats fed raw meat receive ample taurine and other essential amino acids.

Herbal Therapy: Bilberry, a wild blueberry, is well known as a vision improver. Bilberry teas, tinctures and other products improve capillary circulation in the eyes and throughout the body. While not a specific for cataracts, bilberry is an appropriate support therapy and preventive for any eye disease or disorder.

Other herbs that improve circulation and, as a result, help improve vision and eye health are gotu kola, ginkgo, cayenne and ginger.

Chinese medicine treats the liver for all vision problems, an indirect approach that has cured or improved many different conditions. Make liver support part of your pet's vision program by using milk thistle seed, burdock root, dandelion leaf or root and other alterative herbs.

In *Health Through God's Pharmacy,* the Austrian herbalist Maria Treben recommended applying the orange sap of greater celandine *(Chelidonium majus),* a common roadside plant, to the eyelids with a wet finger to treat cataracts, detached retinas, eye fatigue, defective vision and distressed greenness from the eye. The then German writer used it on the daily walks he took with his old German shepherd. One day, as a joke, he applied it to the dog's eyes, and, from then on, the dog sat begging whenever his master used the celandine juice.

Having spent hours chopping this plant and getting its sap all over my hands and arms, not to mention applying its orange juice to my eyelids and occasionally Samantha's, I was startled to read a slew of warnings in American herbals. "Toxic," says *Eastern/Central Medicinal Plants* by Steven Foster and James Duke. "Stem juices highly irritating, allergenic, may cause paralysis."

Greater celandine is widely used in Europe, where doctors routinely use botanical medicines. In his authoritative textbook *Herbal Medicine,* German physician Rudolf Fritz Weiss, M.D., wrote of his extensive experiments with juice from the fresh plant and its effectiveness as a cure for warts. He made no mention of its internal or external toxicity. *The Protocol Journal of Botanical Medicine* (Volume 2, Number 2, 1997) reviewed the application of greater celandine sap to the eye as a treatment for cataracts and indicated that the treatment is safe. It may be that the warnings in American field guides and herbals are based on the plant's chemical analysis; they don't seem to be supported by clinical experience.

Greater celandine tea is a popular eye wash, and many herbalists and their students use it on their dogs and cats. Other eye-friendly eyewash treatments are calendula, chamomile and eyebright teas, and although it sounds uncomfortable, a tiny pinch of cayenne pepper added to the tea increases circulation without causing pain. To brew a tea that can be given internally and used as an eyewash for cataracts, combine equal parts of greater celandine, eyebright and St. John's wort; pour 1 cup boiling water over 2 teaspoons dry tea blend and add a tiny pinch of cayenne; let steep until cool. Filter the tea through fabric or a paper coffee filter, then add just enough unrefined sea salt to make it slightly saline, like tears. Test the tea on your own eyes to be sure it's comfortable. To apply, use an eye dropper or soak a cotton pad with tea and hold it to your pet's closed eyes.

Castor oil is a folk remedy for styes and eye infections; it is also used to treat cataracts. This is a sticky, viscous oil so apply it carefully, one drop in either corner of the eye daily until healed. Cod liver oil is rich in vitamin A and can also be applied as an eye drop as well as added to your pet's food in small amounts.

Homeopathy: Christopher Day recommends *Sulphur* for a cloudy lens, *Conium* for an aged dog suffering an eye injury, *Nat. mur.* for incipient cataracts and several other remedies for cataracts; Richard Pitcairn recommends *Conium maculatum 6x* once a day for four weeks.

Color Therapy: Lemon systemic front followed by two weeks of lemon and yellow on the face, then four weeks of lemon and orange, then six weeks of lemon and red. Also use magenta on the upper chest.

Light Therapy: Just as too much exposure to direct sunlight is blamed for cataracts, so is too little exposure to natural light. Help prevent this illness from developing or progressing by giving your pet many hours of unfiltered natural light every day.

Conjunctivitis

Conjunctivitis or pink eye is a red inflammation of the eyelids accompanied by a mucus discharge and, if the infection is severe, substantial quantities of pus. Sometimes conjunctivitis is caused by long hair that transfers bacteria into the eye, in which case cutting the hair short or tying it up helps prevent infection. Conjunctivitis can be highly contagious; it is more common among rabbits penned together than in those living alone, and, if one dog has it, his best friends may soon take it home.

Herbal Therapy: To prevent conjunctivitis, limit your pet's exposure to infected animals or, if your animal has the disease, keep her from spreading it. In either case, add infection-fighting herbs to her food, such as echinacea and grapefruit seed extract, use any of the eye washes described on page 383, adding 2 drops of grapefruit seed extract per 1/4 cup as a disinfectant and increase vitamin C to bowel tolerance for several days or until the infection clears.

Homeopathy: In *Homeopathic Treatment of Small Animals,* Christopher Day's list of the 22 "most useful" remedies for conjunctivitis reflects the need for proper diagnosis. For example, *Argent nit.* is recommended for intensely red or pink inflammation with profuse pus discharge or granular conjunctivitis with or without clouding of the eye and accompanied by abdominal symptoms. *Euphrasia* is recommended for conjunctivitis caused by traveling with the head held out a car window and aggravated by cold, dry wind; the eyes water profusely and the animal frequently rubs them. If your pet's symptoms exactly match one of the above, try it; otherwise, study a detailed handbook or consult an experienced veterinary homeopath.

Acupressure: Stimulate points LI4 and LI11.

Feathers: See *Bird Care*

Feline Acne: See *Skin and Coat*

Feline Immunodeficiency Virus: See *Viral Infections*

Feline Infectious Peritonitis: See *Viral Infections*

Feline Leukemia: See *Viral Infections*

Flatulence: See *Digestion*

Fleas: See *Parasites*

Hairballs

Gag. Hack. Hawk. Wrenching vomiting noises. Spit. Sometimes the concert includes a deep, yodeling yowl. The end result? A slimy looking mass of hair.

No, it isn't appetizing. Hair balls in cats are more common in long-haired breeds but any cat with insufficient roughage in the diet can have them. Cats swallow hair as they groom themselves, and the hair, unless pushed through the digestive tract, collects in the stomach. When enough accumulates to disturb the system, it gets ejected.

The most popular treatments for hairballs are flavored petroleum jellies, but these are not recommended by holistic veterinarians because petroleum products are immune suppressants and carcinogenic when taken orally. More important, they don't cure the problem.

Nutritional Therapy: Cats in the wild don't spend their afternoons gagging on hairballs, and they swallow not only their own hair but all the fur attached to their prey. To prevent hairballs at home, feed your cat a natural diet with plenty of raw bones, raw meat cut into chunks (not ground), finely chopped wheat grass, minced raw vegetables and, in small amounts, finely grated or puréed sprouting grain. These foods provide ample roughage to push swallowed hair through the digestive tract. To help it move smoothly, add olive, flaxseed or other oil as a lubricant. During shedding season, add well-soaked psyllium to your cat's food; stir 1/4 cup powdered psyllium husks into 3/4 cup warm water and let it stand to form a soft gel. Add 1 teaspoon of this hydrated gel to morning and evening meals. Adding diatomaceous earth as described on page 110 helps prevent the condition as well.

Grooming: Daily brushing is important because hairballs tend to be more serious in cats that neglect their grooming. If your cat enjoys water, wetting him with chamomile tea can be a special treat after brushing. It doesn't prevent hair balls, but it removes dander and smells wonderful.

Hair Conditions: See *Skin and Coat*

Halitosis, Bad Breath: See *Odors*

Heart Disease

Heart disease is tragically common in aging pets. Though dogs and cats don't have heart attacks or atherosclerosis the way people do, weak heart muscle, enlargement of one or both sides of the heart and related circulatory problems cause fatigue, shortness of breath, breathing difficulties and other problems.

Nutritional Therapy: To prevent and help treat heart disease, feed your pet a well-balanced, raw diet. Supplement the diet with high-quality vitamins A, E and C, coenzyme Q10, essential fatty acids and trace minerals. Wilfred Shute was a medical researcher as well as a Doberman Pinscher breeder, show judge and national club president when he and his brother, Evan, demonstrated the effectiveness of vitamin E in treating and preventing heart disease. It is thanks to his efforts that vitamin E is so widely used by veterinarians. Be sure to use a high-quality, natural vitamin E complex and not a synthetic.

Cider vinegar provides essential potassium; make a cider vinegar tincture of garlic or add cider vinegar by itself to food and water. Magnesium is essential to heart health but consult with your holistic veterinarian before adding magnesium supplements in large quantities. Raw bones provide magnesium, calcium, potassium and other minerals in the form most easily assimilated by dogs and cats and in their proper balance; make raw bones (not processed bone meal) your first choice in mineral supplements for heart health.

Selenium, zinc and chromium are also essential for the heart. Feed foods that are rich in these minerals, such as Brazil nuts (selenium), lamb, turkey and beef (zinc) and brewer's yeast or nutritional yeast (chromium) or give appropriate supplements.

Without the amino acid taurine, cats develop heart disease. This is not a risk factor for any cat on a raw-meat diet.

Fish oil supplements help reduce the loss of heart muscle mass in dogs suffering from heart disease, according to a study at Tufts University School of Veterinary Medicine. The condition, called cachexia, results in decreased strength and immune function. Patients receiving fish oil lived longer and had fewer symptoms than those who received a placebo. To provide fish oil, feed your dog fatty fish or use a fish oil supplement.

Herbal Therapy: Garlic, which is both a food and a medicinal herb, is one of the best herbs for the heart. By far the most frequently prescribed herb for heart disease it beautocou hotogr it repairs and strengthens heart muscle and can be used daily for months or years with no adverse side effects. See the dosage chart for herbal tinctures on page 136. If your pet does not improve within a week, double the dosage. Remember that individual needs and variations in tincture quality make specific instructions impossible. Hawthorn berry tincture is safe in large doses, so don't be afraid to increase the amount you use. Consult an herbalist or one of the recommended herb companies for a superior-quality product. The Chinese herb fo-ti protects and dilates blood vessels, increases blood flow to the heart and acts as an adaptogen to correct imbalances.

Cayenne pepper is another heart healer. Add small amounts of cayenne to your pet's dinner or give cayenne in capsules with plenty of food and water. Start with standard-strength cayenne, usually 45,000 heat units, and give a single capsule to a medium-size dog. For small dogs, take the capsule apart, remove about half and close the capsule. Give it to your dog in a piece of food so he swallows it whole, although some dogs really like the taste and enjoy chewing it. Gradually increase the amount of cayenne in food or capsules or increase the heat units (100,000 or more). Hot peppers are a concentrated source of vitamin C and they help eliminate intestinal parasites. Cayenne is appropriate for prolonged daily use.

The herbs gotu kola, ginkgo and ginger all help improve circulation. Bilberry strengthens capillaries. Add their teas, tinctures, powders or capsules to your pet's food on a rotating basis along with fresh minced dandelion greens, watercress and other herbs.

Exercise: Without daily exercise, heart muscles atrophy. Strengthen your pet's heart with regular exercise that is not too strenuous or exciting. Start with short walks and go a little farther each day.

Environmental Factors: Second-hand smoke is a serious risk factor for pets with heart disease, and it actually causes many of the symptoms associated with heart disease. Protect all your pets from it.

Homeopathy: For mild cases of heart weakness, the tissue salt *Calcarea fluorica 6x* (calcium fluoride) can be given daily. If the problem is related to nervousness or excitement, use *Kali phosphoricum 6x* (potassium phosphate).

Crataegus oxyacantha (hawthorn berry) remedies at low potencies such as 1x or 3x are widely used for animals with weak, dilated hearts, breathing difficulty, fluid retention and, in most cases, nervousness or irritability. Give once daily.

In his book of homeopathic remedies for dogs, George Macleod lists 11 remedies for congestive heart failure in dogs; in his handbook for small animals, Christopher Day gives 14 for heart and circulatory problems. For best results, consult an experienced homeopath.

Hands-on Therapies: Therapeutic Touch, massage, TTouch, acupuncture and acupressure are all appropriate therapies. To help improve heart imbalances, stimulate point SP6. In case of heart failure, stimulate the emergency point GV26 as described on page 217.

Color Therapy: Treat cardiac insufficiency with a lemon systemic front followed by magenta and indigo on the upper chest. For additional stimulation, scarlet can be used on the same area.

Flower Essences: Fear, excitement, anxiety and stress can overwork a diseased heart. Help your pet relax with an appropriate remedy, either Dr. Bach's emergency formula or one that fits your animal's situation and personality.

Heartworm: See *Parasites*

Hepatitis: See *Liver Disease*

Hip Dysplasia: See *Arthritis*

Hot Spots: See *Skin and Coat*

Hyperthyroidism: See *Thyroid Imbalance*

Incontinence: See *Urinary Problems*

Insect Bites: See *Parasites*

Influenza: See *Viral Infections*

Jaundice: See *Liver Disease*

Kennel Cough: See *Viral Infections*

Kidney Problems

Like every serious condition, problems such as nephritis (inflammation of the kidney) are easier to prevent than cure. Start with the healthy offspring of healthy parents, feed them correctly and, barring injury, they will live to a ripe old age with fully functioning kidneys.

Now that America's pets are fed from bags and cans, kidney failure has become the second leading cause of death among cats, and an estimated 25 percent of our dogs have some form of the disease.

Kidney failure is difficult to treat because it usually develops slowly, without obvious symptoms, for months or years before being detected. Any disease is more difficult to treat in its advanced stages, and by the time an animal's excessive thirst, weight loss, poor appetite, vomiting and strong urine odor in the mouth and skin receive attention, it may be too late.

If your dog or cat has kidney disease, consult a holistic veterinarian. The following support therapies may be appropriate.

Nutritional Therapy: The quality of protein in the diet is important, so buy the best you can find, preferably meat and poultry that is organically raised in open fields. Most holistic veterinarians recommend a low-protein diet based on white or brown rice, millet or other grains mixed with raw egg yolks, chicken or meat, parsley, grated asparagus, carrots or garlic, unrefined sea salt and unrefined olive, safflower, corn or sesame oil. Whenever you feed your pet cooked grains, be sure to add digestive enzymes.

Glandular supplements are often prescribed, depending on the animal's condition and lab test results along with vitamins, especially B complex and vitamin C. Use high-quality multiple vitamins derived from food sources and mineral supplements that are easy to assimilate. Richard Pitcairn recommends calcium lactate or gluconate or chelated calcium (supplements that do not contain phosphorus), 600 mg daily for dogs and 1,500 mg for cats. Magnesium is another heart-friendly herb and an ingredient in many calcium supplements. Look for a liquid supplement that contains calcium, magnesium and vitamin D, and adjust label directions for your dog's weight or consult a holistic veterinarian for advice.

Herbal Therapies: The kidney-cleansing herbs cleavers and cornsilk are often recommended; in addition to these, Juliette de Bairacli Levy recommends parsley tea and grated parsnips mixed with honey and shaped into balls. Small amounts of wheat grass juice, finely minced wheat grass or green juice powders help heal and deodorize the system. Small amounts of marshmallow tea (1/2 teaspoon to 1 tablespoon, depending on the animal's size) can be added to food twice a day for several weeks.

Hands-on Therapies: Therapeutic Touch and other physical therapies can be very helpful, and acupuncture has successfully treated many cases of kidney failure. At home, stimulate acupressure point SP6. In addition, stimulate the skin by vigorously brushing the skin and coat every day and, on a weekly basis, bathe using gentle soap or brush thoroughly and rinse the animal well with chamomile tea.

Homeopathy: The more serious and long-lasting the ailment, the more important is accurate diagnosis. Consult a veterinary homeopath.

Color Therapy: For acute nephritis, give a turquoise systemic back, magenta systemic front and tonate with scarlet on the lower back. For chronic nephritis, renal sclerosis or uremia, give a lemon systemic back, magenta systemic front and scarlet on the lower back.

Leptospirosis

Once known as lamp post disease because it affected city dogs who inspected urine deposits, leptospirosis is spread through urine by rats and other animals. In people, it causes severe flu-like symptoms that last up to three weeks. In dogs, symptoms include loss of appetite, a tender abdomen, strong-smelling urine that may contain blood, rapid weight loss and internal bleeding that causes death.

Nutritional and Herbal Therapies: As Juliette de Bairacli Levy wrote, "Healthy dogs do not get leptospiral infections; they come to the ones reared by unnatural methods." Keep your pet's resistance high with a well-balanced raw diet and a natural lifestyle.

De Bairacli Levy's herbal treatment for infected dogs is to fast the animal immediately (water only) in a comfortably warm room with a supply of fresh air, dosing him morning and night with disinfecting herbs as described on page 284.

Bacterial infections usually respond quickly to grapefruit seed extract, bee propolis, noni, olive leaf extract, echinacea and other infection-fighting herbs. See the natural immunization programs described on pages 285-286. If your healthy dog is exposed to leptospirosis, his immune system will probably deal with it on its own. If he develops symptoms, dosing him with infection-fighting herbs should stop the illness's progression.

Lick Granulomas

Although they can be caused by a serious bacterial infection in the body, lick granulomas are most often the canine or feline equivalent of feather plucking; see page 362. In dogs and cats, excessive licking creates a shiny pink hairless spot that becomes an infected sore.

The most important treatment for lick granuloma is to boost your pet's overall good health by keeping him well fed, exposed to natural light, active and happy.

Herbal Therapy: Adapt the recommendations given for feather-plucking birds to your pet. In addition, apply aloe vera gel to the sore and add it to your pet's food. Although this probably won't work by itself, you may be able to discourage licking by applying diluted tea tree oil or grapefruit seed extract, full-strength Tabasco sauce, powdered cayenne pepper, echinacea-goldenseal tincture or several drops of a full-strength liquid trace mineral supplement to the sore. All of these help fight bacterial infections while healing the skin, and their taste may deter your pet from licking.

Lipomas: See *Tumors*

Liver Disease

The liver is your animal's busiest filter and its malfunction can be fatal. Hepatitis, cirrhosis, jaundice, hepatic lipidosis and other forms of liver disease all interfere with the removal of toxins from the blood, resulting in nausea, vomiting, loss of appetite, yellowing of the whites of the eyes, fatty-looking stools, diarrhea containing undigested food or abdominal swelling.

Jaundice, which produces the visible yellowing of tissue, can occur for reasons other than liver disease, such as a snake bite, chemical exposure, blood parasites or infection. Your veterinarian's diagnosis is important for proper treatment. As Beverly Cappel-King observes, conventional veterinarians are beginning to realize that not every case of kidney or liver failure is untreatable. Holistic healthcare has saved the lives of many dogs and cats given up for dead by their allopathic veterinarians. Use the resources in this book to locate a knowledgeable veterinarian to supervise your pet's care or to consult with your regular doctor.

The following are often recommended as part of the treatment of liver disease.

Nutritional Therapy: Begin with a short fast to let the digestive system rest. Give clean, pure water, not tap water that may contain impurities or toxins.

Improve the diet and give large doses of vitamin C, 500 to 2,000 mg four times per day depending on the animal's size. Glandular supplements are recommended as indicated by the animal's lab tests. The thymus gland is essential to liver health, and a combination of thymus tissue extracts, beta carotene and a multiple vitamin-mineral supplement has cured hepatitis in humans. To provide this same therapy for your dog, provide a high-quality thymus gland supplement and raw carrot juice daily. Begin with small amounts of carrot juice or grated carrots and increase to 4 to 6 tablespoons per day for dogs. Cats derive usable vitamin A from animal sources such as liver or cod liver oil.

Most veterinarians recommend reducing the amount of fat in the diet and, to some extent, protein. The food's quality is more important than usual and should be organically grown because any chemical residue will stress the liver. Feed only the highest quality, fresh foods to an animal with liver disease.

Feed digestive enzymes with meals and give acidophilus supplements. Cider vinegar can be added in small amounts to food and drinking water. Brewer's yeast and nutritional yeast are good sources of the B vitamins your dog needs, or give a high quality B complex supplement derived from food sources.

Herbal Therapies: Milk thistle seed and the Minor Bupleurum Formula (page 304) are specifics for the liver. All of the alterative or blood-cleansing herbs, such as dandelion, burdock root, red clover, yellow dock and nettles provide additional support. Essiac tea is often prescribed by holistic veterinarians for dogs and cats with liver disease. Herbal reference books list a bewildering variety of herbs for the liver, but these are the most important. Refer to the herbal dosage chart on page 136, follow product labels and adjust them for your pet's weight or ask your veterinarian for recommendations.

Homeopathy: Observe your pet carefully and write down all her behaviors and symptoms before consulting a veterinary homeopath.

Hands-on Therapies: Acupuncture is very helpful in the treatment of liver disorders. At home, use Therapeutic Touch, TTouch, other massage techniques and acupressure to encourage healing. Stimulate acupressure points ST36 and SP6.

Color Therapy: For jaundice, give a lemon systemic front, red on the liver, yellow on the entire abdomen area and magenta on the upper chest and lower back. For a fatty liver, give a green systemic front and red on the liver area. For acute hepatitis, give green and blue systemic fronts, then red over the liver. For chronic hepatitis or cirrhosis, give a lemon systemic front, red over the liver and magenta on the entire abdomen.

In these and other tonation schedules that involve abdominal organs, it's difficult to shine anything on the abdomen of a dog or cat unless the animal cooperates by sleeping upside down. Direct the colored light as best you can, keeping the animal calm and relaxed, and color-charge drinking water to supplement or replace the tonations.

Lyme Disease

Caused by a spiral-shaped bacteria called a spirochete (pronounced SPY-ro-keet) and spread by ticks, Lyme disease can infect humans, farm animals, birds and pets. The Middle Atlantic states, southern New England, Georgia, Wisconsin and California are

America's Lyme disease hot spots, but the infection is spreading geographically.

Lyme disease, named for the Connecticut town in which it was discovered, is difficult to diagnose because its symptoms mimic other illnesses, such as arthritis. Left untreated, it can cause neurological damage and the degeneration of several systems and organs. The primary symptoms of Lyme disease are lameness and joint inflammation, which can develop gradually or paralyze the animal overnight. Sometimes a loss of bladder control in housetrained dogs is caused by advanced Lyme disease.

At Texas A&M University, Colin Young, Ph.D., headed a research team that infected cats with Lyme disease bacteria. When the scientists did "exhaustive work on every conceivable tissue and organ," Young reported, they found increased antibodies and organ or tissue damage. The infected cats didn't show symptoms, just as mice and deer, which are the most common hosts of the ticks that carry Lyme disease, don't show clinical signs of the illness. Do cats really contract the disease? Veterinarians see what they consider to be Lyme disease in cats, but felines appear more resistant than canines or humans. The initial symptoms in infected cats are said to include a fever, fatigue, lethargy and a loss of appetite.

Tick Removal

While tiny Ixodes or deer ticks (black-legged ticks) are most associated with Lyme disease, researchers suspect the larger Lone Star tick and American dog tick of carrying its *Borrelia burgdorferi* bacteria. Every bite should be treated with suspicion. Inspect your pet daily, checking for tiny bumps that might be gorging ticks. Be careful when removing a tick to grasp it with tweezers firmly at the head, as close to the pet's skin as possible, and slowly pull straight back. Never twist, press, burn or apply irritating substances like kerosene to an attached tick because doing so can cause the parasite to regurgitate the contents of its digestive tract, creating a hypodermic effect. After removing the tick, cover the bite with 3-percent hydrogen peroxide, a dilute solution of tea tree oil, diluted grapefruit seed extract or all three. These antiseptics are recommended because they destroy the Lyme disease bacteria on contact.

Nutritional Therapy: To help prevent Lyme disease, feed a well-balanced, raw diet with appropriate supplements. During tick season, increase the animal's vitamin C and trace minerals. To help a dog who's being treated for Lyme disease who has mild joint pain, follow the suggestions for arthritis on page 354-356.

Herbal Therapy: To prevent Lyme disease, do what you can to prevent tick bites; see page 169 for natural tick repellents. During tick season, occasionally dose your dog with grapefruit seed extract, olive leaf extract, maitaki mushrooms, astragalus, bee propolis or other infection-fighting supplements (see pages 285-286) to deter the growth of bacteria in the body. Do this whenever you discover a gorging tick as a preventive measure.

The herbal antiseptic tablets developed by Juliette de Bairacli Levy, which contain garlic, rue, sage, thyme, eucalyptus and wormwood, have reduced the incidence of tick bites, cysts or infections at the bite location and Lyme disease infection in dogs that previously suffered from these problems. Any of the vermifuge programs described on page 402-404 should have a similar effect.

For the past six years, herbalist Pam Montgomery at Green Terrestrial in Milton, New York, has been blending Auntie Lyme tea, which contains nettle, red clover, comfrey, calendula, peach leaf, strawberry leaf, mint, burdock seed and milk thistle seed. These liver tonic and calming ingredients are recommended as an adjunct therapy in the treatment of active cases and as a support remedy for those previously treated for Lyme disease. Although this tea was designed for humans, it is appropriate for dogs who are being treated or have been treated for Lyme. Brew a medicinal strength infusion and add it to your dog's food or drinking water or grind the tea into a powder and add it to food. Using either method, 1 teaspoon of the dried herbs would be appropriate for a 50-to 60-pound dog as a daily dose. Like most herbal blends, this formula is forgiving; there are no adverse side effects if you give more than the amount suggested here. Nettle tincture in large doses for extended periods is part of the human herbal Lyme disease protocol.

Homeopathy: Stephen Tobin, D.V.M., a holistic veterinarian in Connecticut, has published reports in the homeopathic literature of his successful treatment of several hundred cases of Lyme disease. After trying different homeopathic preparations with limited success, he discovered that *Ledum palustre* in a 1M potency given 3 times daily for three days is "about as close as you can get to a specific cure." According to Tobin, this method has cured cats, dogs and horses with recent and established infections, some of which were first treated with antibiotics. In addition, he uses the Lyme disease nosode, a homeopathic preparation of *Borrelia burgdorferi 60x*, as a preventive, giving 1 dose (one dropperful) daily for one week, then 1 dose weekly for one month, then 1 dose every six months. "In the past four years," he reported in 1995, "I have had only two dogs out of over 500 on this regimen that might have contracted Lyme disease, both of which readily cleared with Ledum."

Despite this protocol's apparent success, it doesn't work in every case, as I discovered when Lyme disease paralyzed Samantha two years ago. However, it has made such a difference to so many pets and people that it deserves consideration. Richard Pitcairn suggests five homeopathic remedies for Lyme disease in *Natural Health for Dogs and Cats*, one of which, *Bryonia alba 30c*, matched Samantha's symptoms well, for she lay quietly, unable to move and in great pain. Had she become more limber after moving, *Rhus tox 30c* would have been appropriate; had she been unusually submissive and uninterested in drinking water, *Pulsatilla 30c* might have helped; if she'd had red, inflamed gums, bad

~~breath and a tender joint that would heal with *Mercurius 30c* and if she had a high~~ fever and restless anxiety at the earliest stages, the most suitable remedy would have been *Aconitum 30c*. We continue to dose Samantha with the Lyme disease nosode, and she hasn't had a recurrence, knock on wood, despite occasional bites from deer and dog ticks.

Hands-on Therapies: Therapeutic Touch, TTouch, massage, acupressure and acupuncture help keep an animal's resistance strong. If Lyme disease develops, these treatments can help relieve symptoms and stimulate healing.

Mange: See *Parasites*

Motion Sickness

Some dogs throw up the minute they get into a car or boat. Others wait an hour. Any pet can develop motion sickness, but dogs are the most frequent victims, no doubt because they're taken so many places.

If you want your dog to be a good traveler, take her everywhere so she gets used to the car. Healthy, well-socialized, frequently handled puppies don't get carsick; they can sleep anywhere.

Motion sickness is often related to feeding. We discovered that if we feed Samantha before we drive to New England, she throws up right on the Connecticut border. Two trips taught us to skip breakfast and feed her later. Fast your pet for half a day and give small, not large, amounts of water before departure.

Herbal Therapy: Ginger is the premium antinausea herb recommended for pregnant women, seasick or airsick passengers and anyone who gets carsick. It is most effective when people take enough to feel a heartburn-like sensation in the back of the throat, which can require as many as eight or more capsules. Individual responses vary so widely that it is impossible to convert a human dosage for animals. Fortunately, ginger is well tolerated by pets of all ages so you can experiment safely. Start with 1/2 capsule for very young or small animals or give 1 or 2 capsules to adults. If your pet will swallow pills, follow with juice, water or a small piece of food; if not, give the ginger in a small amount of food. The effects are usually apparent within half an hour and last for several hours. If traveling makes your pet anxious, any of the calming nervines, such as valerian, hops, passionflower or skullcap, will help him relax and sleep.

Flower Essences: Dr. Bach's emergency formula and other flower essences help calm a traveling pet. Apply frequently by mouth or topically, beginning several hours before departure.

Hands-on Therapies: The responses that trigger nausea can be interrupted with any of the physical therapies described in Chapter 7. Massaging the animal's ears, for example, or applying therapeutic touch can help prevent nausea.

Aromatherapy: Aromatherapist Nelly Grosjean recommends giving the animal essential oil of basil 48 hours before departure and placing a bunch of parsley under the animal while traveling.

Nails, Claws, Paw Pad Disorders

Our pets' claws are like our fingernails. They can break, become brittle, split and crack.

Trim your cat's claws often, every week or so, in order to keep sharp claws blunt. If your cat objects, use flower essences or calming herbs to help her relax and massage her ears and paw pads. Grooming can and should be a comfortable, pleasant ritual for both you and your pet. To trim a cat's claws, squeeze the paw pad so the claw extends and cut it with a sharp clipper or toenail trimmer far enough from the quick to prevent bleeding. If bleeding occurs, stop it with yarrow tincture or a styptic powder. With frequent trimming, the quick will retract and you can make the nails even shorter.

Use the same procedure for dogs or file their nails blunt with an emery board or use a rotary grinding drill called a Dremel tool. Ask your trainer, veterinarian or groomer for advice or check pet supply catalogs. If your dog gets sufficient exercise on sidewalks, gravel walks, concrete playgrounds, granite boulders and other rough surfaces, her nails will stay blunt, and you can use a file to smooth them further. Short nails help prevent injury to dogs, for long nails can snag, break or pull. They can also scratch people. Nursing home therapy dogs are required to have short, smooth nails because the skin of some elderly people is so fragile that a scratch resulting from a friendly handshake can result in infection.

Nutritional Therapy: The underlying cause of poor nail health is almost always poor nutrition. Upgrade your pet's diet with raw foods and easily assimilated trace minerals.

Herbal Therapy: Horsetail, which is rich in silica, is a specific for hair and nails. Add horsetail capsules, powder, tea or tincture to food or water. Myrrh hardens nails, claws and hoofs; dilute essential oil of myrrh with 2 parts carrier oil and massage it into splitting, cracking nails or apply myrrh tincture full strength. Any fungal infection involving the nails can be treated the same way or with tea tree oil or grapefruit seed extract. In addition, treat any fungal infection by adding grapefruit seed extract capsules, noni powder, olive leaf extract or acidophilus supplements to food.

Outdoor activity can be hard on a dog's paw pads, causing them to dry and crack.

In summer, hot pavement burns them; in winter, ice and road salt irritate the skin. Pet supply catalogs carry products for toughening, soothing and protecting canine paw pads. Look for products containing natural waxes or apply your own healing salve containing comfrey, calendula and/or St. John's wort. Oil-based salve is so interesting to most dogs that they lick it off as soon as you apply it, but even a few minutes of treatment will improve the skin. Soaking the feet in a solution of 1 teaspoon unrefined sea salt per cup of water heals cracks rapidly. This is because unrefined salt, unlike table salt or road salt, contains trace minerals that strengthen and repair the skin. Liquid trace mineral supplements have the same effect; apply any colloidal trace mineral product directly to broken, cracked, irritated or infected skin. For even faster healing, brew a very strong comfrey tea, add unrefined salt or colloidal minerals and soak your pet's feet in the solution.

Odors

If your pet gets skunked, you have an olfactory challenge, just as you do if he rolls in manure, dead fish or well-rotted mammal parts. Odors caused by sources external to your pet are easy to treat with odor-neutralizing enzyme products. Your pet supply store or mail order catalog stocks several brands. Keep at least a quart on hand for emergencies.

To treat your pet, apply the enzyme liquid, work it in and leave it on for several minutes according to label directions. Use the same type of product on pet stains in the house. The enzyme works by digesting the proteins in vomit, urine, fecal matter, skunk spray and decomposing organic material, literally removing the odor's cause.

The traditional treatment for skunk sprays is a tomato juice bath. This method is still widely recommended because it has worked for many. The secret, they say, is to apply canned tomato juice before doing anything else, like giving the animal a bath or rinsing the coat with water. Let the tomato juice stand for 15 minutes or longer before washing it out. A modern version of the same approach is any ready-to-use vaginal douche product applied full strength and left on the fur for half an hour before washing.

All of these treatments have a following, but the most effective may be a mixture of three common household products. Illinois chemist Paul Krebaum recommends 1 quart of 3-percent hydrogen peroxide, 1/4 cup baking soda and 1 teaspoon liquid soap for just about any malodorous condition. As reported in *Popular Science* magazine, this recipe derived from Krebaum's experience with thiols, the chemicals that give skunk spray, decaying fecal matter and decomposing flesh their distinctive odors. Note that the mixture is volatile if stored; it has to be prepared immediately before using. Combine the ingredients, apply thoroughly and rinse off.

In houses where cats live, litter box odors can be overwhelming. Here the solution is improved hygiene, more frequent changes of cat litter or the use of litters that help control odors. Orange or citrus oil sprays have become popular pet deodorizers, as have air sprays containing lavender oil. You can create similar air treatments at home. To help hide the scent of cat urine, Nelly Grosjean recommends a blend of 6 parts lavender oil, 3 parts terebinth oil, 2 parts lemon oil and 1 part mint oil. Use in a diffuser or spray the blend by hand. Other effective combinations are 5 parts pine oil and 1 part mint oil or 5 parts lavender and 1 part mint. The essential oil of eucalyptus is not sufficient to hide the smell of cat urine, Grosjean reports; the essential oil of exotic verbena repels cats, and none of the mild essential oils combine well with cat odors.

The odors that emanate from within an animal are more challenging to deal with than the external ones, but they can usually be improved. Check with your veterinarian to be sure the odor is not caused by a medical problem, then upgrade the diet. Raw bones and gristle are the first step to improving the teeth and gums, and green foods (wheat grass, other grasses and green herbs) deodorize skin and breath from the inside out. In addition, brush your pet's teeth with a canine or feline toothbrush and a pet toothpaste, plain water or a small amount of sea salt. Pet supply stores sell gauze wipes containing tooth-cleaning chemicals and you can make your own by wrapping your finger with gauze and dipping it in salt water.

Several companies make tablets or capsules containing breath-freshening ingredients for pets. Follow label directions.

As Valerie Ann Worwood noted in *The Complete Book of Essential Oils and Aromatherapy*, peppermint oil is an excellent deodorizer. She recommends rubbing a drop of full strength peppermint oil in a line from beneath the animal's ears down to and into the shoulders as an aid to internal as well as external detoxification.

In addition to brushing your pet's teeth, brush or comb her every day to remove old hair or fur and any debris that might be caught in it. Brushing distributes natural oils that keep the coat healthy. Bathing with soap isn't always necessary; in fact, it can strip these oils from the fur. To freshen your pet's coat, make her less allergenic, improve her smell and leave her looking fluffy, spray or soak her to the skin with an enzyme product appropriate for cats, dogs, birds, rabbits or other animals (check labels carefully) or rinse her with a fragrant herbal tea such as chamomile, lavender or peppermint.

The essential oil flea treatment described on page 170 is another effective coat deodorizer.

Overweight, Obesity: See *Weight*

Pancreatic Disorders

An inflammation of the pancreas, pancreatitis is most common in overweight dogs and cats who eat commercial pet foods, especially those that are low in protein and high in fat or carbohydrates. Its symptoms, which are related to indigestion, may follow episodes of overeating. The pancreas is important in the digestion of fats, and it produces insulin. Animals with chronic pancreatitis can become diabetic as the organ malfunctions.

Pancreatitis is often accompanied by hard abdominal muscles and arching of the back. The symptoms of acute pancreatitis are a loss of appetite, vomiting, frothy diarrhea, blood in the stools, weakness and severe abdominal pain; an animal with chronic pancreatitis usually maintains his appetite but loses weight, passes large, pasty-looking, grayish or pale, fatty-looking stools, is chronically tired and may have a rough coat.

Pancreatitis is easy to prevent. It's a condition that well-exercised, correctly fed dogs and cats simply don't develop. While your pet is still young and healthy, switch to a well-balanced raw diet and keep him active. Regular exercise stimulates all of the body's systems and helps eliminate waste products by stimulating the intestines and lymph system.

Nutritional Therapy: The treatment of pancreatitis is complicated by the need for gradual, not abrupt, changes in diet. If your pet has already suffered acute symptoms, work with a holistic veterinarian to improve the diet without triggering an attack. Otherwise, introduce raw foods and avoid feeding butter, fatty foods and vegetable oils because their digestion stresses the pancreas. Avoid fruits and gradually decrease grain-based foods for the same reason. Give digestive enzymes with meals and supplement with an all-purpose vitamin derived from whole-food sources and a complete trace mineral product that is easy to assimilate. Give additional vitamin C complex with bioflavonoids and vitamin E complex. Glandular extracts may be prescribed, depending on test results.

Feed dogs a variety of pressed vegetables, fresh vegetable juice or puréed vegetables to which you have added enzymes to improve digestibility; do the same for cats, but in smaller quantities. Think of the rainbow and serve yellow corn, green broccoli, white cauliflower, purple cabbage, red peppers and other colors.

Avoid cold foods; serve food at room or body temperature. Serve several small meals instead of a single dinner. Follow the instructions in Chapter 2 for determining food sensitivities and avoid any foods that seem to worsen symptoms.

Homeopathy: Consult a veterinary homeopath for best results. Richard Pitcairn lists six helpful remedies, and George Macleod gives 14; everything depends on individual symptoms.

Color Therapy: For acute pancreatitis, give a turquoise systemic front, blue and indigo on the upper abdomen and lower back, then magenta on the upper chest. For chronic pancreatitis, give a lemon systemic front and on the lower back (pancreas area).

Panleukopenia (Distemper): See *Viral Infections*

Parasites

Bugs and worms are the bane of every animal larger than a gnat. Bees have mites, fish have worms, every mammal in the forest picks up fleas and ticks, mosquitoes and flies are everywhere and so are tiny creatures that lurk in our lakes and rivers waiting for a nourishing home.

Tapeworms, roundworms, hookworms, whipworms, heartworms and other internal parasites thrive in a good host, sucking the animal's blood, absorbing nutrients and causing symptoms such as diarrhea, stomach distention, vomiting, anal itching, arrested growth, pale gums, anemia, weight loss, weakness, fainting or an inability to mount a strong defense against infection.

Giardia lamblia and other microbes that pollute water supplies can cause stomach cramps, diarrhea and other symptoms.

The most important thing to understand about parasites is that there is no escaping them. Unless you seal your pet in a glass jar, he's going to be exposed to something, most likely several somethings, every day. Parasites lurk in the air he breathes, the water he drinks, the food he eats and the ground he walks on. While commonsense precautions are always appropriate (buy the best quality foods you can, keep the kitchen clean, don't board your pet at a flea-infested kennel and bring pure water when your pets travel with you), any attempt to prevent your pet from ever having contact with an internal or external parasite is a waste of time. It's impossible. The only sensible strategy is to focus on the animal's overall health. As mentioned throughout this book, pets fed a natural diet and appropriate herbs and supplements, exposed to unfiltered natural light, exercised often and given a secure, happy, stable home are very poor hosts for parasites.

Intestinal Worms

Nearly all conventional veterinarians and many holistic vets give some type of worming medication to puppies and kittens on the assumption that all young animals are infected. However, this practice is not endorsed by everyone. Veterinary homeopaths like Richard Pitcairn and Larry Bernstein do not treat young animals for worms unless they show signs of infestation because healthy animals slough off their parasites and do not become reinfested. Throughout Francis Pottenger's ten-year nutrition experiment, cats who were fed raw milk and raw meat had few if any fleas, mites or worms while cats in adjacent cages who were fed either cooked meat or pasteurized milk were overrun by parasites. Pottenger's results have been confirmed by everyone who has tested the effects of fresh and raw foods. Regardless of the animal's size or species, if it eats the raw, natural diet on which it evolved, drinks clean water, gets daily exercise, breathes fresh air and is exposed to unfiltered natural light, it is extremely unlikely to attract and keep harmful parasites.

Roundworms can reside undetected in a female dog or cat for years, until her pregnancy awakens them and they migrate to her unborn offspring. This is why puppies and kittens can be born with roundworms even though their mother tested negative. If the mother and her offspring are poor hosts, the roundworms are unlikely to thrive and multiply. Serious roundworm infestations are most likely in the inadequately nourished offspring of unhealthy mothers.

Hookworms can cause anemia by sucking the host's blood. Whipworms can penetrate deeply into all areas of the body, including the lungs. Both can be difficult to eradicate.

Tapeworms attach themselves to the wall of the small intestine. Their presence is usually indicated by the egg sac segments that break off and pass through the large intestine; they look like grains of white rice or small maggots in the animal's stool, around the anus or on bedding.

Chemical worming treatments seldom kill the whole tapeworm; they may cause a sudden release of segments without affecting the attached head, which survives and grows new segments. For this reason and because fleas carry tapeworm eggs, this parasite is difficult to eliminate.

Nutritional Therapy: Vitamin A, which the body manufactures from carotenes, is essential to the prevention of roundworms, which is why carrots have such an established reputation as a deworming vegetable. The foods with the highest vitamin A value include not only carrots but collard greens, beet greens, cress, chard, mustard greens, watercress, spinach, broccoli, red peppers, winter squash, pumpkins and sweet potatoes. Finely grated, these raw vegetables provide both the nutrients that help repel roundworms and the roughage that helps expel them. Even though cats need other sources of vitamin A, carrots are still nutritious and help deter parasites. Feed cats and dogs up to 1/2 teaspoon per 10 pounds of body weight, starting with smaller amounts and increasing gradually. Because lactic-acid fermentation increases the digestibility of vegetables, feeds beneficial intestinal flora and cleanses the digestive tract, making it less hospitable to parasites, press grated vegetables with a small amount of unrefined sea salt (see page 105).

Garlic helps repel tapeworms and roundworms, not because it is toxic to them but because it strips protective mucus from the intestine's wall, exposing the worms to conditions they normally evade. Add fresh or powdered garlic, aged garlic extract or a tincture made of garlic and cider vinegar to your pet's food to give intestinal worms fewer places to hide. Many veterinarians recommend 1 capsule of Kyolic aged garlic extract three times daily for four weeks with or without food for pets up to 35 pounds in weight; use 2 capsules three times daily for large and giant breeds.

With garlic removing a layer of protection, intestinal worms are far less comfortable in the presence of roughage and sharp irritants. Add diatomaceous earth (see page 110) to your pet's food. Another effective irritant is the pumpkin seed. Buy fresh, raw seeds at your health food store or save and dry the seeds of pumpkins you use at home. Store pumpkin seeds in a tightly sealed jar. While preparing your pet's dinner, grind enough to make 1/4 teaspoon powder for each 10 to 15 pounds of your animal's weight. Pumpkin seeds are most effective when freshly ground.

Herbal Therapies: Grapefruit seeds are a natural vermifuge; that is, they kill, weaken and repel parasites. The chopped seeds of fresh grapefruit, oranges, lemons, limes and other citrus fruits can be added to food just like pumpkin seed, above, or you can add grapefruit seed extract to your pet's dinner. For convenience and palatability, use the capsules, which contain debittered powder. As with all supplements, begin with a small dose to be sure your pet tolerates it well, then increase to a maximum dosage of 1 capsule per 10 pounds of body weight for five to seven days.

Corsican seaweed is a traditional parasite treatment. To brew Corsican seaweed tea, simmer 5 to 10 grams (about 1/3 of an ounce by weight) in 2 cups boiling water for 10 to 20 minutes. This makes a truly awful tasting tea, but most dogs and many cats take it willingly when mixed with food. Add a small amount at first, such as half a teaspoon for a cat or a tablespoon for a large dog, then build up to 1/8 cup per day for cats and small dogs and from 1/4 to 1/2 cup per day for medium and large dogs. Continue dosing for one week.

Aloe vera juice and gel are popular supplements for pets; add 1 tablespoon per 20 pounds of body weight (1 teaspoon per 6 or 7 pounds) to food once a day to help repel worms.

Cayenne pepper irritates parasites and helps repel them from dogs, cats, birds and rabbits. Many birds love chile peppers; offer whole fresh or dried chiles or add small amounts of powdered chile to your bird's food. Juliette de Bairacli Levy recommends as much cayenne as possible, as hot as possible, to treat tapeworms. For this purpose, use cayenne of about 45,000 heat units (check labels) in capsules. Begin by giving your pet 1/2 capsule per 50 pounds of body weight. Open the capsule, empty what you don't need and place the capsule back together. Wash your hands after handling cayenne and don't touch your eyes or your pet's eyes until after you do. To prevent gastrointestinal discomfort while your pet becomes accustomed to cayenne, give the partly filled capsule at the beginning of the largest meal of the day. Gradually increase the daily dosage until you are feeding 1 capsule per 25 pounds of body weight twice daily and continue this dosage, in combination with other vermifuge strategies, for at least one week.

Parsley is another plant with vermifuge properties. Fresh parsley can be grated or puréed and added to food the same as carrots and greens. Hulda Clark's pet parasite program, as described in her book *The Cure for All Diseases*, begins with parsley tea (she calls it parsley water) made by cooking a large bunch of fresh parsley in a quart of water for three minutes, then straining. She recommends adding 1 teaspoon per 10 pounds of body weight to a pet's food daily. Parsley water can be frozen in ice cube trays for convenience. Transfer frozen cubes into sealed plastic freezer bags for storage.

The rest of Clark's program for pets uses black walnut hull tincture made from green hulls, which are revered in Europe for their vermifuge properties, wormwood capsules containing 200 to 300 mg of wormwood by itself or in a blend with other herbs and clove capsules containing about 500 mg freshly ground cloves (size 00 capsules). Check product labels and adjust the wormwood dosage accordingly; a size 00 capsule containing powdered wormwood by itself is equivalent to two capsules containing 250 mg wormwood.

During the first week of Clark's program, add parsley water to food as described above. In the second week, continue the parsley water and add 1 drop of black walnut hull tincture per 10 pounds of body weight twice weekly for cats and every day for dogs. In the third week, continue with the parsley water and black walnut tincture and add 1 wormwood capsule per 10 pounds of body weight every day. In the fourth week, continue with the parsley water, black walnut tincture and wormwood and add 1 clove capsule per 10 pounds per day. Continue these dosages indefinitely.

On this program, a 60-pound dog will consume 6 drops of black walnut hull tincture, 6 wormwood capsules and 6 clove capsules per day.

Some pet nutritionists have developed their own versions of Clark's program, adding additional herbs, glandular supplements and other nutrients. This is sensible because the liver is stressed during any type of detoxification. Many have adopted the program for short-term use, which is in keeping with the concept of herbal "courses," in which a schedule is followed for a certain length of time, then discontinued or interrupted. For example, the schedule described here could be given to a dog, cat or other pet for six to eight weeks, then discontinued for one or two months and then resumed. During the interruption, other vermifuge herbs can be substituted, such as chaparral, rue and pau d'arco. Chinese medicine has its own repertory of vermifuge herbs. Any worm-repelling herb can be given in capsules or added to food. It's a good idea to use different vermifuge herbs on a rotating basis throughout the year.

Worming Strategy

After about two weeks of feeding increased amounts of grated carrots, greens, sweet potatoes, pumpkin, other hard-shelled squashes, diatomaceous earth, pumpkin seeds and vermifuge herbs, temporarily increase the amount of insoluble fiber in the diet by adding a small amount of wheat bran to the diet. Soak the bran in water first so it is well-hydrated; use just a pinch for small puppies and kittens and about 1/8 teaspoon per 10 pounds of body weight for larger animals. The bran will further irritate the worms and help sweep them out of the body. Feed the wheat bran for several days, then discontinue. The raw vegetables in your pet's diet will provide ample fiber for normal digestion.

The digestive enzymes found in figs and papaya literally digest the outer coating that protects intestinal worms. These foods are more easily fed to dogs than cats, but some cats love both. Feed either or both of these foods separately, so that their enzymes can reach the worms in a more concentrated form. Feed fresh figs whole or in small pieces; finely chop dried figs and soak them in a small amount of water for an hour before feeding.

Proteolytic enzymes can be given on an empty stomach to digest intestinal worms. Using a product such as Zymex II from Standard Process, give 1 capsule per 5 pounds of body weight up to a maximum of 1 for birds, 3 for cats and 9 for dogs, dosing the animal once per day. Give the capsules with water or a food that does not contain protein; otherwise the enzymes will digest the food's protein and not the parasites.

Wheat germ oil is sometimes recommended as a tapeworm repellent. Buy a high-quality oil and keep it refrigerated or buy high-quality oil in capsules and squeeze the contents onto your pet's food. Use about 1/8 teaspoon per 10 pounds of body weight.

Encourage your pet to drink extra water to help flush toxins and debris from the system. Add water, herbal tea or fresh carrot juice to food.

Some vermifuge programs, such as the one recommended by Juliette de Bairacli Levy, begin with a one- to two-day fast and the use of a purgative laxative such as castor oil or Epsom salts (magnesium chloride). This strategy clears the intestines, removes some parasites, disrupts the worms' environment and increases their exposure to the irritating herbs that follow. De Bairacli Levy also recommends enema treatments of salty tobacco tea to treat roundworms, hookworms and whipworms. See *The Complete Herbal Handbook for the Dog and Cat* for instructions.

Aromatherapy: Blend equal parts of the essential oils of bergamot, caraway, sassafras, wild marjoram and thyme. Give 1 drop per 4 to 5 pounds of body weight twice a day for three days.

Color Therapy: Yellow and lemon systemic tonations over the front of the body, including the abdomen.

Heartworm

Transmitted by mosquitoes, heartworms live in the hearts of their canine hosts, where they can grow nearly a foot long. Before a dog can be infected, it must be bitten by a mosquito that has already sucked the blood of an infected animal. When biting its new victim, the mosquito transfers young parasites (microfilaria), which develop under the skin and then enter the bloodstream. After reaching the heart, they mature and reproduce.

Fatal heartworm infestations are the stuff of science fiction movies, and anyone who has seen live heartworms or even their photographs will do anything to avoid them. For most of America's canine population, this means daily or monthly doses of heartworm preventives that have alarming side effects. The American Veterinary Medical Association has reported that 65 percent of the adverse drug reactions it monitors and nearly half of all drug-related deaths are caused by heartworm prevention medicine.

Because it's a frightening disease, most veterinarians, including many holistic veterinarians in areas where heartworm is epidemic, believe the benefits of chemical prevention outweigh the risks. However, as Richard Pitcairn and others are quick to point out, wild animals like coyotes don't die of heartworm. Instead, they develop a mild infestation and then become immune. The same is true of an estimated 25 to 50 percent of the dogs who live in high-heartworm areas.

Despite the extensive use of heartworm preventive drugs, the rate of heartworm infestation in dogs in any geographical part of the U.S. is the same today as it was in 1982. As Pitcairn remarks, "It doesn't take much contemplation to realize that the path of continued drug use is a dead end road."

Heartworms thrive in America's canine population because our dogs' depleted health makes them good hosts. However, if your dog sleeps indoors or on a screened porch during mosquito season, does not take prescription drugs or receive annual vaccinations, eats a well-balanced, raw diet supplemented with vermifuge herbs (which repel insects as well as internal parasites) and wears natural insect repellents outdoors, he or she is at low risk even if you live in an area with a high incidence of heartworm disease. In North America, the highest rates of infection are in the southeastern Atlantic and Gulf Coast states.

To reduce your mosquito population, use preventive measures. Don't leave old tires lying around; they are favorite mosquito hatcheries. Empty unnecessary barrels, buckets and other water collectors. If you have decorative ponds or fountains, stock them with small fish that eat mosquito larvae. Check organic gardening supply catalogs for products that interfere with the insect's growth cycle. Welcome and encourage bats, which eat prodigious quantities of mosquitoes all night long. To get rid of a bat in your attic, don't panic and call public health officials; they still think, inaccurately, that all bats are rabid. Instead, check your library for books by Melvin Tuttle, who founded Bat Conservation International, or find a pest removal service that knows how to deal with bats humanely. Many garden supply catalogs carry bat houses with instructions for making them attractive to these very special mammals.

Heartworms are diagnosed when their microfilaria are found in a dog's blood. This is usually done with a simple blood smear, but the ELISA test, which involves sending the blood sample to a laboratory, is more accurate. It takes about six months for heartworm larvae to develop into adult worms, which is why veterinarians recommend testing twice a year, in spring and fall.

Homeopathic nosodes are being tested as nontoxic heartworm preventives, but, according to Richard Pitcairn, results are not yet available. There is some evidence in the veterinary literature that heartworm medicine given at the regular preventive dose rather than the far more toxic therapeutic dose may be an effective treatment for infestation, as reported in the March 1993 *Veterinary Forum*. Among herbalists, there is much enthusiasm for plant-based antiparasite treatments, such as Hulda Clark's program, which are said to repel and eliminate heartworms. In the end, each owner must decide on the individual animal's best treatment.

Herbal Therapies: If your dog is diagnosed with heartworms and shows the symptoms of a serious infestation, consult with a holistic veterinarian for the best course of treatment.

Natural heartworm prevention consists of two parts: (1) protecting your dog with nutrition and vermifuge herbs on the inside so the heartworms that enter her bloodstream can't thrive and (2) repelling mosquitoes on the outside so she isn't infected in the first place. All of the strategies described for the prevention of internal parasites are appropriate for dogs who live in heartworm areas, especially the use of black walnut hulls and wormwood.

Mosquitoes are the most thoroughly studied insects in the search for repellents because they transmit so many serious diseases, among them malaria and yellow fever. Citronella, several basils, juniper, rose geranium, rosemary, lemon thyme and cedar have all been shown to have at least some mosquito-repellent properties. Although citronella candles are widely sold, the essential oil of this lemony plant works better, though it fades as the oil evaporates and must be reapplied often. In the June 1994 *Herb Companion*, Arthur O. Tucker wrote that in one experiment, citronella oil was effective against yellow fever mosquitoes for only 1 hour, 18 minutes.

Scientific studies show that mugwort, a roadside weed through most of the eastern U.S. and a cousin of the wormwood, is effective in repelling the yellow fever mosquito when crushed onto clothing, applied as an oil on clothing or burned as a fumigant. Tansy is also highly effective. This "bitter buttons" herb used to be planted near doorways to discourage flies, and it repels other insects as well. Other plants shown to be effective against mosquitoes include yarrow, sweet Annie (annual wormwood), hyssop, German chamomile, bog myrtle, sassafras and sandalwood.

Several of these herbs are available as essential oils, which can be diluted with a carrier oil or diluted with alcohol and added to water. Review Chapter 5 (Aromatherapy) for instructions and sources. The essential oils of wormwood and rue come with warning labels, for they are not recommended for internal use and may cause allergic reactions on sensitive skin. In her book *Herbal Medicine,* Dian Dincin Buchman recommends a blend of equal parts rue, rosemary, basil and wormwood essential oils as an all-purpose insect repellent. She wrote, "This preparation is terrific and has even been used by friends in South and Central American jungles." I have experimented with variations of this blend, adding opopanax myrrh for its tick-repellent properties (see page 169) with good results. These essential oils should be handled with care and be well diluted with alcohol and water or a carrier oil before application to skin or fur. Before walks in the woods I like to spray Samantha and the rest of us with these oils diluted in alcohol and water, but in rainy weather or whenever she goes swimming, a carrier oil keeps them from washing away. Every week we use an eye dropper to dab the essential oil blend on her collar.

Whatever your choice of insect repellent, use it frequently during black fly season, when mosquitoes are everywhere, whenever ticks are active and wherever fleas are abundant. Keep essential oils away from your pet's eyes, nose and mouth. Remember that essential oils should not be applied to a cat's fur; instead, treat a fabric flea collar with diluted essential oils, apply strongly brewed tea made of insect-repelling herbs or rub their coats with fresh herbs.

Mange

The mite that causes demodectic mange lives in the intestinal tracts of healthy animals. It is only when the host's resistance is low that it migrates to the skin and takes up residence in hair follicles. The result is bare patches marked by tiny bumps or pimples, often near the chin or eyes or on the feet.

Healthy pets don't have mange problems, and the way to make your pet healthy is with nutrition, exercise, natural light and a happy home. Dietary changes alone have cured many cases of mange. Vitamins C and E, zinc and lecithin are recommended supplements.

Herbal Therapy: The Chinese herb astragalus and the familiar echinacea are often recommended for dogs with mange.

To make a lemon skin lotion that Juliette de Bairacli Levy uses to treat mange, place at least two dozen lemon skins in a glass gallon jar, cover them with warm water and leave the jar in the sun for several days. If the weather is cool or cloudy, simmer the peels for several minutes in a covered pan and let them steep. If pomegranate rinds are available, put them in with the lemon peels. Squeeze the peels, remove them as they become moldy and add new ones. Bathe the dog thoroughly and apply the lemon peel lotion all over his body, including the tip of the tail and around the toes. Avoid only the eyes and genitals.

Some herbalists apply a garlic tincture of apple cider vinegar or a dilute solution of tea tree oil. There are many possible external applications, but what really matters is improving the animal's health. Mites are best treated from the inside out.

Ear mites, see page 377

Fleas

For every flea you see, the saying goes, there are a hundred hiding. Given the right conditions, fleas can spread quickly through a building, biting dogs, cats, people and even birds in their cages.

The adult flea can jump 150 times its own length, which is about one-tenth of an inch. Leaps of a foot or more are not uncommon, and a flea can jump repeatedly without tiring. In one experiment, a flea jumped 30,000 times without stopping. Fleas can survive for months without eating and survive freezing as well. They are powerful animals and very difficult to eradicate, as pet owners know.

Fleas on a cat or dog can number in the hundreds, and such a large flea infestation has serious health consequences. It can reduce the animal's appetite and interfere with its immune system. Some fleas carry illness, such as the bubonic plague, or parasites, such as tapeworm. Flea bites can cause severe allergies, itching, hair loss and raw sores.

In general, fleas are not attracted to well-nourished, healthy pets, although even they can be overwhelmed if the flea population is sufficiently high. Flea infestations are easier to prevent than cure, so make a quick inspection with a flea comb part of your weekly health check and be ready to act fast if you find fleas to prevent their spread.

Fleas are difficult to eradicate because they lay thousands of eggs, and the eggs can incubate anywhere: on furniture, in carpets, in cracks on the floor and on your pet. Flea eggs usually hatch within two weeks. During the next two weeks to six months, the tiny white larvae molt twice, then they spin a loose cocoon in which they remain for between a week and a year. It is during the larval stage that fleas are most susceptible to nontoxic flea control. Adult fleas are short-lived; it's their constant reproduction that makes them such a nuisance.

Flea-growth inhibitors are available from some pest control services, which treat both houses and outdoor areas. Ask local companies whether they offer this treatment or check natural pet magazines for information.

You can treat your house yourself with an inexpensive powder that disrupts the fleas' life cycle. Although this is not a perfect solution, flea infestations can be eliminated with a blend of 2 parts diatomaceous earth, 1 part baking soda and 1 part cornstarch. The diatomaceous earth scratches the soft skin of flea larvae (it has no effect on adults), the baking soda encourages their dehydration and the cornstarch acts as a carrier.

Diatomaceous earth can irritate the lungs, so wear a pollen mask and keep pets and small children out of the room while you work. Protect computers and electronic equipment with dust covers.

Before treating the carpet, gather all washable items, including your pet's bedding, and put it through your washer and dryer on the hottest possible settings. Add 2 tablespoons of 15-percent tea tree oil solution to the final rinse water.

After vacuuming thoroughly, discard the vacuum cleaner bag. Sprinkle the powder thickly onto carpets and rub it in with a push broom or with your foot. Apply it between mattresses and box springs, into carpeted corners and into sofas and other upholstered furnishings. Once worked into floor cracks, carpet and upholstery, the powder should remain in place. However, vacuuming a treated carpet may cause diatomaceous earth to fly, especially in dry weather, so make a pollen mask part of your housecleaning uniform. Consider your pets, children and lifestyle before using this strategy.

Note: This flea deterrent is not a flea powder. Do not apply it directly on pets. Some books and magazines recommend rubbing diatomaceous earth into fur, but it can scratch and irritate the lungs if inhaled. Even if the animal's face is protected during application, grooming can dislodge the dust in the animal's nose. Treat your pet's living area but use other flea treatments on the animal itself.

Nutritional Therapy: Feed a well-balanced, raw diet. Pottenger's raw-food cats didn't have fleas although they were abundant in adjacent cages.

Herbal Therapy: The internal use of bitter herbs like wormwood and rue helps deter fleas by making the blood taste bitter and less appetizing.

One of the most interesting flea stories was told by James Montgomery, an officer of the Southern Forest Institute, in *American Tree Farmer* magazine. Montgomery returned home from an extended vacation to discover the neighborhood's stray cats in residence in his basement and the entire house infested with fleas. His family physician had long used leaves from the black walnut tree to keep his bird dog kennels free of fleas, so Montgomery spread walnut boughs under furniture, in closets and everywhere. In a few days the fleas were gone. Many advances have been made in insecticides since then, he said, but never found a more effective treatment.

Pennyroyal, a member of the mint family, is an increasingly popular alternative to chemical products. A fresh sprig of this cheerful plant can be rubbed over your pet's fur every day to repel fleas.

Another flea repellent is cedar, better known for its ability to prevent moth damage. Dog and cat cushions stuffed with cedar shavings have been popular for centuries.

Aromatherapy: The essential oils of pine and eucalyptus kill fleas. To make an effective flea shampoo that won't harm your pet, add several drops to a gentle liquid soap or pet shampoo just before applying it to your wet dog or cat. Massage it thoroughly into the fur and skin. Rinse well and repeat. Watch for fleas that climb onto your pet's nose in order to escape the water; pick them off and drop them into a glass of soapy water.

To remove fleas and improve the coat without using soap, use the essential-oil brushing treatment described on page 170.

Herbal flea collars can be "recharged" with pennyroyal oil which, if applied frequently, repels fleas, flies, mosquitoes, wood ticks, chiggers and gnats. To keep flies and other insects away from outdoor kennel runs, mix 1 tablespoon pennyroyal oil with 1 quart water and spray. The essential oil of pennyroyal should never be applied full strength to animals; always dilute it first and keep it away from pregnant pets and women. For additional information about pennyroyal, see page 168.

A few drops of cedar oil on your pet's bedding may help; a little goes a long way, so add just a drop at a time. See page 183 for information about orange oil.

Treating Bites and Stings: See *First-Aid* (Chapter 12)

Parvovirus: See *Viral Infections*

Psittacosis or Parrot Fever: See *Respiratory Illnesses*

Reproduction and Breeding

How many puppies and kittens are born in the U.S. every year? No one knows, but estimates range from 60 to 75 million. Most are the mixed-breed offspring of opportunity, but registered pedigreed babies are born in large numbers to family pets at home, to dogs and cats at commercial breeding farms and to animals belonging to hobby breeders.

Because so many of these puppies and kittens are unwanted and abandoned and because of ethical concerns, breeding has become controversial. Some animal rights activists argue that breeding should be prevented by law, and their efforts have made it illegal for dogs and cats to reproduce in some communities. This is an emotional issue that excites passions on all sides.

Advocates of antibreeding legislation argue that anyone who wants a puppy or kitten should adopt one from a shelter. They point to the declining health of purebred dogs and cats, the disastrous results of inbreeding or careless breeding, the inhumane practices of some breeders and the overwhelming number of homeless animals, all of which are serious problems.

Political activism may be an effective way to improve the lives of brood bitches trapped in puppy mills and improve their breed by preventing the production of their often-defective offspring, but irresponsible breeding is only partly responsible for the tragic state of health in America's dogs and cats. Antibreeding laws can't improve nutritional deficiencies or repair compromised immune systems.

Laws can't solve the population problem, either, for this type of legislation is impossible to enforce. As long as there are pedigreed animals on the planet, there will be fanciers who want them. Antibreeding laws will work only if you can somehow repeal the laws of supply and demand.

It's easy to loathe a nasty person who treats living beings as commodities and abuses them in the name of profit, but irresponsible breeders are often very nice people. They want their children to see the miracle of birth, they believe that Fluffy will make a wonderful mother, they've heard that an animal's personality improves with motherhood, they don't want Buck to have a disfiguring operation, they think neutering makes an animal gain weight and become passive, they don't want to spend the money, they're afraid of the surgery, they had no idea she was in heat, they can sell the puppies or kittens and make a profit and the list goes on and on.

The only solution to the problem of declining health and quality in pedigreed dogs and cats is responsible breeding accompanied by proper care and feeding. Most of the demand for holistic veterinary care in the U.S. has come from breeders wanting healthier puppies and kittens and longer-lived dogs and cats. Pet owners support these trends, but it was America's network of breeders and their clients who first spread the word about natural methods that prevent and cure health problems.

Responsible breeders are the people most aware of a line's genetic problems and the motivating force behind the medical research being done to prevent them. Responsible breeders look everywhere for sound mates for their animals, breed them carefully and infrequently and do everything they can to improve their animals' health.

The details of responsible breeding are beyond the scope of this book, but it is worth repeating the advice given by experts interviewed here and elsewhere: unless your animal is recognized as a superior example of his or her breed in every way and unless you are prepared to spend substantial time, energy and resources finding the ideal mate, preparing for breeding and whelping, finding the right homes for your puppies or kittens and guaranteeing their health and temperament, you should spay or neuter your wonderful pet and enjoy your life together.

Also outside the scope of this book are instructions for dealing with the serious problems that often accompany breeding, pregnancy, whelping, nursing and the care of weak or deformed offspring. Rather than explaining how to deal with medical emergencies, the following section emphasizes their prevention. Juliette de Bairacli Levy has written that if you don't have a goat of your own to produce raw milk for your dogs, you have no business breeding puppies. I won't go that far, but if you feed your bitch canned or packaged dog food, inject her with a dozen vaccines a year, dose her with antibiotics and cortisone, deprive her of natural light, spray her with pesticides and make her swallow toxic chemicals in the name of parasite control, it is misguided to think that any magical herb or supplement will insure a healthy litter.

Breeding

The famous English dog trainer Barbara Woodhouse, Juliette de Bairacli Levy and a host of other experts agree that the best results come from a compatible breeding, in which the animals are introduced in a relaxed setting, have an extended visit and seem fond of each other. De Bairacli Levy is very much opposed to forced matings between unwilling partners, no matter what the blood lines or how "ideal" their combination. Breeding is a stressful activity for which holistic medicine offers many support therapies, including flower essences, calming herbs and all of the hands-on healing techniques described in Chapter 7.

Nutritional Therapy: For at least a year before breeding, both parents-to-be should be fed a well-balanced, natural, raw diet with superior-quality supplements and given a healthful lifestyle of active exercise, exposure to natural light, protection from toxins and a happy, stable home life. Supply ample B-complex vitamins and vitamins C and E to both parents. Remember that synthetic vitamin B reduces fertility; be sure your supplements are derived from whole-food sources. Although not a specific for reproduction, the metabolic antioxidant lipoic acid detoxifies the body and has an overall tonic effect. Its regular use will help any animal attain and maintain optimum health.

Herbal Therapy: Some breeders give their male dogs or cats ginseng, the adaptogen herb renowned for its benefits to the male system. While that's not so important as a healthful diet, ginseng does protect against stress and correct imbalances. Ginseng can be given as a tea, powder or tincture daily or every other day for years; because its effects are cumulative, its short-term use has no appreciable benefits. Other adaptogenic herbs that may be equally helpful are astragalus, schizandra and Siberian ginseng.

When Chinese carp were accidentally fed a blend of green oats and stinging nettle, their reproductive rate increased dramatically. Subsequent research in China, Europe and the U.S. has shown that the blend increases virility, aerobic capacity, muscle strength, testosterone levels, stamina and endurance in humans, horses and other animals. As a result, green oat and nettle blends have become popular supplements. To give this combination to a dog or cat, adjust package directions to the animal's weight and begin adding it to his food at least a month before breeding.

The male's stamina can be further aided with royal jelly (a bee product), given two or three times a day through mating.

For several weeks before her heat cycle, the female can be given raspberry leaf, either as a tea or powder, continuing through pregnancy and delivery. Raspberry leaf is such an important herb for pregnancy that even breeders who know nothing about natural rearing feed it to their pregnant animals.

To help the animals relax and adjust to each other prior to mating, any of the calming nervines can be used, such as chamomile, skullcap, valerian, hops, passionflower or oatstraw. They can be given as teas or, for faster and more effective results, as tinctures. Although dogs tolerate small doses of alcohol tinctures, this is a good time to use low-alcohol or vegetable glycerine tinctures. It wouldn't hurt most owners to take some of these relaxing nervines at the same time.

Herbs to avoid during breeding include aloe vera gel or juice, pennyroyal and wormwood. If you have been feeding aloe vera, using a flea repellent containing pennyroyal oil or using a wormwood-based antiparasite program, discontinue these a week or two before breeding. In addition, avoid angelica, black cohosh, blue cohosh, motherwort and yarrow.

Misalliance

Preventing an unwanted mating sounds simple enough: you anticipate and recognize your female's heat cycle, separate her from resident males, protect her from visiting males and take her outdoors under supervision. Neglect these responsibilities and you have an unwanted mating or "misalliance."

An injection of hormones can prevent conception, but at potential cost to the animal's health. When this strategy is repeated several times, the animal's resistance to uterine infection declines.

Herbal Therapy: The seeds of the wild carrot or Queen Anne's lace (*Daucus carota*) have a long history of use as a "morning after" pill. Some Appalachian women drink a glass of water containing a teaspoon of the previous autumn's seeds whenever they wish to avoid pregnancy, and rural women in Rajastan, India, chew dry seeds for the same purpose. This strategy, which is at least 2,000 years old, was documented by Dioscorides, Hippocrates and other ancient authorities.

Extracts of Queen Anne's lace seeds, which contain estrogenic substances, have been tested on rats, mice, guinea pigs and rabbits. While not all of the experiments gave positive results (a decoction did not prevent rat pregnancies in two studies), the seeds prevented implantation if given before the sixth day of pregnancy in several studies.

According to public and private statements by herbalists and other users, seeds of recently harvested wild carrot are an effective contraceptive. There is no substitute for preventing unwanted matings in the first place, but when an accident occurs, adding ground seeds to an animal's food may be a drug-free way to prevent unwanted puppies or kittens.

Pregnancy

Assuming that the right couple got together and all is going well, here is how to prepare for a healthy litter.

Nutritional Therapy: According to Juliette de Bairacli Levy, healthy pregnant dogs and cats on a raw diet require far less food than their unhealthy counterparts. Feeding double rations in order to nourish the litter as well as the pregnant animal is, in her words, a great mistake. Overfeeding causes sour food deposits to accumulate in the intestines and burdens the bloodstream, which already has to deal with the excretions of the growing litter. Pregnant animals need extra fluids, and clean water should be available at all times. In fact, increased thirst is a common symptom of pregnancy.

Feed your mom-to-be a variety of raw meaty bones, pressed or finely grated vegetables, raw milk, cultured milk dishes, fruits, finely puréed sprouted grains treated with digestive enzymes and other foods. Supplement her diet with superior-quality multiple vitamins derived from food sources, seaweeds such as kelp, colloidal trace minerals and Willard Water. Study Chapter 2 for menu planning.

Wendell Belfield recommends vitamin C supplementation throughout pregnancy to produce healthy, full-size offspring, prevent hip dysplasia, reduce whelping time, enhance nursing and quickly return the mother to her previously firm condition. Use natural vitamin C complex derived from food sources or a good-quality calcium ascorbate with bioflavonoids and rutin, not ascorbic acid. Belfield suggests that as soon as a bitch displays signs of pregnancy, she receive the high adult dose of vitamin C that would normally be given to a working dog: 1.5 grams (1,500 mg) daily for small dogs, 3 grams (3,000 mg) daily for medium dogs, 6 grams (6,000 mg) daily for large breeds and 7.5 grams (7,500 mg) daily for giant breeds. Pregnant cats receive 1 gram (1000 mg) daily. Start with small amounts and increase gradually to these recommendations, giving the vitamin in divided doses during the day. Watch for any sign of diarrhea or loose stool, which is a symptom of vitamin C saturation known as bowel tolerance level. When vitamin C produces this reaction, reduce the dosage until it disappears.

Vitamin E is another aid to effortless delivery and healthy offspring. As Dr. Belfield discovered many years ago, the combination of vitamins C and E enhances conception, increases female fertility, prevents miscarriage, reduces birth defects and eliminates uterine exhaustion during delivery. Use a natural vitamin E-complex supplement derived from food sources, not synthetic vitamin E. Feed 100 IU daily to cats and small dogs, 200 IU to medium dogs, 400 IU to large dogs and 600 IU to giant breeds.

Herbal Therapy: Raspberry leaf is so important that it deserves a page to itself. Juliette de Bairacli Levy was the first to popularize this aid to easy whelping, which she did over 60 years ago. After difficult whelpers began producing normal litters quickly and without effort, including toy and miniature breeds and large headed bulldog type breeds, word spread quickly.

Undiluted raspberry leaf tea can be added to food, which may be the easiest way to serve it. There is no maximum recommended amount; raspberry leaf has no known side effects except that, as de Bairacli Levy noted, at the time of delivery, placentas are often dark green and have an unmistakable raspberry leaf odor.

In case of nausea or morning sickness, a strongly brewed chamomile tea, chamomile extract or ginger can help, but remember not to force food on your pregnant animal. Her body will tell her when it's time to eat.

Additional recommended herbs include cleavers, which is a urinary system tonic; black haw and crampbark, both of which help "quiet" uterine muscles and help prevent miscarriage; blessed thistle leaf in the last three weeks of pregnancy to stimulate the flow of mother's milk; burdock root, which is a tonic herb that strengthens the entire system; chamomile blossoms, which soothe and relax the body; dandelion greens and root, which are excellent sources of easily assimilated vitamin A, calcium, iron and bitter compounds that aid digestion; lemon balm, which is a calming digestive tonic; nettle leaf, which is rich in calcium, iron and other nutrients; oatstraw or oatgrass, which is the young stalks of unripe oats; slippery elm bark, which is rich in mucilage, soothing and nourishing; and strawberry leaf, which is similar to raspberry leaf in its effects, may help prevent miscarriage and treats diarrhea. Any of these herbs can be used in any combination to nourish, calm and protect the pregnant mother.

Fresh herbs can be finely minced and added to food; dried herbs can be brewed as tea and added to drinking water or food or powdered and added to food; fresh or dried herbs can be combined with vegetable glycerine and/or alcohol to prepare tinctures. Low alcohol tinctures are recommended during breeding and the first half or two-thirds of pregnancy.

Grapefruit seed extract, wheat grass, garlic and diatomaceous earth are all appropriate during pregnancy. Wheat grass (or barley grass, rye grass, buckwheat lettuce, sunflower seed sprouts or other greens) should be finely minced.

Herbs to Avoid During Pregnancy: As noted above for breeding, avoid feeding large quantities of wormwood, such as in Hulda Clark's antiparasite program. The tiny amounts used in Juliette de Bairacli Levy's herbal antiseptic tablets are safe and have been used by pregnant animals for half a century with no adverse effects.

Fresh pennyroyal is not a threat to unborn puppies, but the essential oil of pennyroyal is highly concentrated and is known to stimulate uterine contractions. Aloe vera is considered by some to be a possible risk to unborn puppies during the first half of pregnancy. Avoid using the insect-repelling essential oils of wormwood, rue or tansy unless greatly diluted and not until the later weeks of pregnancy. Never give these oils internally.

Other herbs to avoid during pregnancy are those that are recommended during whelping because they stimulate uterine contractions: angelica, black cohosh, blue cohosh, motherwort and yarrow. Because parsley and sage reduce or dry up the flow of mother's milk, these herbs should be avoided during the final month of pregnancy.

Homeopathy: There are dozens of homeopathic remedies for breeding, pregnancy and whelping. Consult a veterinary homeopath for appropriate treatments depending on your animal's condition and symptoms. George Macleod wrote that *Viburnum op. 30c* can be given in the first two weeks of pregnancy to help prevent miscarriage (it is most appropriate for animals with a history of miscarriage) and that *Caulophyllum 30c* should be given once every two weeks with a final dose during the last week of pregnancy. He also recommended that *Arnica 30c* be given twice in the final week of pregnancy to facilitate normal delivery and reduce tearing or injury.

Light Therapy: Give your pet ample exposure to unfiltered natural light, which is essential to the health of the reproductive system. Some of John Ott's earliest discoveries about full-spectrum light involved the reproductive problems of animals raised under artificial light.

Color Therapy: During a normal pregnancy, occasionally tonate with a green systemic front, yellow on the abdomen and magenta on the upper chest and lower back. *Let There Be Light* by Darius Dinshah gives 10 tonation schedules relating to pregnancy and its complications, all of which are appropriate support therapies.

Whelping

This section assumes a safe, speedy, uneventful delivery of healthy, lively, intelligent, curious, alert puppies or kittens, the essential ingredients for which are healthy parents, and appropriate diet, supplements and exercise during pregnancy. There are many reference books that describe whelping emergencies. By the time your bitch or queen is ready to deliver, you should have a small library of well-thumbed books from both holistic and conventional medical authorities on hand.

Nutritional Therapy: About a week before whelping, reduce the daily meat supply and increase the amount of raw milk until your mother-to-be is on a liquid diet. Add a teaspoon of raw honey to each cup of milk. If you don't have access to raw milk, substitute Lactaid-treated goat's or cow's milk and add a digestive enzyme or make fresh yogurt or kefir with Lactaid-treated milk.

Starting about a week before whelping, provide small amounts of chopped dates, figs and extra grated carrots for their mild laxative effect.

Herbal Therapy: Because comfrey so effectively heals tears, cuts and injuries caused during birthing, strengthens muscles and provides important nutrients, add comfrey to food from about a week before whelping to a week after. Chamomile tea or tincture calms and relaxes an anxious mother-to-be. Fennel seed, nettle, raspberry leaf and blessed thistle enrich the flow of milk. Any or all of these herbs can be given during the week preceding birth.

To encourage and strengthen uterine contractions during labor, have on hand a tincture made with blue cohosh, black cohosh, milk thistle seed and pennyroyal leaf (not the essential oil). Combine 3 tablespoons of each herb in a pint jar and cover with vodka, rum, brandy or other 80-proof alcohol or with a combination of vegetable glycerine and alcohol. Use at least 1 part alcohol per 3 parts glycerine because glycerine cannot extract all of the plant constituents alcohol does. Cover the herbs with enough liquid to leave at least a 2-inch margin of liquid at the top. As the dry herbs absorb the liquid, which will take a few days, add more. Keep the jar in a warm place and shake it every day or two for five to six weeks, adding additional alcohol as needed. Strain into amber glass dropper bottles and label "Birth Tonic." This tincture has an indefinite shelf life; stored away from heat and light, it will remain effective for decades.

After contractions begin, mix 1/2 teaspoon honey with 1 dropperful of tincture and feed it to your birthing mother. You could just squirt the tincture into her mouth, but it's pretty awful tasting and she can use the energy honey provides. Repeat every 15 to 30 minutes, as needed. Give the tincture more often if she seems to be tiring or if her contractions seem weak.

As mentioned earlier, large amounts of raspberry leaf during pregnancy may change the placenta's color to green. This does not make it dangerous or toxic; the bitch should be allowed to consume the placenta, for it is rich in the nutrients she most needs.

Sound Therapy: Music for delivery? Absolutely! The soothing sounds of slow Baroque string music by Mozart and other 17th and 18th century composers played at a comfortably low volume will help slow everyone's pulse and relax both you and your pet. Some sound therapists suggest that playing this soothing music throughout the animal's pregnancy will produce more intelligent, coordinated offspring.

Homeopathy: In addition to the recommendations you may receive from a veterinary homeopath, here are suggestions from George Macleod. Should the uterus fail to dilate properly, give one dose of *Caulophyllum 30c* every 30 minutes for a total of four doses. Give a single dose of *Arnica 30c* after whelping to restore tone to the birth canal. *Sepia 30c* in a single dose after whelping prevents straining and uterine prolapse.

One remedy of special interest to breeders is Fading Puppies Syndrome

Homeopathic Preparation. Marina Zacharias, publisher of *Natural Rearing* newsletter, swears by this preparation, which has been used for over 30 years in Europe, where it has successfully treated tens of thousands of puppies and kittens. It can be given to bitches and queens during whelping to prevent exhaustion in them as well as a failure to thrive in their offspring.

Lactation, Nursing

Nutritional Therapy: As high as the female's nutritional requirements are during pregnancy, they are even higher during lactation. Feeding puts a tremendous strain on any nursing mother, especially those with lots of puppies or kittens. Feed the same diet that sustained the bitch during pregnancy, with increased rations, including an early-morning meal of raw cow's or goat's milk with honey. Be sure to include seaweed, for it has been shown to increase the butterfat content in milk in animals.

Dr. Belfield recommends supplementing the puppies' diet with directly administered pediatric vitamin C drops, increasing the dosage after five days and again after ten. After weaning, pups can be switched to a tablet or powder form of supplementation.

Belfield's recommendations. Small breeds: 20 drops per day on days 1-5, 35 drops per day on days 6-10 and 65 drops per day until weaning. Medium breeds: 35, 65 and 100 drops. Large and giant breeds: 65, 100 and 135 drops.

Although bovine colostrum is not a substitute for mother's milk, this food supplement can be given to weaning puppies along with acidophilus and raw goat's or cow's milk or freshly made yogurt or kefir to help keep their resistance strong. The same combination of milk foods, colostrum and acidophilus can help prevent infection after the puppies move to their new homes.

Herbal Therapy: Fennel seed, blessed thistle leaf, fenugreek seed, nettle and raspberry leaf are all said to help increase the flow of milk. Garlic in the mother's food goes directly to the nursing offspring and helps protect them against parasites. In fact, any medicinal herbs can be administered to the kittens or puppies through their mother's milk, including (if necessary) a complete antiparasite treatment.

The mild and calming nervines chamomile, lavender, lemonbalm, oatstraw, skullcap and valerian are all appropriate as they soothe and nourish the nervous system of both mother and babies.

Do not feed parsley or sage during lactation, as these herbs dry up the milk supply, which is why they are designated herbs for weaning. When it's time to decrease the milk supply, begin adding fresh minced or dried parsley and sage to food or brew medicinal-strength teas and add the tea to food or drinking water.

Grapefruit seed extract is such a powerful, natural antibiotic it will help protect the puppies or kittens from pathogens as well as protect the nursing mother from infections such as mastitis. Other infection fighters include vitamin C, astragalus root, echinacea, goldenseal, olive leaf extract, noni and bee propolis. Any combination of these herbs and supplements can be given in place of antibiotics to prevent or treat bacterial, viral and fungal infections (see pages 285-286). Don't assume that your pet and her babies have no natural defenses; they probably don't need any of these infection-fighting herbs. But if they're exposed to a contagious illness or if they show signs of infection, rapid treatment with any of the above can clear it rapidly.

Socialization

In addition to providing a safe environment, the right nutrition and, after their eyes open, exposure to natural light (light through a glass window is better than any electric light and gradual exposure to natural light is recommended whenever conditions permit), give your puppies and kittens the one gift that will help them most throughout their lives: proper socialization. Handle them gently every day so that by the time they're ready for their new homes, they are affectionate, calm and used to being touched.

Individual handling is necessary for socialization. Lift, fondle, massage, hold and carry the babies a little every day. Sing to them, dance with them, talk to them, let them sleep on your lap. Some breeders have puppy parties in which everyone in the house sits on the floor, holds and strokes a puppy for five or ten minutes, then passes it to the next person in the circle. By the time they're eight weeks old, these pups are used to all kinds of people and they've spent so much time having their toes massaged, their ears stroked, their teeth scrubbed and their tummies rubbed that they're as malleable as modeling clay.

Contrast this with breeders who think that socialization means leaving a litter of pups where they can meet people all day long. Someone enters the room and they swarm like a school of fish, jumping and playing. No one picks them up for more than a minute, so all their contact with people is a group activity. When these pups are presented one at a time to prospective buyers, they are shy, apprehensive and frightened. Without their littermates, they don't know what to do. When someone calls them, they hide; when a hand reaches out to pet them, they cringe.

The same is true for birds and rabbits. Very young animals are fragile and should be protected from overhandling and, especially at first, from exposure to more than one or two people. But as they grow stronger and older, the benefits of frequent handling far outweigh the risk of infection or injury. Use common sense. Don't come into the house and go straight to the babies; wash your hands first. If you've been handling other animals, change your clothes, too. Protect the infants from other animals, children and strangers. Be gentle. Give them plenty of uninterrupted rest after handling. But don't neglect this essential part of their nurturing.

Reproductive Organ Problems

Female Disorders

In females, the most common reproductive organ problems are pyometra and metritis, both of which involve the uterus. Pyometra means the presence of pus in the womb; metritis means an inflammation of the womb. Both are prevented by spaying.

Pyometra is most common in older bitches who have either experienced several heat cycles without conceiving or been treated with hormones to prevent pregnancy after an unwanted mating. Symptoms include excessive thirst, a vaginal discharge and, in acute cases, distention of the fluid-filled uterus.

Metritis usually occurs immediately after giving birth and in some cases, just after breeding, when the womb is susceptible to bacterial infection. Symptoms include fever, lethargy, discomfort, thirst, diarrhea, vomiting, poor appetite and a staining uterine discharge.

Mastitis is a mammary infection that sometimes occurs after birth, resulting in a hard breast that is painful, tender, sensitive and hot to the touch. It interferes with nursing and causes the milk to curdle and turn yellow. Left untreated, the breast discolors and becomes reddish purple or brown.

Herbal Therapy: These conditions require medical attention, but you may be able to lessen their severity by dosing the animal at once with appropriately large quantities of grapefruit seed extract, noni powder, olive leaf extract, echinacea, the herbal immunization described on page 285, other infection-fighting herbs or vitamin C.

Male Disorders

Middle-aged male dogs, like middle-aged men, can suffer from benign prostatic hyperplasia (BPH), a gradual swelling of the prostate gland that interferes with urination and sexual function. Prostate problems are most common in intact males and dogs that were neutered late in life. Dogs with BPH have a desperate urge to urinate and great difficulty producing a flow, which comes in fits and starts. Prostate inflammation can also occur in younger dogs that are sexually hyperactive.

Nutritional Therapy: Feed a raw, natural diet with vitamins derived from food sources and a comprehensive trace mineral supplement. Because zinc is important to healthy prostate function, supply additional zinc; adapt label directions to your pet's weight. Pumpkin seeds are rich in minerals and essential fatty acids that benefit the prostate. They are most effective when finely ground just before using. Add 1/4 teaspoon per 10 pounds of body weight to food.

Herbal Therapy: The same herbs that cure prostate problems in men work for dogs. Concentrated extracts of saw palmetto berry are the most widely prescribed prostate medications in Germany, France and other European countries. It is safe to give in large doses over long periods. Start with 1/8 teaspoon tincture per 20 pounds of body weight daily; if symptoms don't improve within a week, add more or try another brand as tincture quality and individual needs vary. As symptoms improve, decrease the dose to whatever level provides continued relief.

Respiratory Illnesses

Sneezing cats, coughing dogs, wheezing birds — any pet can have what looks and sounds like hay fever, asthma, the common cold or bronchitis. These conditions can be caused by allergies, viruses or bacteria. They are least likely to occur in animals with strong immune systems, such as those raised on natural food and in natural light. Common infectious illnesses can and do infect even these animals, but their symptoms usually don't last long and the patient recovers quickly. Changing your pet's diet as described in Chapter 2 is the most important protection you can provide against respiratory problems.

Asthma and Hay Fever Allergies

Pets who develop asthma or symptoms resembling hay fever allergies have often received, in the preceding year, some combination of antibiotics, multiple vaccinations, commercial pet food and cortisone drugs. Respiratory problems are common in breeds with short muzzles or flat faces, such as pug dogs and Persian cats, but anatomy is probably not the sole cause. In addition to the use of steroid drugs and other conventional medical practices, holistic veterinarians and nutritionists have linked these symptoms to blood sugar imbalances caused by excessive carbohydrates (cooked grains) in the diet and mineral deficiencies, especially magnesium deficiencies in dogs and cats.

Environmental and dietary allergens pose a hazard to all pets, and any animal with a respiratory condition is at special risk. Protect your pet from cigarette smoke, food preservatives and other unnatural substances.

Nutritional Therapy: Upgrade the diet. Feed raw meaty bones to dogs and cats; raw bones (not processed bone meal) provide magnesium in the perfect form and proportions for rapid assimilation and mineral balance. Feed birds and rabbits fresh, raw foods such as sprouting seeds, wheat grass, carrot tops and other greens. Give all pets extra vitamin C complex containing bioflavonoids and rutin as well as a complete trace mineral supplement and a multiple vitamin derived from whole-food sources. Once a week, let your pet fast for a day on water only to let the digestive tract rest; fast very small or young animals for half a day. If you suspect a food allergy, use a rotation diet to determine sensitivities.

Herbal Therapy: Add aloe vera, garlic, finely minced wheat grass and other green grasses and herbs such as dandelion to meals. If your pet is being treated with steroid drugs for a skin condition, arthritis or other problem, consult with a holistic veterinarian about gradually replacing the drugs with herbs or other therapies.

Mullein is a specific for asthma. As New York herbalist Robin Rose Bennett has shown, the fastest way to interrupt a human asthma attack is to light a dried mullein leaf, blow the flame out and breathe the smoke. This emergency treatment may be appropriate for pets as well, for it is safe and effective in children. Fresh or dried mullein herb can be added to food or brewed as a tea for use in food and drinking water. Stinging nettle is a specific for hay fever and is appropriate for all respiratory problems. When using an herb to improve respiration, give a pinch of powdered cayenne pepper, Tabasco sauce, fresh or powdered ginger or lobelia tincture (1 drop per 20 pounds of body weight) at the same time. These catalysts help accompanying herbs work faster and more effectively.

The bronchial dilator ephedra or Ma huang (*Ephedra sinica*) is widely used in human hay fever preparations, but it is a powerful herb with serious side effects. Ephedrine, the active constituent in ephedra, increases the pulse and blood pressure and feels like a shot of adrenalin. Humans have died from overdoses. Ephedra can be used safely by dogs, cats and other pets, but only as part of a blend containing relaxing herbs such as chamomile and respiratory herbs such as mullein and only in small amounts for short-term use. To adapt an herbal allergy product that contains ephedra for pet use, assume that label directions refer to a 150-pound person, divide according to your pet's weight (a 75-pound dog would receive half the prescribed amount; a 10-pound cat would receive 1/15) and divide again by half as a margin of safety. To make small quantities easier to measure, crush or grind the pill or capsule and mix it thoroughly with a teaspoon of carrier powder such as Jerusalem artichoke flour, acidophilus or powdered wheat grass juice.

Homeopathy: Consult with a veterinary homeopath to treat your pet's specific symptoms. Accurate prescribing is especially important in chronic conditions; the use of over-the-counter combination remedies or an incorrect single remedy may alter symptoms without curing the ailment.

Hands-on Therapies: All of the therapies described in Chapter 7 are appropriate. Asthma is often triggered by stress and anything you can do to relieve stress symptoms will help prevent wheezing attacks. Therapeutic Touch, Tellington TTouch and massage all relax, soothe and calm an agitated animal as well as reduce future agitation.

Acupuncture is very successful in the treatment of respiratory problems. At home stimulate acupressure point LU7.

Flower Essences: Dr. Bach's emergency formula is always appropriate, for it helps calm the animal. Check descriptions of flower essences for additional remedies that address your pet's situation.

Color Therapy: During an asthma attack, tonate with purple on the face and upper chest, scarlet on the lower back and orange on the upper chest. Between attacks, give a lemon systemic front, orange on the throat and upper chest and magenta on the upper chest and lower back.

For hay fever-type allergies, give a lemon systemic front and turquoise or blue on the face.

Coughing

Coughing is never an illness in itself; it's a symptom that has many possible causes. Coughing might signal the onset of an infectious disease, such as kennel cough in dogs or an upper respiratory infection in dogs, cats, birds or rabbits. Coughing that has lasted for a long time might be caused by allergies, asthma, bronchitis, heart disease, heartworms, periodontal disease, pneumonia, growths or parasites in the throat, a too-tight collar or environmental irritants like cigarette smoke.

If your pet's coughing has an obvious cause, act accordingly. If she's choking on a swallowed object, give the Heimlich maneuver (see page 330) and get her to a veterinarian fast; if he has outgrown his collar, take it off and give him a new one; if she breathes second-hand smoke or other irritants, give her clean air. Otherwise, consult your veterinarian for an accurate diagnosis.

Herbal Therapy: For temporary relief of a sore throat caused by coughing, mix a small amount of raw honey with any of the following herbs finely powdered, brewed as a very strong tea or in a tincture: coltsfoot, mullein, wild cherry bark, thyme, sage, peppermint, licorice root or slippery elm bark. Give small amounts every hour or as often as it is helpful.

Color Therapy: For a dry cough from a throat irritation, use blue on the face and throat. If the cough is related to a heart or lung disorder, give a green systemic front and purple on the upper chest. For a wet cough with little or no fever, give a green systemic front and green on the upper back. If there is a fever, follow a green systemic front with magenta on the upper chest or purple if the fever is high; follow with a blue systemic front and, if the fever is high, blue on the upper back.

Respiratory Infections

Kennel cough (Canine infectious tracheobronchitis), feline viral rhinotracheitis (FVR), feline calicivirus (FCV) and parrot fever (psittacosis) are only a few of the viral and bacterial infections that affect the respiratory systems of household pets.

In conventional medicine, the distinction between viral and bacterial infections is important because antibiotic drugs like penicillin kill bacteria but have no effect on viruses. Such a distinction is not important in herbal medicine, aromatherapy or nutritional therapy, for the same treatments are usually effective against all infectious agents, including fungi, parasites and other microbes.

The following treatments can be used both as a preventive, to protect your pet against an infectious disease to which he's exposed, and to treat an active illness. All of these treatments work best if administered at the first sign of illness, and this requires careful observation because in many cases, early symptoms are overlooked or ignored.

Nutritional Therapy: Vitamin C is the all-purpose infection fighter. Although all pets manufacture their own vitamin C, they don't always make enough. Boost your pet's ability to fight infection with a C-complex supplement; give about 500 mg per 10 pounds of body weight or dose to bowel tolerance until the infection clears.

Herbal Therapy: Use any of the natural immunizations described on pages 285-286.

Hands-on Therapies: All are appropriate.

Homeopathy: Accurate prescribing is important; consult a veterinary homeopath. Remember that eucalyptus and other strong essential oils antidote homeopathic remedies and should not be used while the patient is being treated homeopathically.

Aromatherapy: See the essential oil immunization on page 286. In addition, help your pet breathe by placing several drops of the essential oils of chamomile, eucalyptus, ginger, thyme or lavender, or any combination of these oils, in a diffuser or spray them in the air near your pet.

Birds: For birds with respiratory infections, Nelly Grosjean recommends diffusing a blend of 10 parts eucalyptus, 5 parts pine, 3 parts niaouli or cajeput and 2 parts tea tree oil near the cage for five minutes several times a day. In large parrot rooms, use the following to treat a 15 by 30 foot area: 9 parts eucalyptus, 3 parts pine, 4 parts terebinth, 2 parts tea tree and 1 part each thyme and rosemary. Diffuse approximately 1/2 teaspoon of this blend per hour for three to 12 hours per day for two to three days, then use a maintenance schedule of one to two hours per day for 10 days.

Cats and Dogs: For cats, Grosjean recommends a diffused blend of 20 parts eucalyptus, 10 parts pine, 5 parts tea tree and 2 parts thyme essential oils. For dogs with infectious diseases, use a blend of 8 parts lavandin, 4 parts eucalyptus, 2 parts each thyme, rosemary and wild marjoram and 1 part each mint and cinnamon. These oil blends can be diffused continuously or as desired until the infection clears. The essential oils recommended for cats can be adapted for use with rabbits and other small animals.

Hands-on Therapies: All are appropriate. Stimulate acupressure point LU7 for any breathing problem. In addition, for upper respiratory infections, use LI11 and for sinus congestion, LI4.

Color Therapy: For any respiratory infection resembling the common cold, give a scarlet tonation on the upper body at the first onset of symptoms, then a green systemic front and blue on the face and throat.

Ringworm

Ringworm isn't always shaped like a ring and it has nothing to do with worms (it's a fungal infection like athlete's foot), but its descriptive name is often apt. Ringworm spreads in concentric circles, leaving thick reddened irritated skin and broken hair behind. In cats, which are its primary victims, ringworm causes less irritation and itching. This is a highly contagious infection which can be transmitted to humans as well as other animals. Children are especially vulnerable.

Like a parasite infestation, ringworm infections reflect a stressed or unhealthy host, for a strong animal will not become infected despite exposure. *Important :* Keep the infected animal isolated from other pets and people, especially children, until the infection clears. Wash your hands well after handling or treating your pet.

Nutritional Therapy: Fast the animal for one to two days, feeding water only. Then resume feeding a natural, raw-food diet or begin introducing one after the fast. Zinc, lecithin, cod liver oil and essential fatty acid supplements are often recommended for pets with ringworm.

Herbal Therapy: Most veterinarians recommend clipping the hair around the infestation and disposing of the removed hair carefully so it doesn't spread the fungus. On an animal with a very short coat, that may not be necessary. Fungal infections thrive in damp, dark places, so expose the area as much as possible to air and light.

Shampoo thoroughly with a gentle liquid soap or pet shampoo to which you have added several drops of tea tree oil and grapefruit seed extract. Massage this into the fur and skin before rinsing well. As a final rinse, add 1/2 cup of 15-percent tea tree oil solution and 20 drops grapefruit seed extract to 1 cup water. Apply this all over the animal's body except near the eyes and massage it into the coat.

To visibly infected areas apply 15-percent tea tree oil, diluted grapefruit seed extract or strongly brewed plantain or goldenseal tea several times a day until the infection disappears. If desired, alternate treatments from one to another.

Treat the animal internally with antifungal herbs by adding grapefruit seed extract, noni powder or olive leaf extract, tea or tincture to food.

Homeopathy: Give *Sulphur 6x* once daily for four weeks. As tea tree oil will antidote most homeopathic remedies, begin this treatment several hours after bathing your pet and apply grapefruit seed extract or an antifungal tea to affected areas.

Shedding, Chronic: See *Skin, Coat*

Sinus Congestion: See *Respiratory Problems*

Skin, Coat

By far the most common disorders experienced by America's dogs and cats involve the skin and coat. Hot spots, bare patches, feline acne, dull-looking fur, itching, bumpy rashes, scratching, shedding, bad smells, dandruff, a greasy texture, pigment changes, matting and tangles reflect both nutritional problems and owner neglect.

The key to a lifetime of healthy skin and fur is good nutrition, but be aware that as you switch from commercial pet food to a well-balanced raw natural diet, your pet may get worse instead of better, with flaring hot spots, itching, a greasy coat, unpleasant odors or excessive shedding. What's going on?

Chronic health problems are caused by a number of factors, including the accumulation of toxins in the body. Changing the diet stimulates detoxification, during which the body excretes stored wastes.

If your pet's coat seems to get worse as soon as you change his diet, remember that the skin is an organ of elimination and for a while it may be overworked. Vitamins, herbs and other supplements will help your pet make the transition, which may last for several days or even weeks, depending on his overall condition.

In most pets with minor skin and coat problems, the healing crisis doesn't last long. Shedding may continue — in fact, your pet may shed his old coat completely and grow a gorgeous new one — but other symptoms improve quickly. The advantage to persevering through a healing crisis is that the cure, when it comes, is permanent. Check with a holistic veterinarian for advice, especially if your pet has been given antibiotics, cortisone drugs or other chemicals in the past or if you have any concern or question about his body's reaction to the change of diet.

Grooming: Nothing you do on the outside improves an animal's coat like regular brushing. Brushing stimulates the lymph system, which involves both the immune system and waste removal. It also stimulates the skin, improves circulation, prevents tangling, distributes natural oils through the coat and removes fleas, flea eggs and roaming ticks.

Long-haired dogs and cats require more attention than their short-haired cousins, but all pets benefit from regular grooming. Birds need bathing (see page 360), rabbits can be stroked with a soft brush, most cats love to be brushed with a stiff-bristled hair brush, and dog groomers have more special tools, brushes, combs and scissors than a barber shop. If your dog or cat has long hair, follow your groomer's advice regarding equipment and its use. In addition, brush any pet with a loofa sponge or rough, dry washcloth. It won't remove hair but it will stimulate circulation and smooth the coat.

Frequent shampooing may contribute to coat problems rather than solve them. Soap strips natural oils from the coat and can irritate sensitive skin. Instead of using a pet shampoo or soap, experiment with herbal teas and essential oils. Wet the animal to the skin, let him dry, then brush.

One of the most common skin irritations is an allergic reaction to flea bites. Go over all furry pets with a flea comb once a month during winter months and once a week in the summer or whenever your pet has been visiting animals that might have fleas. Pet supply stores and catalogs sell a variety of metal, plastic and wooden combs with close-together teeth that trap hair and debris. To check for fleas, comb your pet along the neck and chest, then remove hair from the comb on a white paper towel or sheet of white paper. If you don't see any fleas, look for small dark grains that look like sand. These are probably flea feces; you can tell for sure by dampening the paper and moving the grains. If they leave a brownish stain behind, it's the residue of your pet's digested blood.

Check for ticks at the same time. Gently massage your pet all over, feeling for tiny bumps. If you find one, inspect it under a bright light and, if it's a tick, remove it with tweezers. Frequent brushings during tick season help remove ticks that are crawling on fur but it won't dislodge attached ticks. See page 393 for more information on tick removal.

Related Conditions: If your pet has broken hair and tiny skin bumps, the problem might be mange, which is caused by a mite; see page 407. If hair loss occurs in circular patches, it might be ringworm, which is caused by a fungus; see page 425.

Feline Acne

If your cat has small dark bumps around the chin that resemble blackheads, white pimples that contain waxy debris or black flecks within individual hairs, he has feline acne. In some cats, the condition flares, goes away and returns. Symptoms range from just a few small blackheads to severe ulceration.

Conventional diagnosis can require anesthetizing the cat in order to remove a skin sample for laboratory analysis but more commonly a smear sample is taken to check for the presence of yeast or bacteria. In many cases, the finding is "idiopathic," which means no specific cause can be determined. Conventional treatment can include medicated ointments, shampoos and more aggressive therapies, such as anesthetizing the animal in order to express and clean out the infected areas, followed by oral antibiotics.

A large number of veterinarians, groomers, breeders and owners have noticed that feline acne is common in cats who eat commercial pet food out of plastic bowls. Switching from plastic to glass, ceramic or stainless steel will help, but don't stop there: give your pet a natural diet and the condition should clear quickly. You can speed healing by dabbing your cat's chin with a 15-percent solution of tea tree oil or diluted grapefruit seed extract once a day or gently clean the area with a dilute solution of calendula tincture or a similar herbal wash. Cats dislike tea tree oil, so try the other remedies first.

Skin Allergies

Persistent itching, scratching, patchy hair loss and inflamed skin are all symptoms of allergies that may be complicated by bacterial infections. Conventional treatment with steroids, antibiotics, tranquilizers and antihistamines may suppress symptoms for a while, but the condition usually returns. In addition, drugs may cause new problems. Cushing's syndrome, Addison's disease, liver disease, kidney failure and autoimmune disorders have all been linked to the long-term use of drugs for skin conditions.

If your pet has been taking prescription drugs, consult with a holistic veterinarian for advice on whether and how to discontinue the medication. Don't just stop abruptly; some drugs have to be tapered off gradually.

Vaccinations often worsen skin and coat allergies. Consult a holistic veterinarian before vaccinating a pet with skin problems. In the case of required vaccinations such as rabies, homeopathy can reduce the side effects.

Another contributing cause of skin allergies can be a hormone imbalance. See page 435 for the side effects of spaying and neutering, which may include skin disorders; please note that this side effect is easy to correct and should not be a deterrent to the surgery.

The adrenal glands play an important part in skin health. In addition to providing herbs and supplements that support adrenal function, be sure your pet receives ample exposure to natural light. Fluorescent lighting is especially likely to disrupt the normal function of glands and organs that affect the skin and coat.

Nutritional Therapy: If your pet has inflamed, irritated skin, begin with a fast. Let the animal's digestive tract rest for a day or two on water only. For dogs and cats with serious hot spots and related allergic symptoms, follow the water fast with several days of liquid fare such as raw juices, raw milk diluted with water or small quantities of raw meat blended with water. Introduce solid foods gradually toward the end of the fasting week.

Feed your pet once or twice a day, not all day long. Remove food after 15 to 20 minutes and omit between-meal snacks.

Most skin conditions respond well to a complete change in diet. Stop feeding dry or canned food and switch to a natural diet of fresh raw food. Study Chapter 2. The simple removal of chemical dyes, preservatives and additives from the diet has stopped allergic reactions in many dogs, cats, birds and rabbits; replacing canned and packaged "complete" foods with fresh raw or growing foods supplies essential nutrients that convenience foods lack.

Supplements are important because most pets with allergies have impaired digestion and need help assimilating nutrients from food. Digestive enzymes, cider vinegar, hydrochloric acid, bitter herbs and acidophilus are all likely to help, as described in earlier chapters. Give your pet a multiple vitamin from whole-food sources, such as Congaplex by Standard Process (give 1 tablet per 10 pounds of body weight). Supplement with additional vitamin C and E complex, an all-purpose glandular supplement (or follow your veterinarian's recommendations based on your pet's blood profile), a comprehensive mineral supplement containing trace minerals, small amounts of additional zinc (Standard Process zinc liver chelate, for example) and a variety of oils to provide essential fatty acids (EFAs). Avocado, fatty fish, fat from organically raised meat and poultry, EFA supplements and small quantities of borage seed, evening primrose, flaxseed, olive, cod liver and other oils on a rotating basis will improve your pet's coat, especially if they are given with digestive or enzyme supplements. If the animal isn't able to digest these fats, they only make the skin and coat feel greasy.

Antioxidants are an allergic pet's allies. Fresh carrots and green plants are important sources, as are vitamins A, C and E, the mineral selenium and lipoic acid. Avoid synthetic vitamins and use mineral supplements that are both comprehensive (essential and trace elements) and easy to assimilate (colloidal liquids, powders or chelated tablets crushed or ground before serving). Adjust human product dosages for your pet's weight.

Willard Water concentrate improves the assimilation of nutrients and by itself improves skin and fur. Add it to drinking water and apply it topically.

If the coat lacks proper pigmentation, add extra kelp or other seaweeds as well as small amounts of unrefined sea salt and colloidal trace minerals to the diet. Glandular supplements also help correct pigmentation problems.

Liquid (colloidal) trace mineral products can be applied full strength to hot spots, irritated areas and healing wounds. Another source of trace minerals is unrefined sea salt. In addition to adding small amounts to your pet's food, add 1 tablespoon of unrefined salt to 2 quarts water or herb tea as a rinse and work it into the skin. For open sores and healing wounds, use a more concentrated solution, such as 1 tablespoon salt per cup of water or tea. A female German Shepherd in Samantha's obedience class suffered from a sore that wouldn't heal despite repeated trips to the veterinarian. Her owner applied this salt solution and the sore improved the same day.

Bee propolis tincture or liquid extract is another helpful supplement. Add 1 drop per pound of body weight twice daily for 10 days, then half that amount once daily for two additional weeks. For convenience, remember that there are 60 drops in a teaspoon. Alternatively, bee propolis capsules or tablets can be added to food; adjust label directions for your pet's weight.

Apple cider vinegar is recommended for dogs and cats with skin problems although dogs tend to accept it more readily than cats. Cider vinegar is recommended for pets with any condition that resembles eczema, but it helps clear all skin conditions because it improves digestion.

Herbal Therapy: Add up to 1 tablespoon aloe vera juice or gel to your pet's food for each 20 pounds of body weight; that is about 1 teaspoon per six or seven pounds. Start with smaller amounts and increase gradually. Aloe vera helps improve digestion and the animal's overall health. In addition, apply aloe vera juice or gel to hot spots and areas of irritation to soothe and heal them. This therapy helps speed the clearing of feline acne.

Brew a very strong chamomile tea and apply it to irritated skin. Chamomile soothes and reduces inflammation. In addition, use this tea as a rinse after or instead of shampooing.

Licorice root and yucca contain natural cortisone and help relieve inflammation; licorice is a specific for the adrenal glands, which are often stressed or depleted in pets with chronic coat problems. Use licorice in small amounts (1/4 to 1/2 the usual recommended quantities) for long-term use or follow a schedule such as the one described on page 434 for hormone balance.

Wheat grass, other grasses, bitter herbs such as dandelion, flowers such as calendula and chamomile, fresh green herbs such as chickweed or plantain and the most skin-friendly herb of all, comfrey, help clear skin allergies. Comfrey can be added fresh, dried or in tea or tincture to food or applied to skin irritations; see page 147 for notes on this herb's safety. Goldenseal powder can be mixed with water or aloe vera juice or gel and applied to hot spots.

For an all-purpose skin and coat supplement, combine equal parts of dried burdock root, cleavers, dandelion, garlic, kelp, horsetail and nettles. Grind these ingredients well in a spice or coffee grinder. Add 1/4 teaspoon per 10 pounds of body weight to food per day.

Homeopathy: There are literally hundreds of homeopathic remedies for skin and coat problems. Accurate diagnosis is essential in the treatment of chronic conditions. Carefully document your pet's symptoms and behavior before consulting a veterinary homeopath by phone or in person.

Aromatherapy: A 15-percent solution of tea tree oil can be sprayed or dabbed onto hot spots, irritated areas, feline acne and flea bite areas. However, cats dislike its turpentine fragrance, so consider this an emergency treatment for felines.

Treat areas of hair loss with a blend of 12 parts St. John's wort oil (an olive oil infusion of St. John's wort blossoms, not an essential oil), 6 parts wheat germ oil, 3 parts essential oil of lavender or lavandin and 1 part each rose geranium and rosemary essential oils. The pressed oil of wild rose hips has a dramatic healing effect on skin and hair; use it as a carrier oil or apply it directly to open sores and inflamed skin.

The essential-oil brushing treatment described on page 170 improves the condition of dull, dry coats.

Hands-on Therapies: All are helpful because they improve circulation, stimulate the elimination of toxins and correct imbalances. Stimulate acupressure point LI11 for any allergic symptoms; for dry, itchy skin, press SP6 or LU7.

Color Therapy: For moist or weeping skin conditions, give a turquoise systemic that includes affected areas until signs of drying appear, then also tonate with indigo. For dry or scaly conditions, give a lemon systemic and orange on affected areas.

Smells: See *Odors*

Spaying and Neutering

Although the surgical sterilization of dogs and cats is by definition unnatural, the spaying of females (removal of the uterus and ovaries) and the castration of males (removal of the testicles) is widely recommended by holistic veterinarians and natural health care experts. The term "neutering" describes either spaying or castration, but most people use it in reference to castration.

Juliette de Bairacli Levy firmly opposes surgical sterilization and pleads with pet owners to allow dogs and cats to sire puppies or kittens "at least once in their lifetime so that they can survive on earth through their offspring when the time comes for them to die." This is a valid argument, but in North America, where tens of millions of dogs and cats are euthanized every year because no one wants them, it is difficult to support. Tracing the female offspring of the one-time litter of a single dog or cat is an eye-opening exercise. If Fluffy's kittens or puppies include four females, each of which gives birth at the age of one year to a single litter containing four females, within five years Fluffy's female offspring will number 1,024; after six, 4,096; and after seven, 16,384. Add all the males from these litters, and Fluffy has produced a population explosion.

Overpopulation is one reason to spay and neuter, but just as important is the deterioration of America's domestic pet gene pool. Surgical sterilization is the only guarantee that common genetic defects won't be passed to new generations. Unless your dog or cat is truly a superior example of the breed and likely to produce superior puppies or kittens when mated after careful research on your part to an equally superior partner, he or she should be prevented from reproducing.

Every medical decision measures risks and benefits both for the animals involved and the people who care for them. For most Americans, the benefits of spaying and neutering far outweigh the benefits of life with an intact dog or cat. In *The New Natural Cat,* Anitra Frazier wrote that most catteries that have a male for siring purposes keep him confined where it will be easy to clean the pungent urine he sprays to mark his territory. As Frazier explained, "Once you've smelled the urine of an unaltered tom, it's not something you'll easily forget." Spraying is a natural behavior that can't be trained away, and no litter product can disguise it. A single intact male can regularly service the six to twenty females who reside in his cattery as well as the outside cats who come to him for stud service. If the male doesn't have anyone to service, says Frazier, he is likely to become tense, nervous and out of sorts.

Intact toms who are free to roam are compelled by their hormones to seek receptive females and to fight for the opportunity to mate with them. They often have torn ears and other injuries; fights are inevitable and sometimes fatal.

When female cats come into heat, they don't spray the house but they are high strung, nervous, jumpy and too distracted to eat. Most are extremely vocal as well. Going through repeated heat cycles without being allowed to mate takes a toll; intact females who aren't bred are often thin and less resistant to disease. For example, cystic ovaries are common in cats that come into heat more than twice a year because their unfertilized eggs remain in position; they are not discarded by the body.

Similar behaviors and health problems are seen in intact dogs. Intact males are notorious for mounting everything including furniture and people's legs; they tend to be more aggressive and difficult for novices to control and they are more likely to roam, disappear, get hit by a car, get into fights or be exposed to illnesses in other strays. Bitches in heat have their own personality changes and health stresses and of course require owner supervision and care to avoid unplanned mating.

Problems involving the reproductive organs are common in unaltered dogs and cats, including testicular cancer, breast cancer, false pregnancy, continual heat and uterine infections such as pyometra.

When is the best time to spay or neuter? Veterinarians used to be taught to wait until males were past puberty because neutering earlier was believed to increase the danger of urethral obstruction; however, several recent studies show that prepuberty castration does not cause lower urinary tract disorders or urethral obstruction. Similarly, some veterinarians recommend waiting until the female has experienced at least one heat cycle before spaying, but the incidence of breast cancer is lowest in females spayed before their first heat.

In recent years, "pediatric" neutering has become popular in large animal shelters and among some breeders. Advocates of the practice, in which 6- to 14-week-old puppies or kittens are spayed or neutered, argue that it limits unwanted pregnancies, decreases the incidence of genetic disorders, improves the animal's chances of sale or adoption and assures breeders that pet-quality animals won't be bred. Opponents cite increased risks from anesthesia and subsequent urinary incontinence, obesity, vaginal infection, dermatitis, growth and weight deficiencies and behavioral changes. Although at least one study showed no significant differences between cats whose surgery took place at seven weeks and those who were operated on at seven months, many veterinarians believe there isn't sufficient scientific data to determine whether early-age sterilization is completely free of long-term side effects.

An obvious advantage to waiting until age seven months to one year, at which age most of America's dogs and cats are spayed and neutered, is that your pet will have several months of excellent nutrition and natural care before surgery, preparation that reduces the risks of adverse side effects and speeds healing.

Richard Pitcairn notes that spaying can cause complications when performed to resolve prolonged heat cycles, cystic ovaries, infections and other medical problems. He prefers to treat these conditions with improved nutrition and other holistic methods so that the animal can be spayed when healthy and not during an active infection or chronic illness.

In *The Very Healthy Cat Book*, Wendell Belfield recommends that cat owners have their pets tested for feline leukemia before surgery because the stress it causes can activate the illness in animals who carry the virus but have no symptoms. If the test shows the presence of the virus, he says, you should not operate. "My regular clients who test before neutering and who maintain their animals on a good supplement program never have deathly sick cats after surgery," he wrote. Many holistic veterinarians have observed that surgery-related deaths are highest in animals fed commercial pet food without supplementation. As described on page 297, Belfield has found that vitamin therapy eliminates the feline leukemia virus, removing this risk factor from feline surgery.

One significant difference between altered dogs and cats and their intact counterparts is size. Altered animals are almost always larger and heavier because removal of the testes and ovaries changes the body's fat metabolism. Without testosterone from the testes or estrogen from the ovaries, more fat is deposited in the body's tissues. Feeding your pets a well-balanced natural diet and keeping them physically active helps prevent excessive weight gain. Overweight animals should not be placed on "lite" brand low-fat, high-carbohydrate pet foods. Their lack of essential fatty acids and good-quality protein combined with their high grain content and chemical preservatives makes these foods the opposite of what dogs and cats are designed to consume. Raw foods, nutritional supplements and an active life will help your pet stay fit.

Nutritional Therapy: Every pet should be on a healthy diet. A well-balanced, natural raw diet will prevent common problems in your spayed or neutered pet. In addition to a good multiple vitamin derived from food sources and a comprehensive mineral and trace element product, consider giving your pet a raw multiple glandular supplement to supply the building blocks of natural hormones no longer produced by the body and to help compensate for the fact that pet dogs and cats seldom consume the prey animals on which their species evolved and which are a rich supply of glandular substances. Nonprescription glandular supplements, most of which are derived from beef cattle, do not contain the hormones produced by the pituitary, thyroid, adrenal and other glands, for those are extracted for pharmaceutical use, but the remaining glandular tissue provides important nutrients not available in other foods. There are several glandular and organ supplements on the market for both human and pet use. Consult a holistic veterinarian or pet nutritionist or buy different types and feed them on a rotating basis. Adrenal and liver support is especially important for spayed and neutered animals.

Sex hormones influence the production of adrenal cortisone, which governs the production of antibodies in the lymph glands, a crucial part of the immune system's natural defenses. Nutritional supplements can compensate for this lack, especially a multiple vitamin-mineral program that emphasizes pantothenic acid, which is one of the B-complex vitamins, and vitamin C complex.

Herbal Therapy: Licorice root is a specific for the adrenal cortex. One of its ingredients, glycyrrhetinic acid, or GA, mimics the adrenal hormone aldosterone, which is involved in salt and water metabolism. Very large amounts of GA in people can cause pseudoaldosteronism, a potentially serious condition that causes headaches, lethargy, fluid retention and elevated blood pressure. However, small amounts given intermittently provide important support to the adrenal glands without adverse side effects. In Europe, where licorice root is commonly prescribed for the treatment of ulcers, deglycyrrhized licorice or DGL prevents fluid retention and blood pressure elevation. Many U.S. pharmacies now stock DGL products next to their antacids and digestive aids. While deglycyrrhized licorice can help prevent bloating and indigestion in your pet, it cannot provide the adrenal gland support for which licorice is renowned. Be sure to use whole root extracts, tinctures or powders for this purpose.

A commonly recommended protocol adapted for pet use is to give 1 dropperful of licorice root tincture once daily to small animals (up to 20 pounds) and twice daily to larger animals for four weeks, then cut the dosage in half for one week, then give the lower amount every other day for a week and discontinue the herb altogether for four to six weeks before repeating. Any of the adaptogen herbs such as ginseng, ashwagandha or schisandra can be given in addition and without interruption. All of these herbs help correct hormonal imbalances.

As they age, some surgically altered animals, especially male cats and female dogs, develop urinary tract infections or incontinence. Considering that most of these animals have spent their entire lives eating commercial pet food, nutrition no doubt plays a role. So does the lack of natural hormones. The change from dry to fresh food may be all your neutered cat needs to resume normal urinary function but you can give him small amounts of any adaptogen herb and occasional licorice root as well.

Spayed bitches who urinate in their sleep (look for damp bedding and wet thighs) are often treated with synthetic female hormones to strengthen the urinary tract's muscle tone and alleviate this problem. Diethylstilbestrol (DES), which is commonly prescribed for spayed dogs, has well-documented side effects in humans, including cancer in the offspring of women who took it in minute amounts during pregnancy. Owners familiar with its history have misgivings about giving the drug to their dogs year after year. In healthy spayed animals, as in healthy menopausal women, the adrenal glands and liver take over the ovaries' biological function by continuing to produce small amounts of estrogen until old age. A natural diet and the use of herbs and supplements that support the adrenal glands, liver and overall hormone balance can often be used instead of prescription drugs.

When hops cultivation began on a large scale for beer brewing, hops pickers who worked in the fields for several weeks noticed certain changes. Women's menstrual cycles arrived prematurely, young girls menstruated at an earlier age and men experienced a lessening of sexual desire. These centuries-old observations have been validated by scientific research showing that the fresh plant has estrogenic effects. Tinctures made from fresh hops, which are available from herb shops, can be used for female hormone regulation in both spayed and intact animals and to reduce the ardor of sexually hyperactive males. Dried hops offers little or no hormone regulation but is valued for its nervine and sedative properties.

Chasteberry or vitex *(Vitex agnus castus)* stimulates the pituitary gland, which, among other functions, regulates and normalizes hormone production. This herb is a specific for the female system. Dong quai *(Angelica sinensis),* widely known as the "female ginseng" although it benefits both male and female systems, exerts a regulating and normalizing influence on hormone production through its positive action on the liver and endocrine systems. Its bitter taste and pungent smell may make it impossible to give in a tea or tincture, but powdered dong quai in capsules can be hidden in strong-smelling food or given to cooperative pets directly. Other herbs with estrogenic properties include pomegranate seeds and black cohosh.

Wild yam root (*Dioscorea villosa* and related species) has an important place in medical history as the original source of diosgenin used in the production of contraceptive pills and as the base of many steroidal drugs. Its steroidal saponins help produce both progesterone and cortisone; progesterone is an important precursor for cortisol, LH (luteinizing hormone), aldosterone and estrogen. Long before its pharmaceutical discovery, wild yam was valued by herbalists for its ability to normalize hormone production and balance the ratio of progesterone and estrogen. A liver tonic herb, wild yam activates and stimulates liver activity, and its steroidal saponins are used by the liver in the generation of sex hormones. Long used by Chinese herbalists, wild yam is prescribed in Oriental medicine for problems associated with the spleen, kidneys, liver and lungs in both men and women. Wild yam creams are widely sold as a natural hormone replacement therapy.

To use wild yam cream, adapt the label instructions to your pet's weight or apply small amounts to the bare skin of any furry animal, male or female, to help support the liver, adrenal glands and hormone balance and to help alleviate the symptoms of arthritis and other chronic conditions. Typical instructions recommend applying a small amount (start with 1/8 teaspoon for most dogs) once per day to a different body part each time, such as the abdomen one day, an arm pit, ear or foot the next; after applying the cream, sit or play with your pet to prevent her from licking it off. Some instructions note that the faster the cream is absorbed, the more the body needs. Every few days return to the bare skin of the abdomen and watch the clock. According to the absorption theory, when the cream takes a full five minutes to be absorbed, the body has sufficient progesterone stores, and less frequent and smaller applications can be used to maintain that level. Adjusting the dosage for individual animals this way may help prevent unwanted side effects.

Follow the dosage chart on page 136 for the long-term use of dong quai, ginseng, ashwagandha, schisandra and other adaptogen herbs. Give whole root licorice in courses as described on page 435. Make or buy a tincture of estrogenic herbs such as fresh (not dried) hops, chasteberry, pomegranate seeds and black cohosh and dose the combined remedy according to the chart on page 136, or give these herbs separately, one or two per day. You will find many hormone-balancing herbs in products designed for menopausal women, any of which can be given to spayed pets. Adapt label directions for your animal's weight.

Spraying: See *Urinary Problems*

Stomach Problems: See *Digestion*

Surgery

If your pet is scheduled for elective surgery, such as spaying, neutering or dental pro-phylaxis (tooth cleaning), there are several things you can do ahead of time to insure that the operation goes well and the patient recovers quickly.

First, improve your pet's diet, physical exercise and exposure to natural light. These simple steps increase stamina, healing and resistance to infection.

Nutritional Therapy: Beginning two weeks before surgery, increase vitamin C, using a high quality vitamin C complex such as ester-C calcium ascorbate with bioflavonoids and other C-complex nutrients or vitamin C derived from food sources, *not* ascorbic acid. Give 1,000 mg (1 gram) vitamin C per 20 pounds of body weight, divided into two or three doses during the day; if this dosage produces loose stools, reduce the amount until this side effect disappears. Continue vitamin C at this or a larger dosage (just below bowel tolerance) until one week after the surgery.

Beginning three weeks before surgery, give the animal a good-quality vitamin E complex derived from natural food sources, *not* synthetic vitamin E. Give 800 IU vita-min E per day to cats and small dogs, 1,000 IU to dogs weighing 15 to 35 pounds, 1,200 IU to large dogs weighing 40 to 85 pounds and 1,500 IU to giant breeds. Discontinue vitamin E supplementation seven to ten days before the surgery because vitamin E thins the blood. After surgery, resume the recommended dose for an additional week. If your pet's breed is known for bleeding problems, have a blood test done before surgery and, if your animal has a clotting disorder, follow your holistic veterinarian's recommenda-tions regarding supplements.

Beginning two weeks before surgery, provide additional vitamin A by giving dogs fresh, raw carrot juice or pureed carrots, 1/8 to 1/4 cup per 10 pounds of body weight divided into two or three servings during the day. For cats, and dogs who don't like car-rots, give additional liver or a vitamin A supplement; give 10,000 IU per day to cats and medium size dogs and twice that amount to large and giant breeds. Continue these sup-plements until the day before surgery and then for at least a week after surgery.

Beginning one week before surgery, stop feeding garlic, as garlic is a natural blood thinner that helps prevent clotting.

Flower Essences: Beginning two or three days before surgery, place several drops of Dr. Bach's emergency formula or yarrow flower essence in the animal's water and, twice a day, in his or her mouth, behind the ears and on the abdomen. At the same time, prac-tice Therapeutic Touch, massage the ears and project positive, healing thoughts, pictur-ing your healthy pet making a fast recovery. After surgery, use either of the recom-mended flower essence formulas several times a day while your pet recovers.

Before Surgery

On the day before surgery, feed the animal an early dinner (late afternoon) and do not provide food after 6:00 p.m. Withhold water after 8:00 p.m. Continue treating with flower essences and Therapeutic Touch. Do the same before leaving the house and again at the veterinary clinic.

After Surgery

Greet your dog with Dr. Bach's emergency formula and a hug. Wait two or three hours before giving food or water, then provide ample clean water to help clear traces of anaesthetic from the system. When your pet is hungry, give a soft food such as yogurt, soft fruit or pureed meat.

Herbal Therapy: Apply any healing tea to the wound, such as a strong infusion of calendula blossoms or plantain leaf with a few drops of grapefruit seed extract and a pinch of unrefined sea salt. Because comfrey will cause the skin to heal rapidly, it's a good idea to wait until stitches are removed so that they aren't embedded under the skin's surface. After that, use a comfrey tea, poultice or salve to speed healing. Vitamin E, rose hip oil and aloe vera all promote rapid healing without scarring; apply any of these every few hours at first, then two or three times a day.

Calming nervine herbs like chamomile, valerian or skullcap may help your pet relax and sleep.

Homeopathy: After surgery, if your pet is groggy, nauseated or slow to wake up, give a single pellet or tablet of homeopathic *Phosphorus 30c. Arnica 30c* is the all-purpose follow-up treatment for surgery; give 1 pellet or tablet every 4 hours for a total of 3 treatments. If the skin is red or irritated or if there is a discharge of fluid or pus around the wound or its stitches, give 1 pellet or tablet of *Apis mellifica 6c* every 4 hours until the condition clears; withhold food for at least 10 minutes before and after treatment.

Color Therapy: If bleeding resumes, tonate with indigo on the affected area until bleeding stops. For all surgical wounds, give a turquoise systemic to include affected areas, then green and magenta on those areas.

Teeth and Gums

Dental problems and gum disease are serious problems for an estimated 50 to 85 percent of America's dogs and cats, but that's a reflection of their cooked food diets. Animals who eat raw food are unlikely to have receding, inflamed, swollen or bleeding gums.

Nutritional Therapy: Calcium and other minerals are essential to the health of teeth and bones. In addition to trace-mineral supplements, fresh, raw bones are important sources of essential minerals and they provide exercise for the jaws and help clean teeth.

Rabbits need a constant supply of hard items to chew to keep their teeth from growing too long. Clean hardwood, roots like carrots and parsnips and other chewable items are essential to their health.

Vitamin C is known for its ability to improve gum health and it improves the assimilation of essential minerals. Give your pet a good-quality multiple vitamin derived from food sources plus additional vitamin C complex so that the animal receives 250 to 500 mg vitamin C per 10 pounds of body weight.

The supplement coenzyme Q10, usually abbreviated COQ10, is often recommended for tooth and gum problems in dogs and cats. Adapt label instructions to your pet's weight.

For pets with infected gums (gingivitis), give 1 drop of bee propolis tincture per pound of body weight twice daily for two months, then half that amount twice daily for two months.

Some people are reluctant to feed their pets apple cider vinegar because they fear its acidity will harm teeth, but that won't happen. Cider vinegar has a number of health benefits and does not cause dental problems; in fact, its addition to the diet usually improves digestion and thus supports health in the mouth.

Keep your pet's teeth and gums clean and stimulated by brushing them with a pet toothbrush and an appropriate canine or feline toothpaste, plain water or the tooth powder described below or simply use a dry brush. If that doesn't work well, wrap gauze around your finger and massage the teeth and gums with your finger.

Herbal Therapy: All of the green grasses (wheat, barley, rye, kamut and other grains) and green herbs help improve the condition of diseased gums. Add finely minced fresh greens to your pet's food whenever possible.

Make your own tooth powder for dogs or cats with equal parts activated charcoal powder, powdered clay and powdered peppermint leaf, chamomile blossom or any deodorizing herb. Alternatively, combine equal parts baking soda and clay, then add 1 drop of essential clove or aniseed oil to each tablespoon. A drop of blood root tincture can be substituted for or added to these essential oils as it is a specific for dental plaque. Add a small amount of cayenne pepper to improve circulation in the gums.

Echinacea tea or tincture can be used topically and given orally to help clear gum infections; see next page.

Aromatherapy: To improve the breath, combine equal parts essential oil of caraway, cumin and coriander and add this blend to food according to the dosage chart on page 174. Alternatively, if the animal will accept it, add peppermint oil.

Tea tree oil is a specific for gum infections in people. If your pet has a gum infection, you can help disinfect it by rubbing a 15-percent tea tree solution (be sure it is made with vodka and not rubbing alcohol) into the gums. The main disadvantage to this approach is the taste and odor of tea tree oil, which most dogs and cats find objectionable. Diluted grapefruit seed extract, which tastes very bitter, works as well. Either of these or echinacea tea or diluted echinacea tincture, another unpleasant-tasting but effective disinfectant, can be applied with a bare finger, toothbrush, gauze wipe or eyedropper. Many veterinarians, like many dentists, recommend antibiotics for patients with severely infected gums, but many serious gum infections in pets have cleared within two to three weeks with the daily application of disinfecting essential oils or herbs and the internal use of any of the herbal immunizations described on pages 285-286.

Thyroid Imbalances

Thyroid imbalances are widespread in America's pets, especially hypothyroidism (low or underactive thyroid) in dogs and hyperthyroidism (high or overactive thyroid) in cats. Holistic veterinarians blame the frequent use of combination vaccines, commercial pet foods and cortisone drugs for these conditions.

Experienced veterinarians often recognize thyroid problems at a glance. Hypothyroid dogs often have a dull-looking coat with greasy-feeling skin that has a pronounced odor that clings to your fingers when you rub it, a low energy level and a groin rash that looks like tiny black dots. Hyperthyroid cats often lose weight despite a normal appetite and become nervous and irritable. For several days they may be hyperactive and have a rapid heartbeat, then lethargic, apathetic and uninterested in food, play or grooming.

If your pet has an under- or overactive thyroid, work with a holistic veterinarian as these conditions require careful monitoring. The following suggestions apply to healthy pets.

To Prevent Thyroid Problems

- Feed a well-balanced natural, raw diet and occasional raw glandular supplements as described on page 100.

- Give your animal ample exposure to natural light, for malillumination is a contributing cause of all glandular problems.

- The mineral iodine is essential to thyroid health and one of its richest sources is seaweed. Supplement your pet's food with small quantities of kelp and unrefined sea salt to prevent deficiencies.

- The adaptogen herbs astragalus, ashwagandha, ginseng, fo-ti, Siberian ginseng and schisandra help balance hormone production throughout the body. Any of these herbs can be given in small amounts as a general tonic; blends containing these herbs and kelp, raw glandular extracts and the amino acid tyrosine are popular supplements for improved thyroid health.

- Essiac tea, described on page 302, has been used as a support therapy in the treatment of thyroid disorders in people. Many pet owners give their dogs and cats Essiac tea from time to time as a blood-cleansing tonic and to help maintain hormone balance.

Toxoplasmosis

Toxoplasma protozoa infect birds and mammals, including humans, throughout the world. An estimated 50 percent of America's human population, many of our dogs and livestock and most of our cats are infected with the protozoa.

Toxoplasmosis is usually a minor infection that goes unnoticed in people except those with impaired immune systems, such as AIDS patients, cancer patients who have received chemotherapy or those who take immunosuppressing drugs after organ replacement. In addition, the parasite can cause terrible problems in unborn children. If a woman who has never been infected contracts toxoplasmosis while pregnant, her child may be born prematurely, die or have serious brain damage or other defects.

In cats, which are unusually good hosts for the parasite, it may cause symptoms such as diarrhea containing blood or mucus, fever, liver inflammation and respiratory distress or no symptoms at all. Infected cats usually recover quickly on their own and develop a strong immunity that protects them from future infection. During the month that follows infection, the animal passes oocysts, which are egglike structures that spread the parasite to other hosts after a day of development in the animal's feces outside the body or in cat litter or soil. The cat will continue to pass oocysts until it develops immunity, usually after two weeks, but if the immune system is suppressed by cortisone drugs, this natural immunity is delayed.

Although cats are not the most common source of infection for people, they are the most common pet source. Most people obtain their toxoplasma protozoa from infected raw or undercooked meat. Cats do the same except that their source is usually mice and other prey animals. Cats and people can also pick it up from the feces of infected animals or from soil or cat litter contaminated by infected feces within the last year.

Health warnings are appropriate for pregnant women and seriously ill people who have cats. If you are planning a family, have your doctor perform a simple blood test to determine whether the prospective mother is immune to toxoplasmosis. If so, your cats pose no danger to your future children. If you aren't immune but your cats are, you are similarly protected because they won't be shedding oocytes.

But if you and your cat are both susceptible, there is a risk, especially if you feed your cat raw meat as recommended throughout this book. Women contemplating pregnancy and patients with impaired immune systems have to weigh the risks. Have someone else clean the cat box or wear rubber gloves and wash them with disinfectant soap after disposing of litter and droppings in a sealed plastic bag. Keep the litter box clean and disinfect it regularly with a 15-percent solution of tea tree oil, grapefruit seed extract, chlorine bleach or boiling water. You may decide to board your cat with a friend or relative or, if you keep the cat, feed her cooked meat and keep her indoors and away from animals that might carry the infection so she won't contract the parasite. This is, unfortunately, not nearly so good for your cat as a fresh, raw diet but after your child is born, you can resume her regular fare.

Handle meat in your kitchen with sensible precautions, disinfecting everything it touches, and avoid eating raw or undercooked meat at home or in restaurants.

Many pregnant women are warned to give their cats away because of the danger of toxoplasmosis, but it affects only a fraction of one percent of American births. The risk is small and with common sense, even smaller. Pregnant women and people with compromised immune systems need not abandon their feline companions in the interests of good health.

Travel

Household pets are homebodies. They're happiest and most secure when everyone follows the same routine every day. Travel, whether it's yours or theirs, can be disruptive.

Animals who make the easiest adjustment to travel are those who are used to it from an early age. If your pet thrives on adventure and is a well-behaved travel companion, shared vacations can be fun and rewarding. Let common sense be your guide about where to go and how to get there. If your pets don't travel well or it's impossible to include them, your choices for their temporary care are usually a boarding kennel, a stay at the home of a friend or relative or visits from a pet sitter. Of these three options, the pet sitter is often the most comfortable and least stressful for the animal because it means staying at home and eating familiar food.

Pet sitting is becoming a popular business for people of all ages. Check local newspaper ads or ask your groomer, veterinarian or obedience trainer for a referral. Wherever you leave your pets, be sure their caretakers understand when and how to feed them and have clear instructions in case of emergency. To help your pets relax while you're away, the sitter can use Dr. Bach's emergency formula or add calming nervine herbs to their food. The more he or she can maintain your pets' regular routine, the easier it will be for the animals to adjust.

Directories of hotels, motels and other facilities that accept pets are sold in pet supply stores, bookstores and by mail. Check the catalogs listed as resources for Chapter 1 and look for ads in pet magazines. Even facilities with a "no-pets" policy may accept dogs or cats on an individual basis, especially if they stay in a portable crate or kennel and you can document their good behavior. Therapy animals who visit hospitals and nursing homes, for example, are sometimes welcomed at resort hotels or bed-and-breakfast inns that don't usually accept pets.

Transportation is always a concern. Is it better to drive or fly? I know many people who routinely ship animals by air, think nothing of it and report only good results. Many airline personnel are both animal lovers themselves and have received special training for the humane storage and handling of animals shipped as cargo. I worked for five years as a flight attendant, have made long trips with my own cats and am familiar with most U.S. airlines' animal shipping policies and survival records.

While it is true that most animals shipped by air arrive safely, cargo holds are not the same as passenger compartments; their temperature swings can be extreme and they receive less oxygen at altitude. During hot summer months, ground temperatures can be stifling, and a pet trapped in a cargo hold during an air traffic delay can suffer severe stress. Pets can and do die in cargo holds from hyperthermia. Add all the unfamiliar noises and sensations, and it has to be a frightening experience.

My personal rule of thumb is that if I can't take my pet in the cabin with me, she doesn't fly. For my cats, this has meant booking flights on airlines that accept pets whose carriers fit under the seat with sufficient room inside for the animal to turn around. If Samantha were a small dog, she could fly with me, but she's a Lab and she isn't a seeing eye, hearing ear or other type of service dog with public transportation privileges. If we want to take her with us, we drive instead.

Many people dose their pets with tranquilizers before leaving home, but oversedation is the most frequent cause of death in pets being transported by air. Dr. Arthur V. Tennyson of the American Veterinary Medical Association advises veterinarians not to prescribe a tranquilizer or other sedative for animals about to travel by air except in unusual circumstances. Despite their frequent use, very little is known about the effects of sedation on animals enclosed in cages and transported at high altitude. Once aloft in the dark, closed hold, most animals relax on their own, making the sedative superfluous. Tennyson does not recommend any form of sedation — herbal or chemical — for traveling animals. I believe the risk from natural sedatives is minimal, especially herbs like valerian and chamomile, because they do not affect physical coordination, but flower essences can be used with no adverse side effects of any kind. For a review of flower essences helpful to traveling pets, see Chapter 8.

If it is necessary to ship an animal by air, do some research first. What is the most direct flight? Stopovers and transfers are difficult because they lengthen the trip and can expose animals to very hot or cold ground temperatures. Can someone accompany the animal? If you can't go yourself, a friend who can take your cat or small dog in the cabin is the next best thing, but even then things may not go as planned. A friend of my stepdaughter's volunteered to carry her cat from New York to California but when she got to the airport, an airline employee said that the cat's carrier wasn't large enough to allow the cat to turn around; she would have to be placed in a larger container and shipped in the hold as cargo. Had my stepdaughter been there, she would have tried to convince the employee that the cat had plenty of room (which was true), taken a later flight with a new cat carrier or left the cat with whoever was seeing her off, but she was 3,000 miles away. Fortunately, in most cases cabin travel is uneventful for animals and their human ticket holders, but it's a good idea to plan for contingencies.

When pets are shipped as cargo, it helps to have a responsible person on board to remind the flight crew that there's a pet in the hold (it doesn't hurt to send a photo to the cockpit to remind them) and to rescue the animal if there's a long delay between connecting flights, the flight gets cancelled after it leaves the gate, the plane makes an unscheduled landing because of mechanical problems or late arrival causes the travelers to miss their connecting flight.

Is the departure city, connection city or arrival city in the middle of a heat wave, blizzard, hurricane warning or other hazardous weather? These are additional factors to consider as you prepare your pet for travel. So is your pet's health. If the animal displays any symptoms of illness or has a condition like chronic arthritis that limits his mobility and causes discomfort, don't subject him to the stresses of travel.

Pets can and do adapt to travel by car, boat, train, airplane, hot-air balloon and motorcycle, but these trips are always easier if their human companions are present and they aren't subjected to extremes of temperature, deprived of oxygen, confined for long periods, exposed to deafening sounds and badly frightened along the way.

Tumors

Lipomas are benign fatty tumors that feel like firm bumps in or just below the skin. They occur in all animals, including humans. Lipomas are not usually serious, although if they grow large enough to interfere with an animal's motion or breathing, they may require surgical removal. In some cases, fat deposits may become cancerous, although this is unusual.

Lipomas are associated with diets that are high in fat. For example, birds who eat nothing but fatty seeds and cats or dogs who eat a commercial diet that contains rendered animal fat may develop these tumors. As long as the body absorbs excess, indigestible fat, the tumors are likely to grow.

Nutritional Therapy: Switch to a natural diet that emphasizes raw food and supplement the diet with digestive enzymes. Dogs, birds and rabbits can be given fresh fruit, raw vegetables and green herbs and grasses; cats, which are carnivores, need more meat but can be offered fruit and pureed vegetables to which digestive enzymes have been added as well as finely minced wheat grass or other green herbs. If a cat craves a fruit or vegetable, it probably provides something the animal needs.

Blend together 2 tablespoons each olive oil and wheatgerm or flaxseed oil, 10 drops carrot oil and 10 drops evening primrose or borage seed oil. Supplement the diet with 1 teaspoon of this blend per 15 pounds of body weight per day plus a pinch of unrefined sea salt and add this to food with digestive enzymes.

In addition, feed a good-quality multiple vitamin derived from whole food sources, additional vitamin B6 (25 mg per 15 pounds of body weight, such as B6-Niacinamide from Standard Process, Inc.), 1 teaspoon apple cider vinegar tincture of fresh garlic (see page 140) per 15 pounds and a trace mineral supplement.

Herbal Therapy: All of the alterative or blood-cleansing herbs are appropriate. Essiac tea, which is often prescribed by holistic veterinarians as a support therapy for serious illnesses, helps clear benign conditions as well; see page 302. Violet leaves are a traditional treatment for all types of tumors; add a violet leaf infusion or finely minced fresh leaves to food and apply a violet leaf poultice or compress to the tumor.

Hands-on Therapies: Acupuncture and Therapeutic Touch are highly recommended.

Color Therapy: Lemon systemic and indigo on the affected area. Occasional orange tonations may help reduce the size.

See also *Cancer,* **Chapter 11.**

Uremia: See *Kidney Disease*

Urinary Problems

Urinary tract infections, bladder stones, bladder infections, spraying and urinary incontinence are common problems in America's dogs and cats. Like most disorders, they are easier to prevent than to treat, and they are least likely in pets fed a natural diet combined with a healthful lifestyle.

Bladder Infections, Bladder Stones, Feline Urologic Syndrome

The catch-all diagnosis, Feline Urologic Syndrome, or FUS, encompasses inflammations of the bladder and urethra, the formation of bladder stones and blockages of the urethra, especially in males. Similar conditions develop in dogs. Symptoms of bladder infection or inflammation include increased frequency of urination with reduced output, blood in the urine, extreme discomfort with straining, partial or complete blockage of urine or an enlarged and hardened bladder full of accumulated urine.

Stones or gravel in the urine are common in older pets, male and female. Overly alkaline urine causes urinary salts to crystallize into tiny, sharp stones instead of staying in solution. If your pet attempts to urinate and is unable to, stones may be blocking the urethra.

Obviously, serious symptoms require immediate veterinary care, but minor conditions can be treated at home. In addition to using any of the following therapies, protect your pet from exposure to tobacco smoke, which tends to worsen urinary tract problems.

Nutritional Therapy: Many holistic veterinarians have observed a connection between the long-term use of dry commercial pet foods and urinary disorders. To prevent problems or improve minor symptoms, switch your pet to a well-balanced natural diet emphasizing raw foods and appropriate supplements as described in Chapters 2 and 3. This single step may resolve all of your animal's urinary difficulties.

Feed your pet only twice a day and don't leave food out for more than 20 minutes. Too-frequent feeding creates more alkaline urine which is conducive to gravel or stones. If your pet isn't hungry, put his food away and wait 12 hours. In addition, fast your pet one day per week by withholding food and feeding only water. These simple steps will improve digestion, correct the pH of the urinary tract and help restore normal urination.

Ample fluids are essential. Give your pet unlimited access to clean water and encourage him to drink. In countries where withholding water is a common practice to reduce cleanup chores in breeding kennels, bladder and kidney problems are widespread. That's not surprising; it's completely unnatural to keep water from thirsty animals. Add water to the morning meal and place a few grains of unrefined sea salt on your pet's tongue to encourage him to drink. Even in a pet with urinary incontinence, this is an important strategy. Flushing the system well is a first step toward healthy urinary function. Add Willard Water extract to your pet's water for improved nutrient assimilation and to boost his resistance to infection.

If your pet is not already taking vitamins and minerals, start at once. Give a multiple vitamin derived from whole-food sources, colloidal or chelated minerals, a comprehensive trace element supplement and digestive enzymes. In addition, for two or three weeks give 250 mg vitamin C complex per 10 pounds of body weight twice daily or dose to bowel tolerance. Vitamin C improves the acid-alkaline balance and, according to Wendell Belfield and other authorities, prevents and dissolves kidney stones despite the widespread belief that it causes these problems. In fact, the connection between vitamin C deficiencies and urinary tract stone formation has been suggested in the medical literature since 1946. In *How to Have a Healthier Dog*, Belfield described a 10-year-old female terrier whose X-rays showed bladder stones. Because the dog wasn't in distress and because of her age, the owner decided against surgery and instead dosed her with 500 mg vitamin C daily. Six months later, while the dog was being operated on for a uterine condition, the veterinarian examined the bladder and found no sign of stones. Belfield also reported that Dr. Geoff Broderick, known for his successful treatment of cataracts with vitamin A, used 8 grams of ascorbic acid (vitamin C) daily in divided doses on a small-breed dog to dissolve a large bladder stone. The treatment took four months and caused no adverse side effects.

When stones irritate the bladder's lining and cause hemorrhage, the urine contains blood and in some cases pus as well. A bacterial infection may produce bladder inflammation without the presence of stones. Both conditions are called cystitis, and vitamin C helps prevent them. For best results, use a natural vitamin C complex or calcium ascorbate with bioflavonoids and other C-complex constituents from whole-food sources.

Raw, unpasteurized apple cider vinegar is appropriate for all urinary tract infections; add it directly to food or put small amounts in your pet's drinking water. If your dog or cat dislikes the taste but will take pills, use an eyedropper to fill an empty two-part gelatin capsule with cider vinegar and immediately give it to your pet. However you administer cider vinegar, start with small amounts and build up to 1 teaspoon per 10 pounds of body weight daily. Cider vinegar can be used to make tinctures for pets; although vinegar does not dissolve all the constituents that alcohol does, it makes most of a plant's medicinal components easy to assimilate. Pour cider vinegar over any of the herbs recommended for urinary tract problems, let the jar stand for a few weeks and use the resulting tincture to dose your pet with beneficial herbs and cider vinegar at the same time.

When a bacterial infection causes cystitis, cranberry juice can be part of the cure. This folk treatment used to be discounted by physicians, but research has shown that cranberry juice prevents bacteria from adhering to bladder walls. In recent years, cranberry juice capsules have become popular supplements. Capsules are much easier to administer to pets than full-strength, unsweetened cranberry juice, but cranberry juice or cranberry juice concentrate can be added to drinking water or food in small amounts. Birds, on the other hand, may enjoy whole cranberries. Add them to your bird's food whenever they're in season. Shop for organically grown cranberries for your bird, make a cider vinegar tincture of cranberries for any pet or look for organically produced cranberry juice concentrate in bottles or capsules. Most cranberry bogs, the swampy areas in which the plants are grown, are heavily dosed with pesticides and other chemicals.

Cod liver oil serves two purposes in keeping the urinary tract healthy. It is a rich source of vitamins A and D, and it provides internal lubrication. Check the label and give enough cod liver oil to provide 2,500 IU vitamin A per 15 pounds of body weight daily for several weeks.

Provide a good quality vitamin B-complex supplement derived from whole food sources and adapt its label directions for your pet's weight. Brewer's yeast and nutritional yeast are rich sources of B vitamins.

In addition to using a comprehensive mineral and trace element supplement, give your dog or cat plenty of soft raw bones for their calcium and magnesium. Low calcium diets used to be recommended for patients with kidney stones, but this actually makes the problem worse. Magnesium helps prevent the reformation of stones. Bones supply calcium, magnesium and other minerals in ideal proportions and in a form that is easy for dogs and cats to assimilate. If your pet is unable to digest bones, give him small quantities until his digestion improves and temporarily give a supplement containing calcium and magnesium, for both minerals are necessary for either to work well. If supplementation is necessary, use calcium lactate from Standard Process. Bruce West, M.D., who has extensive experience with nutritional therapies, recommends this product as the most easily digested and utilized calcium/magnesium supplement and explains that its ratio of calcium to magnesium (5:1 instead of the more commonly prescribed 2:1) "has proven time and again to be correct."

A nutrition-based veterinary protocol for urinary tract infections combines three Standard Process products, Congaplex, Arginex and Cal-Amo, all of which are derived from organically raised whole-food sources. Give 1 tablet of each to cats, 3 each to small dogs and 3 to 6 each for medium and large dogs. Arginex contains arginase, a urea-metabolizing enzyme, Cal-Amo contains acid forming chloride salts and Congaplex is a food concentrate from vegetable and animal sources. For information about Standard Process products, see the resources for Chapter 3.

Herbal Therapy: There are many herbs for the urinary tract. Parsley, cleavers, buchu, dandelion, nettles, cornsilk and horsetail are all diuretic and tonic; that is, they stimulate the flow of urine and have a healing effect on the urinary system. Any of these herbs can be added to food as fresh, chopped plants, dried powders, teas or tinctures. Uva ursi is often called a diuretic herb but it is really a urinary disinfectant and a specific for cystitis. Uva ursi is most effective as a tincture or extract. Uva ursi tea, best brewed as a decoction because the leaves are so tough, is very bitter and astringent. The dry herb is difficult for animals to digest.

One way to use these herbs for the urinary tract is to combine three or four in a powder or tincture for daily use in food. Use the blend for three to five weeks, then switch to another combination for three to five weeks. Another method is to vary the herbs every day. Parsley and dandelion are well tolerated and so helpful that many herbalists give them to their pets daily, freshly chopped in spring and summer, dried or in tinctures in winter.

The herbal dosage chart on page 136 can be used as a general guideline for the total amount of urinary tonic herbs to give your pet daily.

Any bacterial infection can be treated with the herbal immunizations described on pages 285-286.

Hands-on Therapies: Therapeutic Touch, acupuncture and acupressure are highly recommended for urinary tract infections, while veterinary chiropractic is not.

Homeopathy: Because accurate prescribing is essential in the treatment of chronic conditions, observe your pet carefully and write down all his symptoms and behaviors before consulting a veterinary homeopath in person or by phone.

Color Therapy: For difficult urination and possible obstruction, give a green systemic back and scarlet on the lower back. For cystitis or blood in the urine from bladder inflammation or infection, give a green systemic front and indigo on the lower abdomen.

Urinary Incontinence, Spraying

Spraying is common in intact male cats because that's how they mark their territory. The older a cat is when neutered, the more likely he is to continue spraying, although neutering reduces this behavior in most cases. In cats neutered in adolescence, spraying is unusual but sometimes coincides with a move, the arrival of a new pet or person to the household or other stressful conditions. Cats sometimes spray or urinate outside the cat box when the litter is not regularly changed or cleaned.

Don't assume that spraying or urinating away from the cat litter box is a behavioral problem; it may be medical. If the cat box is scrupulously clean and you have a box for each cat in the household so overcrowding isn't a problem, have your veterinarian check the animal for a bladder, kidney or urinary tract problem.

Stress incontinence (urinating in moments of fear or excitement) and sleep incontinence (loss of bladder control when unconscious) are common in dogs. Urination is a sign of submission, which is why submissive males and females urinate when someone or something frightens them. Dog owners who yell at or punish their pets for having accidents in the house can be the unwitting cause of these mishaps. If your dog is still being housebroken and you respond to his or her submissive urination with anger, ask a good trainer for help before you make things worse.

Pets who are easily frightened and urinate under stress can be helped with calming herbs such as valerian, hops, chamomile, oatstraw and other nervines. Flower essences, as described in Chapter 8, treat emotional issues and can help your animal cope with stress, as can massage, Therapeutic Touch and physical manipulations described in Chapter 7.

Stress or sleep incontinence in spayed bitches is often diagnosed as a symptom of doggie menopause and treated with synthetic hormones. In addition to feeding your dog a natural diet, consider the hormone-balancing herbs described on pages 434-436 as an alternative therapy. The Standard Process supplement Vasculin is recommended for muscle and nervous system support in dogs and cats with sleep incontinence; give 1 tablet per 7 to 10 pounds of body weight, up to 9 daily for large dogs.

Even though a well-watered dog urinates more, withholding water does not cure urinary incontinence. Diuretic herbs and increased fluids are helpful to human patients with this problem because they tone and nourish the urinary tract, and this approach works just as well in animals. Give your pet large quantities of water with diuretic herbs as described above from morning through early afternoon, give her active physical exercise, take her for frequent walks and arrange for someone to take her out during the day when you aren't home, walk her where she can urinate in comfortable surroundings, give her a late walk just before bed and be patient.

Homeopathy: There are several remedies that help spraying cats, dogs with submissive urination problems and incontinent animals. Consult a veterinary homeopath for correct diagnosis and treatment.

Flower Essences: Flower essences are most helpful in the treatment of urinary problems that may have an emotional foundation, such as spraying or stress incontinence. Study Chapter 8 or consult a flower essence practitioner.

Color Therapy: For urinary incontinence due to sphincter weakness, give a lemon systemic front and orange and green on the groin area.

Hands-on Therapies: Therapeutic Touch can help any pet with any problem. Acupuncture can be used to treat most urinary problems, and all massage therapies help soothe stressed animals.

Related Conditions: Advanced Lyme disease can cause loss of bladder control; see page 393. Older intact males who have trouble urinating may have an enlarged prostate; see page 420.

Viral Infections

Viruses are minute particles that reproduce within living cells. Too small to see under a light microscope and too small to be trapped by filters, they infect plants, animals and microorganisms. In people, viruses cause the common cold, influenza, measles, mumps, chickenpox, herpes, poliomyelitis, rabies and other diseases. In dogs and cats, the list includes distemper, chorea, feline panleukopenia, feline immunodeficiency virus (FIV), feline infectious peritonitis (FIP), feline leukemia (FeLV), feline viral rhinotracheitis (FVR), influenza, kennel cough, parvovirus and rabies. Viruses also infect birds and rabbits.

Whenever you know your pet has been exposed to a contagious virus, take preventive measures by dosing him with extra vitamin C and antibiotic herbs as described on pages 285-286. Viruses have an incubation period, during which you can help your pet resist infection. Whenever your pet is exposed to a virus, take preventive measures for a week to 10 days, avoid overtiring your pet or subjecting her to unnecessary stress and be ready to consult your veterinarian if symptoms develop.

Distemper

The canine distemper virus is as widespread among dogs as the common cold virus is among humans. Both are airborne germs that land just about everywhere. Although dogs are exposed to it all the time, few develop the illness, for viruses need the right conditions and a good host in order to multiply and cause illness. There is much to be gained by keeping your pet's resistance strong with a natural diet and lifestyle. Dogs who contract canine distemper have a brief fever and lethargy six to nine days after exposure, then appear normal for up to a week, after which they are suddenly ill with a hot, dry nose, fetid breath, fever, shivering, lethargy, loss of appetite, severe eye inflammation with a thick, sticky discharge from the eyes and nose, malodorous diarrhea, lung congestion and skin eruptions on the abdomen or groin area. Distemper used to be called "the husk" because of the persistent dry cough it often produces. Most animals become listless and seek a dark, quiet place in which to rest undisturbed.

Because distemper is caused by a virus, antibiotics are ineffective in its treatment. So, according to Richard Pitcairn, is the administration of fluids and other drugs; in fact, as he observed in *Natural Health for Dogs and Cats,* conventional treatment may increase the likelihood of encephalitis, a severe inflammation of the brain or portions of the spinal cord that often develops after apparent improvement or recovery. Dogs are usually euthanized at that point because conventional treatment is almost always ineffective. Like other holistic veterinarians, Pitcairn has witnessed many successful recoveries in distemper cases treated with homeopathy and nutrition.

Juliette de Bairacli Levy, whose herbal therapies have saved the lives of animals around the world, considers distemper "easy to treat, speedy to cure and devoid of any aftereffects or complications." The first English edition of her herbal handbook for dogs, published in 1955, included 50 reports from breeders who used her distemper cure. The 1992 edition of *The Complete Herbal Handbook for the Dog and Cat* has room for only four, but she has received hundreds more. For a lengthy and detailed description of the herbal treatment of distemper as well as other canine and feline diseases, add her books to your collection.

Remember that dogs fed a well-balanced raw diet and who live a healthful lifestyle with plenty of exercise and exposure to unfiltered natural light are less likely to become seriously ill with canine distemper than other dogs who have the disease.

Whenever your pet is ill, keep him in a comfortable warm, quiet place isolated from other animals and with an ample supply of clean water and some exposure to fresh air.

Nutritional Therapy: Fasting is an important first step in the natural treatment of the acute phase of any viral infection. Check your healthy pet with a rectal thermometer from time to time so you know her normal resting body temperature and take her temperature twice a day, morning and evening, whenever she shows signs of illness. Fast your pet as soon as you notice a fever a degree or more above normal; withhold food and give her plenty of clean water containing Willard Water extract and a pinch of unrefined sea salt to help compensate for the loss of important minerals. To help prevent dehydration, offer her water several times a day or squirt water into her mouth. From time to time place a tiny pinch of unrefined sea salt in her mouth.

In 1967, a veterinary journal published Wendell Belfield's protocol for canine distemper, 0.5 grams of intravenous vitamin C per pound of body weight twice daily, and his paper inspired other veterinarians to use this simple therapy with remarkable success. Its main disadvantage is that it requires hospitalization, but veterinarians experimenting with oral vitamin C found that frequent doses work well and can be given by the animal's owner at home. Whenever your pet develops a fever, withhold food and dose her with 250 mg of vitamin C per 15 pounds of body weight every two hours during the day, then let her rest undisturbed through the night. Continue this regimen until after her temperature returns to normal. Well-nourished adult dogs can fast for as long as a week, though most recover in just a few days. If symptoms recur, repeat the treatment. If you have any questions about your pet's condition or your ability to treat her effectively at home, consult a holistic veterinarian.

Herbal Therapy: At the same time that you are fasting your pet and administering vitamin C, use any of the herbal immunizations described on pages 285-286. Grapefruit seed extract, echinacea, noni and other antibiotic herbs can be given to your pet in capsules, by squirting tinctures diluted with water into her mouth with an eye dropper or needle-free syringe or by mixing powdered herbs, tinctures, crushed tablets or the contents of capsules with honey and shaping it into small balls. The honey can be refrigerated to make it easier to handle, or let your pet lick it off a spoon. Raw, unpasteurized, unfiltered honey is the one food that's appropriate during fasting; because it is predigested, it makes no demands on the animal's digestive system and is a source of energy, enzymes and other nutrients. *Note:* Do not give a fasting animal any herb or supplement whose label says it must be taken with meals.

After the animal's temperature returns to normal, begin feeding small quantities of soft or liquid foods warmed to room or body temperature, such as slippery elm bark or oats blended with freshly made yogurt, kefir, raw goat's or cow's milk, vegetable broth containing digestive enzymes or small amounts of raw meat mixed with water. Add a pinch of unrefined sea salt to every serving to help restore minerals lost from diarrhea. As your pet's appetite and energy return, resume normal feeding. Continue supplementing with vitamin C and disinfecting herbs for a few days after the fever breaks and give large doses of acidophilus and probiotic supplements for several days to help restore normal intestinal bacteria.

Aromatherapy: Disinfecting or antibiotic essential oils can be given to pets whenever they are exposed to or develop an active infection. See the natural immunizations on pages 285-286.

Homeopathy: Carefully observe your pet's symptoms and consult a veterinary homeopath by phone or in person.

Hands-on Therapies: Therapeutic Touch is appropriate for any illness or infection. Acupuncture boosts the immune system and helps an animal resist infection. All of the physical therapies described in Chapter 7 help a healthy animal stay that way.

Color Therapy: Treat any unexplained fever with a green and blue systemic front followed by magenta on the upper chest and lower back or, if the fever is high, use purple on these areas. If the fever persists, give a yellow systemic front and continue as above.

Hard Pad, Brain Distemper (Canine Encephalitis)

Far more common in Europe than in North or South America, hard pad is believed to be caused by a virus and is usually linked with canine distemper; some, including de Bairacli Levy, consider it a form of distemper. Diarrhea, a watery discharge from the nose and eyes, fever, hot inner ears and discharge from the ears are common symptoms, followed much later by a leathery thickening of the foot pads and in some cases the nostrils. This last stage is usually accompanied by obvious symptoms of encephalitis, which is an inflammation of the brain and spinal cord that produces staggering, constant whimpering and unpredictable, irrational behavior.

The same therapies apply as for canine distemper. De Bairacli Levy describes additional treatments in her *Complete Herbal Handbook for the Dog and Cat*, emphasizing garlic, green herbs and, for brain conditions, skullcap.

Feline Panleukopenia (Feline Distemper, Infectious Enteritis)

Like canine distemper, this highly contagious feline virus strikes quickly. Believed to be spread by body fluids, feline panleukopenia is a leading cause of death in young kittens, killing them within 24 to 48 hours. It destroys the white blood cells that protect the body from infection, leaving it vulnerable to secondary infections that produce alarming symptoms about a week after exposure to the virus. Symptoms include a very high fever, severe depression, dehydration, extreme thirst and, in most cases, vomiting.

Recognizing feline distemper in its earliest stages is essential. Call your veterinarian immediately because this illness works fast. As soon as you realize your cat has a fever, withhold food, give him plenty of water and dose him with vitamin C, grapefruit seed extract, echinacea tincture and/or whatever infection-fighting herbs you have on hand. Review the herbal immunizations on pages 285-286 and give small amounts every 10 to 15 minutes, which may reduce your pet's likelihood of vomiting everything he swallows.

Richard Pitcairn describes two homeopathic treatments for emergency use. If the cat is weak, depressed, cold, has diarrhea and vomits after drinking water, give *Veratrum album 6c* every 4 hours for 24 hours or until symptoms improve. If the cat is limp, extremely lethargic and apathetic, craves cold water and vomits 10 to 20 minutes after drinking, give *Phosphorus 6c* every 4 hours for 24 hours or until symptoms improve. If the cat is already very ill and close to death, lying comatose and hardly moving with cold-feeling ears and feet and a bluish nose, administer camphor by holding a small dab or open container of Tiger Balm, Vicks Vaporub or a similar ointment under the cat's nose for a few breaths. Repeat this every 15 minutes until the cat responds, then apply other therapies. As Pitcairn reminds his readers, discontinue the camphor and remove it from the room before treating with homeopathy.

All of the support therapies described for canine distemper are appropriate, but feline distemper is a serious condition that should be treated by a veterinarian if at all possible.

Feline Immunodeficiency Virus (FIV)

Called Feline AIDS because of its resemblance to acquired immunodeficiency syndrome in people and linked to a retrovirus similar to the human AIDS virus, FIV, which was discovered in 1986, depresses the immune system and leaves the body vulnerable to opportunistic infections. It is believed to be transferred only through bite wounds, not from casual or close physical contact, making it most common in intact tom cats who are free to wander.

Like human AIDS patients, cats with FIV have a bewildering assortment of symptoms and conditions, most of which are normally short-lived, minor illnesses but which, because of the animals' impaired immune system, are now major, chronic and life-threatening.

Prevention is the key to dealing with FIV. Cats fed a well-balanced raw diet with appropriate supplements are usually not affected even when exposed. Although conventional veterinarians believe that frequent vaccination improves immunity and offers protection, holistic veterinarians claim the opposite, warning that annual revaccinations weaken the immune system and make a cat more susceptible. Vaccines are not the only substances your cat should avoid, they say; guard against exposure to pesticides, heavy metals, environmental pollutants and other toxins, including flea dips, tick sprays and chemical flea collars.

There is no simple treatment for a cat weakened by the feline immunodeficiency virus. Consult a holistic veterinarian if your cat has this condition.

Feline Infectious Peritonitis (FIP)

First diagnosed in 1963, FIP is a deadly virus that kills most of the cats that develop its symptoms. It is a disease of youth, for an estimated 90 percent of its victims are less than three years old. There are two serious forms, wet and dry FIP, and a less serious third type. In wet FIP, the cat accumulates fluid and develops a distended chest or belly, loses his appetite, develops a fever and loses weight. Breathing becomes labored as fluid collects in the chest cavity and lying down becomes uncomfortable. Dry FIP is more difficult to recognize; various organs such as the lymph nodes, kidneys, spleen, liver, eyes and central nervous system can be attacked, destroying tissue and leading to death. Weight loss, fever, lethargy and the malfunction of affected organs are the most noticeable symptoms. Anemia, diarrhea and vomiting can accompany either wet or dry FIP. The third type, a subclinical FIP, manifests as a mild upper respiratory infection.

FIP is highly contagious and affects male and female cats of every breed. Caused by a caronavirus, FIP may infect cats through the mouth or respiratory tract or it may be carried by fleas and other parasites. Pregnant cats may spread the virus to their offspring.

Holistic veterinarians have long suspected a link between FIP and the feline leukemia vaccine, for many of their FIP patients were vaccinated a few weeks before developing symptoms. One theory is that affected cats were already carrying the FIP virus and the vaccine's temporary suppression of their immune systems gave the virus an opportunity to develop. Another is that the two viruses are directly related, one being a mutant strain of the other.

FIP is difficult to control because cats are infectious before symptoms develop, not after. Other cats in the household will not be helped by the infected cat's isolation, for a visibly sick cat no longer sheds the virus. Because the virus can survive for nearly a month on floors, water bowls and other surfaces, disinfecting these areas helps prevent the spread of viruses the cat shed when the illness first developed.

Holistic veterinarians warn against treating FIP with antibiotics or cortisone drugs, for these ineffective therapies only weaken the animal. Nutrition, homeopathy, herbs and other natural methods may or may not eliminate the virus but, if used in time, they often restore sick cats to their normal appearance and behavior. Provide a natural diet, give the animal extra vitamin C and disinfecting herbs and treat whatever symptoms develop. Cats with FIP may have a fever, cold symptoms or intestinal distress and vomiting, all of which can be addressed with natural methods.

According to Wendell Belfield, it can take up to two years to eliminate FIP from a contaminated cattery or multi-cat household. By eating an improved diet and taking large doses of vitamin C and other supplements, cats can develop a resistance to the virus. New cats entering a household or cattery should be isolated and put on a vitamin program for 60 days before being introduced to other residents. Belfield recommends maintaining cats on a good supplement program and checking their gums frequently; pale gums are a sign that the animal may have FIP, the feline leukemia virus or both.

The most advanced stage of this illness is the accumulation of fluid in the chest and abdomen, a condition which is usually fatal. Richard Pitcairn recommends two homeopathic remedies for cats with advanced FIP, *Arsenicum album 6c* if the animal is anxious, chilly, thirsty and restless or *Mercurius sulphuricus 6c* if it has extreme difficulty breathing and has to sit up because of fluid in the chest. Give either remedy once a day for four weeks. If the animal gets better, maintain this treatment as long as improvement continues.

After Wendell Belfield successfully treated two cats with advanced FIP by removing their enlarged spleens and giving them intravenous vitamin C, other veterinarians did the same and their patients recovered. There is always hope for FIP patients, but this is definitely an illness worth preventing.

Feline Leukemia (FeLV)

Caused by a retrovirus similar to those that cause AIDS in people and FIP in cats, feline leukemia is spread through body fluids from one cat to another, usually by way of bites, grooming and shared water or food bowls. Mother cats can infect their young during pregnancy or nursing.

Juliette de Bairacli Levy reports that although this disease is unknown in the wild, it is found in caged felines in zoos around the world. An estimated 70 percent of America's cats have been exposed to FeLV, and only a few develop symptoms. In those who become ill, however, feline leukemia is a very serious and contagious illness. Most common in multi-cat households in cities or urban areas, feline leukemia used to be considered untreatable and incurable, and animals testing positive for the virus were routinely euthanized. Feline leukemia is a serious illness with a long list of possible symptoms, but it is neither incurable nor untreatable.

The most common symptoms of feline leukemia are weight loss, lassitude, colorless gums and the faded, tired look of anemia. In addition, cats with FeLV often have a fever, dehydration, immune suppression, bleeding disorders, kidney inflammation and deterioration, arthritis, open sores at body orifices, inflammatory bowel disease or persistent bladder infections. Some cats develop skin growths, cartilage deposits, skin disorders, paralysis, urinary incontinence, pupils of unequal size, spontaneous abortions, stillbirths, kittens that fail to thrive despite the best of care and tumors or cancer.

The same nutritional therapy that successfully prevents other viruses helps a cat resist FeLV infection; feed your cat a natural diet with large amounts of vitamin C and infection-fighting herbs such as those described for herbal immunization on pages 285-286. As described on page 297, vitamin C alone has cleared many cats of the FeLV virus.

Wendell Belfield has written that the anemia associated with feline leukemia may be induced or exacerbated by exposure to lead and that a buildup of lead in the body predisposes a cat to FeLV infection. Cats are exposed to lead from paint, plumbing, food cans and other sources. Vitamins C and E, zinc, calcium, iron, magnesium, kelp and other seaweeds, wheat grass and other green plants help prevent the absorption of lead and are inexpensive insurance against this heavy metal.

All of the support therapies described for canine distemper at the beginning of this section are appropriate.

Influenza

Do animals get the flu? Influenza viruses affect animals around the world. Most are unique to a species, such as influenza that affects only birds or camels, but flu viruses can mutate and move from one species to another. Much of today's virology research focuses on the farming practices of Southeast Asia, where viruses that wouldn't otherwise spread from birds to people do so by way of the pigs that share fish ponds with ducks. New strains of influenza develop in these ideal conditions and spread from Southeast Asia to the rest of the world.

The symptoms of influenza in dogs are the same as for people, with upper respiratory distress, vomiting, diarrhea, body aches, fever, apathy and a loss of appetite. It is widely assumed that dogs can't catch human diseases, but Wendell Belfield has noticed that whenever there is an outbreak of flu among humans, some dogs from infected families catch the flu themselves.

Flu outbreaks sometimes happen when many dogs are brought together for field trials, dog shows and other events. Well-fed dogs taking vitamin and mineral supplements show a strong resistance to this type of infection, and any dog that succumbs to the flu can be treated with the natural immunizations described on pages 285-286.

Kennel Cough (Canine Infectious Tracheobronchitis)

Like the flu or the common cold in humans, kennel cough is caused by not one but several viruses and it is often complicated by bacterial infections. Dogs in animal shelters, boarding and breeding kennels, dog shows, pet stores and grooming salons are at risk because the virus spreads rapidly, especially among young dogs under stress and in close physical contact.

Symptoms appear a week to 10 days after exposure and the primary symptom is the dry, hacking, gagging cough for which the illness is named. Some dogs have a watery discharge from the eyes and nose; others lose their interest in food. Kennel cough is not usually serious, again resembling the common cold in humans, but in weak or susceptible animals it can lead to more serious complications. Keep your dog on a well-balanced, natural, raw diet with appropriate supplements to keep his resistance high.

If your dog is exposed to kennel cough, use any of the natural immunizations described on pages 285-286 to prevent infection.

Nutritional Therapy: If your dog shows kennel cough symptoms, fast her for one to three days while administering 500 mg vitamin C per 10 pounds of body weight. In addition to water, honey and infection-fighting herbs, give her 1/4 teaspoon cod liver oil per 15 pounds of body weight once a day, 1/2 to 1 cup of freshly made carrot juice twice a day and the contents of a punctured 50 or 100 IU vitamin E complex capsule or an equivalent tablet three times a day. After a one- to three-day fast, introduce solid foods slowly and continue the vitamin therapy for five to seven days.

Herbal Therapy: Use any of the herbal immunizations described on pages 285-286 to prevent or treat kennel cough. To reduce the presence of air-borne viruses and bacteria, spray the air around infected dogs with dilute grapefruit seed extract or other disinfectants. This is an appropriate treatment for dogs who have been exposed to kennel cough as well.

If your dog is fasting, combine the herbs with honey; otherwise, combine them with food. Honey by itself is soothing to the throat, as are peppermint, licorice root, sage, pine needles and mullein. Brew any of these as a strong tea, combine herbal tea or tinctures with honey or use an herbal cough syrup made with wild cherry bark, horehound, licorice root, comfrey root, mullein, coltsfoot, slippery elm bark or peppermint.

Aromatherapy: Mix 1 drop each eucalyptus and lemon essential oils or 1 drop each eucalyptus and thyme essential oils with 1 tablespoon honey. Add 1 tablespoon warm water, mix well and give by the teaspoon to help soothe your dog's throat. Repeat as needed throughout the day. Check the essential oils chart on page 174 to determine the maximum daily dosage for your dog's weight.

Additional Therapies: All of the support therapies described for canine distemper are appropriate.

Related Conditions: Bronchitis can be brought on by cold weather or sudden drops in temperature. The same therapies are appropriate.

See also *Coughs.*

Parvovirus

Named for its tiny size (parvo means small), the parvovirus belongs to a strain of viruses that infect cattle, pigs, rodents and cats. Prior to 1980, parvovirus was unknown in dogs, but in that year it began making headlines around the world for quickly killing thousands of dogs wherever it spread.

Throughout the 1980s, Juliette de Bairacli Levy received reports from followers of her Natural Rearing (NR) philosophy documenting the virus's spread through Australia, New Zealand, Europe and North America. Even when canine parvovirus rates were at their peak, NR dogs were unaffected, demonstrating the strong resistance of unvaccinated animals on a natural, raw diet, given ample daily exercise and protected by medicinal herbs. De Bairacli Levy agrees with those who theorize that parvovirus is a mutation of the canine distemper virus by way of the ailment known as hard pad. Whatever its history, parvovirus is difficult to eradicate from infected surfaces, which can be literally anything an infected dog has touched or breathed on.

One type of parvovirus affects the heart and is especially dangerous to puppies six to nine weeks old. Affected pups huddle away from the light, breathe painfully, suffer intestinal cramps, collapse and usually die. The other type is a severe intestinal disorder that produces deep exhaustion, vomiting so violent that it ruptures internal blood vessels, rampant and malodorous diarrhea or a fever of 104° F. or higher. Dogs with parvo typically sit by their water bowls but are unwilling to drink; they become severely dehydrated and emaciated, and their sunken eyes seem unable to focus.

When dogs or puppies recover from parvovirus on their own, which many do, their recovery is dramatic and rapid. These animals avoid food and water and sleep in a dark corner for a day or two, then their thirst and appetite return, their diarrhea disappears and their mouths smell clean.

Nutritional Therapy: The best way to protect infant puppies from parvovirus is to maintain their mother's perfect health, beginning before her puppies are conceived, with the best natural foods and a natural lifestyle. Antibodies in her milk protect her puppies, and any antiseptic herbs she is fed pass through to them as well. During weaning and the transition to their new homes, pups can be fed freshly made yogurt or kefir, acidophilus supplements and bovine colostrum, which, although not the same as mother's milk, is a partial substitute. Small amounts of bee propolis, vitamin C and antiseptic herbs can help puppies resist not only parvovirus but every other type of infection during this time of stress.

A well-balanced, raw natural diet with appropriate supplements, active exercise, exposure to natural light and a safe, stable environment is your best insurance against parvovirus for dogs of all ages. Parvovirus is more difficult to treat than to prevent, especially in dogs fed commercial pet foods and weakened by multiple vaccinations.

If parvo infects your puppy or dog, your veterinarian can help with intravenous vitamin C. Wendell Belfield wrote that when his first parvovirus case appeared in 1980, his usual dose of 0.5 gram of intravenous sodium ascorbate per pound of body weight was ineffective. He gave the dog two grams per pound and the year-old spitz recovered. He used the same therapy on the next dozen cases, along with fluids and medication to offset the animals' vomiting, diarrhea and dehydration. After 48 hours, during which the dogs began to recover, they received a multimineral tablet and protein concentrate in addition to vitamin C. All of his patients went home within five days.

It is difficult to administer large doses of vitamin C at home, but you can give the animal as much liquid vitamin C as she will swallow from an eyedropper or needle-free syringe in addition to infection-fighting herbs and honey.

To combat dehydration, brew a strong tea of sage leaves and barley or oats; pour 1 cup boiling water over 1 tablespoon dried sage or 3 tablespoons fresh sage and 1 tablespoon barley or oats, let stand until cool and strain. To 1 tablespoon tea add 1 teaspoon raw honey, 1 teaspoon glucose or sugar, 1/8 teaspoon unrefined sea salt, 5 drops of grapefruit seed extract and 500 mg of liquid or powdered vitamin C complex. Give this combination to the puppy every two to three hours.

As Richard Pitcairn instructs, dehydration can also be prevented with an enema; simply give the same mixture through the other end. Warm the liquid to body temperature (test it on your wrist to be sure it isn't too hot), raise the animal's hindquarters and, using a simple bulb syringe or an infant's enema, slowly inject the liquid. Wait a few minutes before lowering the body so that the liquid is retained and absorbed.

Additional Therapies: All of the support therapies described for canine distemper are appropriate.

Warts

Warts are small benign (not cancerous) growths that protrude from the skin. According to many holistic veterinarians, they are most common in dogs and older animals who are fed a commercial diet and receive frequent vaccinations. In fact, homeopaths consider warts an expression of vaccinosis. While warts are not usually dangerous or life-threatening, they can bleed when scratched or injured and they usually reflect an underlying state of less-than-optimum health.

Nutritional Therapy: Warts often clear after an animal's diet is improved. Feed fresh, raw foods with appropriate supplements for your pet's size and species.

Herbal Therapy: There are almost as many folk cures for warts as there are herbs. The juice of fresh dandelion, milkweed, greater celandine and other herbs with a juicy sap have long been used for this purpose, as has the milky juice of unripe papaya fruits. Dab a small amount of fresh juice onto the wart three times daily and let it dry. In addition, add finely minced raw dandelion greens, fresh or powdered horsetail, any tea or tincture made with alterative (blood cleansing) or adaptogen (balancing) herbs and powdered kelp or other seaweeds to your pet's food.

Supplement your pet's food with multiple vitamins and minerals. In addition, apply vitamin E from a punctured capsule and/or castor oil to the wart three times daily.

Homeopathy: The first remedy most veterinary homeopaths recommend for warts is *Thuja 30c*. Give a single treatment and wait one month. At that time, if the wart has improved or begun to disappear, no further homeopathic treatment is necessary. If it has not improved, Richard Pitcairn recommends a single dose of *Causticum 30c*, a mineral remedy, for warts that tend to bleed easily or *Silica 30c* for very large warts, especially those over old vaccination sites.

Aromatherapy: Apply a drop of full-strength lavender oil to the wart once or twice daily, dilute the essential oil of lemon or cypress with an equal amount of carrier oil or apple cider vinegar and apply it twice daily or combine 2 parts lemon oil with 1 part cypress oil and mix with 4 parts cider vinegar for application twice or three times daily.

Hands-on Therapies: Therapeutic Touch alone may clear warts, and acupuncture stimulates the body's cleansing mechanisms. Consult with a veterinary chiropractor or myotherapist before using those therapies.

Weight Control

Overfed, underexercised, overweight dogs and cats are everywhere in America. Obesity is a serious problem, for it reduces an animal's mobility, worsens other illnesses and shortens the lifespan.

Nutritional Therapy: Correctly fed and exercised animals aren't overweight, they don't break into cupboards or garbage cans stealing whatever they can find and they aren't obsessed about food. The first step in helping your pet lose weight and get into shape is changing him over to a well-balanced, natural diet with appropriate supplements. Give your dog or cat raw, meaty bones to chew on; they'll keep him busy, provide essential nutrients and satisfy his craving for large portions. Study Chapter 2 for menu planning guidelines. Give birds and rabbits fresh, whole foods as well.

Exercise: Feeding the right food is only half of the solution. The other half is increasing your pet's exercise and her exposure to natural light. If your dog enjoys the company of other dogs, find a place where she can romp and play with like-minded canines. Make exercise fun and interesting; don't take the same monotonous walk every day. Your dog might enjoy agility training, scent tracking, field work or simply running off-lead in a safe yard or pasture. Walk your dog in different terrains, up and down hills, with many changes of pace and scenery.

Take your underexercised cat or rabbit outside whenever you can, either in a safe, fenced garden or on a leash attached to his harness. Nature is an exciting, fascinating place to be. Let your indoor pet explore the outdoors whenever possible.

Increase your pet's exposure to natural light, for malillumination contributes to obesity and lethargy.

Play with your dog, cat, bird or rabbit every day and make your play time an exercise hour. Use whatever toys your pet enjoys to encourage him to run, jump or stretch his wings.

As with any exercise program, start slowly. If your pet is middle-aged, elderly or not in the best of health, consult your veterinarian before doing anything strenuous. If you usually walk your dog around the block, start extending your trip while you watch for signs of overexertion. Use common sense. If your pooch tires easily, let her rest; if the weather is hot, go in the morning or evening and take water along to keep her cool. Every day you can go a little farther until you are both enjoying a good workout.

The worst way to exercise your dog is to take her on long weekend hikes or runs with no preparation. Give her daily workouts that lead up to long outings; it takes time for a dog to build up muscle tone, endurance and stamina. Don't limit her exercise to monotonous, flat surfaces like sidewalks, paved roads or athletic field tracks. And if your dog begins to limp or shows any sign of muscle strain or injury, don't insist that she continue. Injuries, however minor, should be attended to at once. See pages 233-237.

Underweight Pets

Chronically underweight pets may have a condition that requires medical attention; consult your veterinarian.

See also *Appetite, Loss of.*

Worms: See *Parasites*

Zoonosis

Zoonosis refers to any illness (zoonotic infection) that can be transferred from an animal to people. Rabies, ringworm, parrot fever and toxoplasmosis are some of the most common zoonotic diseases, and parasite infestations are often included in the definition because fleas and worms can be transferred from pets to people.

Zoonotic diseases are uncommon in households where dogs, cats, rabbits, birds and other pets are fed a natural, raw diet, exposed to unfiltered natural light and exercised daily. The humans most at risk from zoonotic disorders are those in poor health, the elderly and the very young. Common-sense precautions are always appropriate: maintain your pets' good health, keep a clean house, supervise small children when they play with animals, educate yourself about the risks of zoonotic diseases and use the methods described throughout this book to prevent and treat infectious illnesses. ✒

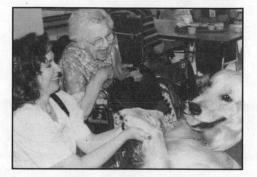

Volunteering
with
Your Pet

WHENEVER THEY ENTER a nursing home or hospital, heads lift, faces smile and hands reach out. The pets are here! Long banned from healthcare facilities, dogs, cats, birds, rabbits and other pets are being welcomed with open arms, and for good reason. Science has shown that visits from pets enhance and enrich lives everywhere, but for those deprived of pet contact, the opportunity to scratch a furry ear can have stirring consequences, as when unresponsive nursing home residents speak or laugh for the first time in months or when people with Alzheimer's disease reminisce in detail about pets they used to have. Even brief contact with a caring animal has been shown to lower blood pressure, cheer the depressed and motivate the apathetic.

Nursing homes with resident dogs have lower death, infection and staff turnover rates than those without. In recovering heart attack patients, the most significant difference between those who survive and those who die is pet ownership. Elderly pet owners experience less psychological distress, fewer doctor visits and less depression than those without pets. The beneficial effects of pets, well documented in professional journals, outweigh other factors, such as marital status, family relationships, religion, community activity, exercise and diet. Even at their most disabled, people respond in measurable, positive ways to the presence of animals.

Thanks to the efforts of national and local organizations, volunteers are able to receive training, screening and liability insurance that make their visits safe as well as fun. Dogs and other pets are tested for friendly personality, calm temperament, good disposition, polite manners and handler control. Pets must be well groomed and in excellent health. Their owners learn how to approach and interact with people whose health is fragile and who may have difficulty hearing, seeing or reaching the animals.

In addition to visiting nursing homes and hospitals, called Animal-Assisted Activity in the vernacular of social scientists, some pets are used in Animal-Assisted Therapy. Under the supervision of a physical therapist, speech therapist, psychologist or other health professional, the pet works with individuals on a regular basis, motivating extra effort and results. A dog stands still while a patient performs arm exercises while brushing him, someone in speech therapy gets to pet a cat as a reward for articulating words or sounds, someone who refuses to exercise gets up and walks because the prize is a friendly animal's greeting at the end of the hall and, in small groups, children who have never cooperated learn to do so while tossing a ball to an attentive canine.

Shari Lashinksy, activities director at a large New York nursing home that receives monthly visits from a team of dogs and an occasional rabbit, put it best. "These pets are magic," she told a television news crew filming a visit. "They reach people in ways that we as fellow human beings simply can't. There are residents in my facility who literally do not respond to anything we as activities directors or visiting relatives or concerned friends or caring staff can do, no matter how hard we try. But whenever a dog visits, they wake up, become animated, reach out, talk, reminisce, have long conversations and are truly transformed."

Many of the animals who make regular visits to schools, hospitals, nursing homes, retirement homes and other facilities are registered with national organizations that provide training, testing and insurance coverage for pets and handlers. If you are at all interested in participating in this rewarding activity, please take advantage of the benefits these organizations provide. Since she was two years old, Samantha and I have visited nursing homes, hospitals, schools, retirement homes and other facilities as part of the Hudson Valley Humane Society's Visiting Pet Program. With its director, Dolores Schaub, and Shannon, her very special Doberman Pinscher, we joined national therapy organizations, attended advanced therapy dog training classes, read every book and article we could find and sponsored a series of workshops and seminars for the public and our program's members. We owe much of our knowledge to Delta Society trainer and evaluator Elizabeth Teal, who has spent years educating pet owners and health care professionals about the benefits, responsibilities and risks of Animal-Assisted Therapy and Animal Assisted Activity.

Done correctly, pet visitations are wonderful; done badly, they can injure, infect, frighten or even kill. Lawsuits, once unheard of in this type of volunteer activity, are becoming common. Please protect yourself, your pet and the people you plan to visit by learning safe handling techniques before you start making visits.

For information about national and international organizations supporting these activities, see the Resources for this chapter in the Appendix. ◈

Chapter

15

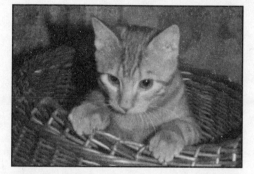

Saying
Goodbye

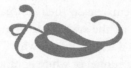

THEY'RE OUR BEST FRIENDS, our favorite companions. They entertain and amuse us, shape our routines, get us out of the house and enrich our lives in more ways than we can count. We wish our favorite pets could live forever.

It happens that way in daydreams, but in real life there comes a time when illness, old age or an accident intervenes and we're forced to say goodbye.

"It's helpful to remember that dogs, cats and other creatures don't view death the way we do," says companion animal behavior counselor and trainer Elizabeth Teal. "We go through life with all kinds of emotional baggage including a fear of dying, but animals don't share that fear. They don't have the emotional attachment to their bodies that we do. That's one of the reasons they can overcome adversity and heal faster than we do. I believe that the reason many of our pets struggle to stay alive in the final stages of illness is their awareness of our desire to keep them with us."

Pet owners often turn to holistic medicine when conventional treatments fail. "For many people," says veterinarian Larry Bernstein, "homeopathy, vitamins, herbs and other natural therapies are a last resort. It's exciting to read about pets whose lives were saved by holistic methods, but it's a mistake to assume that every animal will respond. Natural therapies can extend and improve the quality of the lives of many animals who are seriously ill, but they are not a magic cure. It takes a long time for a chronic disease to become sufficiently advanced to incapacitate an animal, and by then it may be too late for any therapy to make a difference. Sometimes, as difficult as this is for the humans involved, it's simply time for a beloved pet to leave this life."

According to Teal, one of the greatest gifts you can give your pet is permission to die. "The most important advice I can give to people whose animals are in the process of dying," she says, "is to let them go. If you beg an animal not to die or pray that it won't die, the animal may struggle and even increase its pain in order to stay with you. That's a terrible burden to place on any creature who's terminally ill."

Dogs, cats, rabbits and most birds have far shorter lifespans than human beings. As a result, pet owners often outlive not one but several companions. Over time, some have developed rituals that help them release their animals, rituals derived from religion, mythology, legends, intuition or the owner's imagination. Some find comfort in an image of their pets in heaven or the spirit world, where they are forever youthful, vibrant, alert and alive. Others picture a tunnel of white light and encourage their pets to take it to the next realm. For some, it's a simple matter of thanking the animal for a lifetime of companionship and affection.

"These are very personal and individual matters," says Teal. "There isn't any set formula. Whatever helps you release, honor and respect your companion will bring a sense of peace to both of you. I know many, many dogs, cats and other pets who relaxed into a tranquil, final sleep as soon as their human companions gave them permission to die. That's all they were waiting for. I have found this to be true of animals who were in great pain and about to be euthanized, injured animals at the site of an accident and those who were dying in other circumstances."

Euthanasia

Of all the decisions a human companion ever has to make, the most difficult can be whether and when to plan an animal's death. In response to requests from clients, veterinarian Chris Duke addressed this issue in a 1997 Knight-Ridder newspaper column. According to Dr. Duke, there are six important questions that must be answered before a final decision can be made.

1. Can the animal walk on its own? If it can walk, how much pain does it suffer?

2. How well does the animal see and hear? What are the prospects that incapacitating vision and hearing problems can be reversed?

3. Is there serious and irreversible kidney, heart, pancreas, liver or brain damage?

4. Whatever the animal's condition, is there any veterinary treatment that is likely to be effective at this stage of the animal's illness?

5. Is incontinence, a lack of urinary or bowel control, a serious problem?

6. Is the owner ready to release the animal?

While holistic veterinarians might answer some of these questions differently from their conventional colleagues, these six points provide a foundation for evaluation and communication. Decisions about euthanasia should be made jointly between pet owners and their veterinarians and, at home, among family members. Most people say they would use euthanasia to end an animal's suffering in cases of severe pain or incapacitation. There is no simple formula that applies to every case. It is necessary to weigh all of the economic, emotional, logistical and practical considerations affecting the animal, the primary caretaker and everyone else in the family.

If and when you decide to end your pet's life, discuss the procedure with your veterinarian. Some veterinary clinics make house calls so the animal can die peacefully at home. Some provide a special room, counseling and emotional support. The more attached you are to the animal, the more painful this final moment can be. You may want to have a friend or relative with you and cancel plans for the rest of the day.

The Importance of Grieving

People who aren't attached to animals have a difficult time understanding the grief experienced by bereaved pet owners. "It's only a cat," they say. "Get another one." They don't understand that a pet can be truly irreplaceable or that its departure can be as devastating and traumatic as the death of a fellow human being.

Bereavement counselors agree that the best way to deal with the loss of a pet is to honor the animal's memory. One good way to do this is with a funeral, memorial service or private gathering of friends and family in which you tell stories, share memories, look at photographs and relive adventures. If you aren't able to arrange such a gathering, consider phoning a bereavement counselor. Delta Society maintains a referral list of counselors; see the Resources for Chapter 14 in the Apppendix. Many humane societies, veterinarians and animal hospitals provide this service or can refer you to a bereavement counselor.

"Grieving over a pet is no longer a social tabu," says Teal. "It is important to mourn the loss of animals, for these are intelligent beings whom we love and cherish. Talking about your pet is one of the best things you can do. Call friends who knew your animal or who have lost pets themselves. Describe your companion to anyone who will lend a sympathetic ear. Write a letter to your pet. All of these things will help you move through this time of adjustment."

Be ready to return the same kindness to others. Whenever a friend's pet dies, express your sympathy. Send a card describing what you most enjoyed or admired about the animal, or write about something you and the pet did together. The more personal the message, the more meaningful it will be. Encourage your friend to talk, and respond with compassion and support.

Whenever a pet dies, someone will suggest that the family immediately get a new puppy or kitten. Doing so has helped some people recover from the loss of a beloved pet, but it is not appropriate advice for everyone. Mourning takes time. When a human dies, the formal period of mourning typically lasts a year. Where pets are concerned, many people need three to six months or more to adjust. All the experts agree that no one should adopt or buy a puppy, kitten or other pet until he or she feels ready to do so. It is a serious mistake to surprise someone who has recently lost a pet with the gift of a replacement animal.

The experts also warn against trying to replace an animal with his or her exact duplicate. No matter how similar they may be in appearance, no two animals are identical. Their personalities, responses and behaviors are certain to be different, and the result can be stressful for both the new pet and his confused or disappointed owner. The only sensible way to bring an animal into your life is after careful consideration as described in Chapter 1 and with a sense of acceptance and a willingness to allow your new pet to be himself.

Pets in Mourning

When a pet dies, pay special attention to other animals in your household during the weeks that follow. If two animals are attached to each other, the death of one will have a noticeable effect on the other. In a study of 189 dogs and cats whose companion animals died, researchers found that most of the cats and nearly half of the dogs actively sought out and stayed in areas where their departed friends had slept or spent time. The sleeping patterns of more than half of the animals changed and half of them ate less than usual or abstained from food. "These are significant findings," Teal explains, "for they indicate that the animals went through an emotional change after the death of a close friend."

The flower essences described in Chapter 8 can help grieving animals and their owners deal with loss. Borage essence is the primary treatment for depression in animals, but Dr. Bach's emergency formula and other flower essences may be helpful as well. Sometimes a fasting animal can be encouraged to eat by placing small amounts of food in different rooms, especially those which the departed animal favored. Therapeutic Touch is always appropriate.

Talk to your surviving pet. "I can't emphasize this enough," says Teal. "Our pets need emotional support from us just as we need it from them. Acknowledge that your animal misses her companion. Express your sympathy without imposing your own grief on her. Your pet may need more or less time than you do to deal with the loss. It takes anywhere from one to six months for most dogs and cats to recover from the death of a close companion, and the average is about six weeks. Neither of you may be functioning very well, but try to make extra time for conversation with your animal during the weeks that follow the loss of her friend."

Rainbow Bridge

The following essay, "Rainbow Bridge," has been printed in many pet books and magazines, and it has brought comfort to thousands of bereaved pet owners. Its author is unknown.

Just inside of heaven is a place called Rainbow Bridge. When an animal who has been especially close to someone dies, that pet goes to Rainbow Bridge. There are meadows and hills for our special friends so they can run and play together. There is plenty of food, water and sunshine, and our friends are warm and comfortable.

All the animals who had been ill and old are restored to health and vigor. Those who were hurt or maimed are made whole and strong again, just as we remember them in our dreams of days and times gone by. The animals are happy and content, except for one small thing. They each miss someone very special, someone who had to be left behind. They all run and play together, but the day comes when one suddenly stops and looks into the distance. His bright eyes are intent; his eager body begins to quiver. Suddenly he runs from the group, flying over the green grass, his legs carrying him faster and faster.

You have been spotted. And when you and your special friend finally meet, you cling together in joyous reunion, never to be parted again. The happy kisses rain upon your face; your hands again caress the beloved head, and you look once more into the trusting eyes of your pet, long gone from your life but never absent from your heart.

Then you cross Rainbow Bridge together.

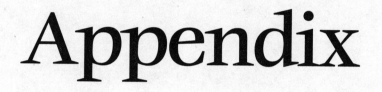

Appendix

Appendix

Home Health Assessment for Your Pet

Copy this form. Evaluate your pet every three or six months and keep the results to document your animal's health.

Date: _____ Pet's Name _____ Age ____ Weight _____

Body Temperature _____ Pulse _____ Respiration Rate _____

If you and your pet are comfortable with your use of a pet thermometer, record the animal's temperature, pulse (heartbeats per minute) and respiration rate (full breaths per minute) when he or she is calm and well-rested, not immediately after exercise or eating.

In general, the smaller the animal, including those of the same species, the faster and higher the pulse, respiration rate and body temperature. Some animals on raw, natural diets have lower resting temperatures than their counterparts of the same breed and size on commercial diets, and individuals vary. It's a good idea to record your pets' baseline vital signs so you know what's normal for each animal.

The following evaluation refers to the coat and teeth of dogs, cats and rabbits, but it applies as well to the feathers and beaks of birds. Adjust the form as necessary for your pet.

This evaluation was inspired by and adapted from a similar health assessment published by Bob and Susan Goldstein in their *Love of Animals* newsletter.

Normal Vital Signs
Typical ranges for resting animals

	Temperature (degrees Fahrenheit)	Pulse (Beats per minute)	Respiration (Breathing rate)
Dogs	100.5 to 101.5	70 to 120	10 to 30
Cats	100.5 to 101.5	110 to 130	20 to 30
Rabbits	103.1	180 to 220	35 to 40
Canaries	110 to 112	500 to 1,000	60 to 100
Parrots	108 to 110	150 to 300	25 to 40

Section A: Overall Health

Using a scale from 1 to 5, with 1 = not healthy and 5 = very healthy, rate your pet in the following categories.

	Not Healthy			Very Healthy	
1. Eyes (1 = oozing, itchy; 5 = bright, clear)	1	2	3	4	5
2. Ears (1 = discharge, malodorous; 5 = clean)	1	2	3	4	5
3. Teeth, gums (1 = diseased, unhealthy, 5 = strong, clean, no coating on tongue)	1	2	3	4	5
4. Fur, coat (1 = dull, bare spots, drab, excessive shedding; 5 = glossy, shiny, feels good)	1	2	3	4	5
5. Skin (1 = red, irritated; 5 = clear, clean)	1	2	3	4	5
6. Weight (1 = obese, severely overweight or anorexic, severely underweight, 5 = trim, fit)	1	2	3	4	5
7. Energy level (1 = no energy, dislikes activity; 5 = alert, lively, abundant energy)	1	2	3	4	5
8. Mental health (1 = depressed, phobic, anxious; 5 = happy, well-adjusted)	1	2	3	4	5
9. Ease of movement (1 = moves slowly, great pain, restricted mobility; 5 = no impairment)	1	2	3	4	5
10. Overall health rating (1 = very poor health; 5 = abundant good health)	1	2	3	4	5
11. Home situation last six months (1 = upheaval, divorce, loss of home, difficult move, death in family, including loss of close animal companion; 5 = stable home life)	1	2	3	4	5
12. Exercise (1 = no exercise, sedentary; 5 = active daily exercise in fresh air, sunlight, excellent muscle tone)	1	2	3	4	5
13. Diet (1 = supermarket-brand dry or canned food; 5 = home-prepared, well-balanced raw food)	1	2	3	4	5

TOTAL points Section A: _____

Section B: Conditions

14. Circle any that apply. Annual revaccinations (count required rabies vaccination as 1 condition; count additional combination vaccines in adult animal as 2 conditions). Use during the past year of any of the following: antibiotics, cortisone drugs, chemical heartworm preventive, internal flea-repellent drug, chemical flea treatment or flea collar, exposure to newly installed outgassing carpet or building materials with pronounced chemical odor, exposure to chemically treated lawn or garden or daily exposure to cigarette smoke or automobile exhaust.

MULTIPLY the number of conditions x 4   Total: _____

15. List any current chronic or frequent condition that is not life-threatening, such as arthritis, hip dysplasia, chronic flea infestation, overweight, skin irritations, vomiting after meals, indigestion, chronic ear infection, etc.

MULTIPLY the number of conditions x 5   Total: _____

16. List any potentially life-threatening diseases or conditions, such as heart disease, cancer, kidney or liver disease, diabetes, severe obesity, etc

MULTIPLY the number of conditions x 10   Total: _____
TOTAL points Section B: _____

Scoring Section

Your pet's age rounded to nearest year   _____
(maximum 20 points for birds over 20 years)
Plus points from Section A + _____
SUBTOTAL: _____
Minus points from Question 14 – _____
Minus points from Question 15 – _____
Minus points from Question 16 – _____

FINAL TOTAL: _____

What Your Pet's Score Means

20 or less: Time is of the essence. Improve your pet's food and water, adopt all the strategies you can to upgrade your pet's condition, consult a holistic veterinarian and follow as many of the strategies described here as you can in order to improve the length and quality of his or her life.

21 to 30: Your pet needs help to interrupt his or her decline. Follow the advice above and expect improvement.

31 to 44: Your pet may look normal but is probably susceptible to infections and other health problems. Focus on improved nutrition, find the right treatments for both obvious and minor conditions. Your pet's overall health should improve soon.

45 to 64: Above average. Your pet is doing well overall. By making a few improvements and changes, you can insure an even longer, happier life together.

65 and above: Congratulations! Your companion is enjoying the best of health. Follow the advice of holistic veterinarians and you will enjoy each other for a long time to come.

Recommended Reading and Resources

Chapter 1: Peace in the House

Pet Selection and Training

Bauman, Diane. *Beyond Basic Dog Training.* New York: MacMillan and Company, 1991. Obedience training for the thinking dog.

Benjamin, Carol Lea. *Second-Hand Dog.* New York: Howell Book House, Inc., 1988. How to live with an adopted dog.

Burmaster, Corally, editor. *The Clicker Journal Collection.* Leesburg, Va.: Coldstream Publications, annual volumes (1995, 1996, etc.). Reports and letters from novice and experienced clicker trainers.

Caras, Roger. *The Roger Caras Dog Book.* New York: M. Evans & Company, 1992. Practical information about breeds, well-told stories.

Cargill, John, and Marjorie Hudson. "Temperament Tests as Puppy Selection Tools." *Dog World,* April 1994.

Clothier, Suzanne. *Understanding Puppy Testing.* Stanton, N.J.: Flying Dog Press, 1996. Convenient booklet describes the history, purpose and methods of testing. Excellent introduction, score sheets, interpretation guidelines.

Hanna, Jack. *Jack Hanna's Ultimate Guide to Pets.* New York: G.P. Putnam's Sons, 1996. Entertaining introduction to dogs, cats, birds, rodents, rabbits, reptiles, fish and other pets.

Hunthausen, Wayne. *Dogs, Cats & Kids* videotape, 1996. Teaches children 5 to 12 years old how to play with pets safely, read dog and cat danger signs and what to do when threatened by stray animals. Available from Pet Love Partnership, below.

Kilcommons, Brian, and Sarah Wilson. *Good Owners, Great Dogs*. New York: Warner Books, 1992. Excellent, comprehensive, practical, easy to understand, highly recommended. Video of the same title available from Direct Book Service, below.

Kilcommons, Brian, and Sarah Wilson. *Childproofing Your Dog*. New York: Warner Books, 1994. Common sense advice for dog-owning parents.

Kilcommons, Brian, and Sarah Wilson. *Good Owners, Great Cats*. New York: Warner Books, 1996. Practical advice, terrific stories, great photos.

Monks of New Skete. *The Art of Raising a Puppy*. Boston: Little, Brown & Company, 1991. Detailed information on puppy testing, growth, development, where and how to get a puppy, training, problem solving. By the authors of *How to Be Your Dog's Best Friend*, also recommended.

Pryor, Karen. *A Dog and a Dolphin 2.0: An Introduction to Clicker Training*. North Bend, Wash.: Sunshine Books, 1996. Easy clicker training for puppies and dogs, clicker tips, games, resources.

Pryor, Karen. *Don't Shoot the Dog! The New Art of Teaching and Training*. New York: Bantam Books, 1985. The classic book on positive reinforcement, also called operant conditioning. Not a dog training handbook but an entertaining review of effective training strategies for all animals, including humans.

Wilkes, Gary. *Click! & Treat Training Kit*. Mesa, Ariz.: Gary Wilkes, 1995. Handbook, video and clickers.

Recommended Magazines and Newsletters

To find a monthly, bimonthly, quarterly or annual publication devoted to your favorite breed, check with your breed's national club as well as ads in all-breed magazines. To locate national breed clubs, call or write the American Kennel Club or check with local breeders. Breed magazines often feature photos and articles about the breed, its rescue organizations, training tips, activities, health concerns and practical advice.

A.K.C. Gazette, American Kennel Club, 51 Madison Avenue, New York, NY 10010. Phone 1-919-233-9767, fax 1-233-3627. Monthly magazine considered "the official journal for the sport of purebred dogs."

Bird Talk, Fancy Publications, P.O. Box 57347, Boulder, CO 57347. Phone 1-800-365-4421, fax 1-303-604-7455. A monthly magazine dedicated to better care for pet birds.

Caged Bird Hobbyist, published by Pet Business, Inc., 7-L Dundas Circle, Greensboro, NC 27407. Phone 1-910-292-4047, fax 1-910-292-4272. Bimonthly magazine for bird hobbyists.

CatFancy, P.O. Box 52864, Boulder, CO 57347. Phone 1-800-365-4421, fax 1-303-604-7455. Online http://www.catfancy.com or www.petchannel.com. Monthly magazine.

Cats, PJS Publications, Inc., Box 56886, Boulder, CO 80322-6886. Phone 1-800-829-9125. Online http.//www.catsmag.com.

The Clicker Journal, Corally Burmaster, 20146 Gleedsville Road, Leesburg, VA 22075. Current and back issues, collections of stories about clicker training.

Critters USA, Fancy Publications, Inc., P.O. Box 6050, Mission Viejo, CA 92690. Phone 1-714-855-8822, fax 1-714-855-3045. Annual guide to buying and caring for small animals.

Dog Fancy, Fancy Publications, Inc. P.O. Box 57347, Boulder, CO 57347, Phone 1-800-365-4421, fax 1-303-604-7455. Monthly all-breed magazine for dog lovers.

Dog World, PJS Publications, 29 N. Wacker Drive, Chicago, IL 60606. Phone 1-800-361-8056 or 1-312-609-4340, fax 1-312-236-2413, e-mail dogworld3@aol.com. World's largest all-breed magazine, published monthly. Check classified and display ads for breed clubs, breed magazines, rescue organizations and other sources of information for specific breeds.

Gun Dog, Stover Publishing Company, Inc., P.O. Box 343, Mt. Morris, IL 61054-0343. Phone 1-800-800-7724 or 1-815-734-1108. Bimonthly magazine of upland bird and waterfowl dogs. See also *Retriever Journal* and *Pointing Dog Journal,* Wildwood Press, P.O. Box 968, Traverse City, MI 49685-0968. These are examples of dog magazines targeted to specific activities.

Natural Rearing Breeders Directory, P.O. Box 1436, Jacksonville, OR 97530. Phone 1-541-899-2080, fax 1-541-899-3414, e-mail ambrican@cdsnet.net. Network of dog and cat breeders who feed a natural diet and use holistic therapies.

Rabbits Yearbook, yearBOOKS, Inc., 1 TFH Plaza, Neptune, NJ 07753. Combination book/magazine. Wide pet store distribution. The same publisher prints yearbooks on other types of pet (birds, cats, dogs, reptiles, etc.) and publishes the monthly magazines *Tropical Fish Hobbyist* and *Reptile Hobbyist* at P.O. Box 427, Neptune, NJ 07753-0427.

Resources

Acme Pet's List of Canine Clubs, e-mail acmepet@acmepet.com, online http://www.acmepet.com/canine/ civic/k9 club. html. Links and listings for national and regional breed clubs, national, international and regional organizations.

Alpine Publications, Inc., Blue Ribbon Books, P.O. Box 7027, Loveland, CO 80537. Phone 1-800-777-7257. Publishes books about dogs, puppies, activities, specific breeds. Send for catalog.

American Kennel Club, Inc., 51 Madison Avenue, New York NY 10010, 1-212-696-9231. Source of information about dog breeds, breed clubs and U.S. rescue groups listed by breed.

American Rabbit Breeders Association, Inc., P.O. Box 426, Bloomington, IL 61702. Phone 1-309-827-6623. International organization, provides information about all breeds of rabbits and cavies.

American Temperament Test Society (ATTS), P.O. Box 397, Fenton, MO 63026. Phone 1-314-225-5346. Tests adult dogs for temperament and gives the TT (Temperament Test) title to dogs judged appropriate for their breed, sex, condition (intact or neutered) and training. Puppies from TT-tested parents are unlikely to have aberrant personalities.

Breed Manual Publications, 3370C Jackson Drive, Jackson, WI 53037. Phone 1-414-677-3122. Publisher of *The Cocker Spaniel Owner's Medical Manual* and other references.

Cat Claws, Inc., 1004 West Broadway, Morrilton, AR 72110. Phone 1-800-783-0977 or 1-501-354-5015, fax 1-501-354-4843. Products for cats.

Dick Neville's Pages, e-mail rneville@hsc.usc.edu, online http://www-hsc.usc.edu/~rneville/mastlink.html. Home page featuring links to various topics including breed descriptions and rescue.

Direct Book Service, Dog & Cat Book Catalog, P.O. Box 2778, 701B Poplar, Wenatchee IA 98807-2778. Phone 1-800-776-2665 or 1-509-663-9115, fax 1-509-662-7233, e-mail dgctbook@cascade.net, online http://www.dogandcatbooks.com. The most comprehensive dog and cat reference catalog imaginable. Books, videos, head halters, clicker kits, information on grooming, training, breeding, specific breeds, art, murder mysteries, everything. Free catalog.

Howell Book House, 800 Third Avenue, New York, NY 10022. Extensive line of books about dogs, breeds, training and activities. Send for catalog.

National 4-H Council, 7100 Connecticut Avenue, Chevy Chase, MD 20814. Phone 1-301-961-2800, or contact your county's Cooperative Extension Office. Information about rabbits and how to raise them.

OTR Publications, P.O. Box 481-D, Centreville, AL 35042. Dog books, including books about unusual or rare breeds. Send for catalog.

Pet Love Partnership, c/o Pronto Connections, 820 North Orleans, Suite 300, Chicago IL 60610. Phone 1-800-784-0979. Distributor of Wayne Hunthausen's *Dogs, Cats & Kids* videotape.

Quadratech, Inc., 10804 La Cienega Blvd., Inglewood, CA 90304. Phone 1-800-649-0780 or 1-310-568-1893, fax 1-310-649-0782, e-mail osa4env@aol.com. Manufactures Flush It cat litter.

RC Steele, 1989 Transit Way, Box 910, Brockport NY 14420-0910. Phone 1-800-872-3773 or 1-716-637-1408, TTD 1-800-468-8776. Pet supply catalog, excellent selection, wholesale prices, everything from crates and leashes to scratching posts and litter boxes. Free catalog.

Sunshine Books, 44811 S.E. 166th Street, North Bend, WA 98045. Phone 1-800-47-CLICK or 1-425-888-3737, fax 1-425-888-9836, e-mail pryork@dontshootthedog.com, online www.dontshootthe-dog.com. Publisher of Karen Pryor's clicker training books, videos and training kits.

TFH Publications, 1 TFH Plaza, Neptune, NJ 07753. The world's largest publisher of books about pets, including guides to the selection and care of ferrets, gerbils, guinea pigs, hamsters, hedgehogs, mice, pot-bellied pigs, rabbits and rats.

Wilkes, Gary, 2753 E. Broadway, Suite 101-125, Mesa, AZ 85204. Phone 1-602-649-9804, fax 1-602-649-4259, e-mail wilkesgm@aol.com.. Click & Treat training kit, books, videos, workshops and seminars on clicker training.

Celeste Yarnall, 9875 Gloucester Drive, Beverly Hills, CA 90210. Phone 1-310-278-1385, fax 1-310-278-3499. Author of *Cat Care, Naturally*, breeder and feline consultant.

Pet Registries

One of the best ways to protect your pet against loss is to provide a permanent method of identification and file that information with a pet registry service. Then keep your records up to date, notifying the registry whenever you move, change your phone number or change "notify if found" names and numbers.

AKC Companion Animal Recovery, 5580 Centerview Drive, Suite 250, Raleigh, NC 27606-3394. Phone 1-800-252-7894, fax 1-919-233-1290, e-mail found@akc.org, online http://www.akc.org/car.html. All companion animals permanently identified by microchip or tattoo are eligible for enrollment. Established June 1995.

National Dog Registry, P.O. Box 116, Woodstock, NY 12498-0116. Phone 1-800-NDR-DOGS (1-800-637-3647), 1-914-679-2355, e-mail ndr@ifam.com. Founded in 1966, America's oldest and largest animal recovery registry has enrolled over 6,000,000 dogs, cats, goats, horses, birds, rabbits and other species identified by tattoo, microchip or leg band (permanent identification only) in the U.S., Canada, Mexico and Puerto Rico. NDR maintains a 95 to 98 percent recovery rate of registered animals lost in these and other countries. Will contact all other registries when animals found with permanent identification are not registered with NDR.

National Pet Registry, 5713 Corporate Way, Suite 100, West Palm Beach, FL 33407. Phone 1-800-477-9130, e-mail information@nationalpetregistry.com, online http://www.nationalpetregistry.com.

Chapter 2: Food Is Everything

Recommended Reading

Anderson, Nina, Howard Peiper and Alicia McWatters. *Super-Nutrition for Animals!* East Canaan, Conn.: Safe Goods, 1996.

de Bairacli Levy, Juliette. *Cats Naturally.* London: Faber and Faber, 1991. Natural Rearing, raw diet and herbs for cats.

de Bairacli Levy, Juliette. *The Complete Herbal Handbook for the Dog and Cat.* London: Faber and Faber, first published in 1953, revised edition, 1991. The Natural Rearing classic.

Billinghurst, Ian. *Give Your Dog a Bone.* Lithgow, N.S.W. Australia: Ian Billinghurst, 1993. Excellent, practical guidelines for feeding a raw bone-based diet.

Frazier, Anitra, and Norma Eckroate. *The New Natural Cat.* New York: Plume/Penguin Books, 1990. Nutrition and natural remedies for cats. Revised edition of a groundbreaking work, highly recommended.

Kenton, Leslie and Susannah. *Raw Energy.* New York: Warner Books, 1984. Out of print but worth searching for; raw food research on people and animals.

Kirschner, H.E. *Live Food Juices.* Monrovia, Calif.: H.E. Kirschner Publications, 1957, 1991. A healing classic.

Love of Animals newsletter: See Phillips Publishing in Resources, below.

McKay, Pat. *Reigning Cats & Dogs.* Pasadena, Calif.: Oscar Publications, 1992. Natural diet for dogs and cats.

Natural Pet magazine: See listing in Resources, below.

Natural Rearing newsletter: See Ambrican Enterprises, below.

Pitcairn, Richard, and Susan Hubble Pitcairn. *Natural Health for Dogs & Cats.* Emmaus, Penn.: Rodale Press, 1995. Comprehensive guide to nutrition, homeopathy, conditions.

Plechner, Alfred J., and Martin Zucker. *Pet Allergies: Remedies for an Epidemic.* Los Angeles: JP Enterprises, 1986. Food sensitivities and allergies in dogs and cats.

Pottenger, Francis M., Jr. *Pottenger's Cats: A Study in Nutrition.* La Mesa, Calif.: Price-Pottenger Nutrition Foundation, 1983. The famous raw food experiment. Additional information about the project was provided by Pat Connolly, curator of the Price-Pottenger Nutrition Foundation.

Schoeneck, Annelies. *Making Sauerkraut and Pickled Vegetables at Home.* Vancouver, B.C., Canada: Alive Books, 1988. Lactic acid fermentation how-to book.

Volhard, Wendy, and Kerry Brown. *The Holistic Guide for a Healthy Dog.* New York: Simon & Schuster, 1995. Scientific approach to raw diet, lots of charts and graphs.

Wigmore, Ann. *The Hippocrates Diet and Health Program.* Wayne, N.J.: Avery Publishing Group, 1984. One of many books by the woman who made wheatgrass famous.

Yarnall, Celeste. *Cat Care, Naturally.* Boston: Charles E. Tuttle Co., Inc., 1995. Natural diet for felines.

Yarnall, Celeste. *Dog Care, Naturally.* Boston: Charles E. Tuttle Co., Inc., 1998. Natural diet for canines.

Resources

AkPharma, Inc., Pleasantville NJ 08232. Phone 1-800-257-8650. Manufactures Lactaid, a milk-digesting enzyme, and Beano, which improves the digestibility of beans. Both products are sold in health food stores, pharmacies and supermarkets.

Alive Books, P.O. Box 67333, Vancouver, BC, Canada V5W 3T1. Publishes *Making Sauerkraut and Pickled Vegetables at Home,* other books on nutrition and *Alive,* Canada's largest circulation health magazine.

Cat Claws, Inc., 1004 West Broadway, Morrilton, AR 72110. Phone 1-800-783-0977 or 1-501-354-5015, fax 1-501-354-4843. Cat products, including dehydrated tuna flakes to flavor any food for cats.

China Prairie Company, Ettersburg Star Route, Garberville, CA 95542. Phone toll free 888-373-7401, phone or fax 1-707-986-7281, e-mail cpc@asis.com, online http://www.chinaprairie.com. Avicultural nutritionist Fred Bauer publishes an online newsletter of natural bird care. Catalog of natural, live-food diet and supplements for birds.

Eden Foods, 701 Tecumseh Road, Clinton, MI 49236. Phone 1-800-248-0301 or 1-517-456-7424, fax 1-517-456-6075. Imports Lima brand unrefined, sun-dried Atlantic sea salt from France; Lima salt is sold in health food stores.

Gold Mine Natural Food Company, 3419 Hancock Street, San Diego, CA 92110-4307. Phone 1-800-475-FOOD, fax 1-619-296-9756. Unrefined sea salt, Japanese salad presses, organic grains.

Grain and Salt Society, 273 Fairway Drive, Asheville, NC 28805. Phone 1-800-867-7258 or 1-704-299-9005, fax 1-704-299-1640. Imports Celtic unrefined sea salt from France.

Imhotep, Inc., P.O. Box 183, Ruby NY 12475. Phone 1-914-336-2070 or 1-800-677-8577. Manufactures ProSeed grapefruit seed extract liquid, capsules, ear wash and other products.

International Yogurt Company, 628 N. Doheny Drive, Los Angeles CA 90069. Supplies health food stores with kefir grains, yogurt starter and yogurt supplements.

Jaffee Bros. Natural Foods, P.O. Box 636, Valley Center CA 92082. Phone 1-619-749-1133, fax 1-619-749-1282. Raw carob powder, organically grown nuts and dried fruits. Excellent quality.

Pat McKay, Inc, 396 W Washington Blvd, Suite 600, Pasadena, CA 91103. Phone 1-800-975-7555 or 1-818-296-1120, fax 1-818-296-1126, e-mail patmckay@earthlink.net, online http://home.earthlink.net/~patmckay/. Full line of nutritional supplements and raw foods for dogs and cats and home of Oscar Publications, publisher of books by Pat McKay.

Natural Lifestyle Supply Company, 16 Lookout Drive, Asheville NC 28804. Phone 1-800-752-2775. Organic seeds, grains, Japanese salad presses.

Natural Pet, P.O. Box 420234, Palm Coast, FL 32142-0234. Phone 1-800-735-9335. Publishes *Natural Pet* magazine, which features holistic health care. Highly recommended.

New England Cheesemaking Supply Company, P.O. Box 65, Ashfield, MA 01330. Phone 1-413-628-3808. Kefir culture, Bulgarian yogurt culture and several cheese starter cultures.

Nutri-Biotic, P.O. Box 238, Lakeport CA 95453. Phone 1-800-225-4345 or 1-707-263-0411, fax 1-707-263-7844, online nutribio@pacific.net. Nutri-Biotic grapefruit seed extract liquid, capsules, tablets, nasal spray, ear drops, Jungle Juice insect repellent and other products.

PetNutrition, 577 Humbolt, Denver, CO 80218. Phone 1-800-494-2659. Freeze-dried or frozen raw meats, enzymes, food-source vitamin/mineral supplements.

Phillips Publishing, Inc., 7811 Montrose Road, Potomac, MD 20854. Phone 1-301-424-3700. Publishes *Love of Animals* newsletter by Dr. Bob and Susan Goldstein, emphasizing natural care for pets.

Price-Pottenger Nutrition Foundation, Inc., P.O. Box 2614, La Mesa, CA 91943-2614. Phone 1-619-574-7763, fax 1-619-574-1314. Publisher of *Pottenger's Cats.*

Prozyme Products, Ltd., 6600 N. Lincoln Ave #312, Lincolnwood IL 60645-3633. Phone 1-800-522-5537, fax 1-847-982-1310. Manufactures Prozyme enzyme powder.

Safe Goods, 283 East Canaan Road, East Canaan, CT 06024. Phone 1-860-824-4301. Publisher of *Super-Nutrition for Animals* by Nina Anderson.

The Sprout House, 7023 McLennan Ave., Van Nuys, CA 91406, phone 1-800-SPROUTS, fax 1-818-989-2468, e-mail info@SproutHouse.com. Organically raised grains and seeds, sprouting supplies.

Celeste Yarnall, 9875 Gloucester Drive, Beverly Hills, CA 90210. Phone 1-310-278-1385, fax 1-310-278-3499. Author of *Cat Care, Naturally* and *Dog Care, Naturally,* distributes raw food and nutritional supplements for pets by mail.

Chapter 3: Supplements for Pets

Recommended Reading
See also the Recommended Reading list for Chapter 2.

Belfield, Wendell O., and Martin Zucker. *How to Have a Healthier Dog.* New York: New American Library, 1981. Vitamins, minerals and canine life cycles.

Belfield, Wendell O., and Martin Zucker. *The Very Healthy Cat Book.* San Jose, Calif.: Orthomolecular Specialties, 1983. Vitamin/mineral program for optimal feline health.

Jacobsen, Roy M. *Aqua Vitae.* Fargo, N.D.: Christopher Lawrence Communications, 1987. Willard Water's history and uses.

Ley, Beth M. *Dr. John Willard's Catalyst Altered Water.* Fargo, N.D.: Christopher Lawrence Communications, 1990.

Resources

Ambrican Enterprises, Ltd., Marina Zacharias, P.O. Box 1436, Jacksonville, OR 97530. Phone 1-541-899-2080, fax 1-541-899-3414, e-mail ambrican@cdsnet.net. Source of nutritional supplements, for dogs and cats. Publisher of *Natural Rearing* newsletter, which emphasizes raw food and natural remedies.

Ameriflex, Inc., 232 NE Lincoln Street, Suite G, Hillsboro, OR 97124. Phone 1-800-487-5463 or 1-503-640-0810. MinerAll 72, a liquid colloidal trace mineral supplement.

Bioforce of America, P.O. Box 507, Kinderhook, NY 12106. Phone 1-518-758-6060. Imports Biostrath and Animastrath liquid yeast from Switzerland; superior products.

Bricker Labs, 18722 Santee Lane, Valley Center CA 92082. Phone 1-800-BRICKER. Distributes Colostrex brand colostrum supplements in tablets, capsules and liquid.

Gardens Alive, 510 Schenley Place, Lawrenceburg IN 47025. Phone 1-812-537-8651. Diatomaceous earth.

Holistic Pet Center, P.O. Box 1166, Clackamas OR 97015. Phone 1-503-656-5342 or 1-800-788-PETS. Diatomaceous earth and holistic pet supplies.

L&H Vitamins, 37-10 Crescent Street, Long Island City NY 11101. Phone 1-800-221-1152, fax 1-718-361-1437. Large mail order catalog of vitamins and supplements. Sells Willard Water extract, food-source vitamins.

Mezotrace Corporation, 5184 Winnemucca Blvd., Winnemucca NV 89445. Powdered trace minerals for pets and people.

Nutrition Coalition, 2417 12th Avenue South, Moorhead, MN 56560, phone 1-800-447-4793 or 1-218-236-9783, fax 1-218-236-6753. Willard Water extract, colostrum supplements.

Pet Sage, 4313 Wheeler Avenue, Alexandria, VA 22304. Phone 1-800-PET-HLTH or 1-703-823-9711, fax 1-703-823-9714, e-mail info@petsage.com, online http://www.petsage.com. Books, supplements, pet health products.

Pet's Friend, Inc., 5871 N. University Drive, Suite 720, Tamarac, FL 33321. Phone 1-800-868-1009 or 1-954-720-0794, e-mail petsfriend@zim.com. Gland-organ concentrates, digestive enzymes.

Springtime, Inc., 10942-J Beaver Dam Road, P.O. Box 1227, Cockeysville, MD 21030. Phone 1-800-521-3212 or 1-410-771-8430, fax 1-410-771-1530. Natural supplements and food concentrates for dogs, horses and people.

Standard Process, Inc., 1200 West Royal Lee Drive, Palmyra, WI 53156. Phone 1-800-848-5061 or 1-414-495-2122, fax 1-414-495-2512. Product information available to licensed healthcare professionals only, not retail customers. Highest quality vitamin, mineral, glandular and food supplement products, all from organically grown whole-food sources. Formulas recommended for pets include Allerplex for allergies, Catalyn or Cryofood multiple vitamin-mineral tabs, Ligaplex for connective tissue, Lactic Acid Yeast and Zypan for digestion, Vasculin for muscle and nervous system support, Diaplex for diabetes and others. Ask your holistic veterinarian for product recommendations (veterinary protocols brochure available from the manufacturer). Available at some health food stores and mail order companies, including the Vitamin Shoppe, below, and Ambrican Enterprises, above. Health Alert (P.O. Box 22620, Carmel, CA 93922-2620. Phone 1-408-372-2103), which sells Standard Process products by mail, publishes a description of 56 Standard Process products and their uses.

T.J. Clark & Company, 1145 N. 1100 Street West, St. George, UT 84770. Phone 1-800-228-0872 or 1-801-634-0309, fax 1-801-634-0308. Liquid colloidal trace minerals.

Vitamin Shoppe, 4700 Westside Avenue, North Bergen, NJ 07047. Phone 1-800-223-1216 or 1-201-866-7711, fax 1-800-852-7153. Large mail order catalog of nutritional supplements, sells food-source vitamins, including Standard Process products. For Standard Process price list, which does not appear in the catalog, phone customer service.

Whiskers Holistic Pet Products, 235 E 9th Street, New York, NY 10003. Phone 1-800-944-7537, 1-212-979-2532, fax 1-212-979-0075, e-mail healthypet@msn.com, online http://choicemall.com/ whiskers.

WonderPet International, Inc., 7811 Montrose Road, Potomac, MD 20854. Phone 1-800-705-5559. Earth Animal Internal Powder developed by Dr. Bob and Susan Goldstein, publishers of *Love of Animals* newsletter (contains high-sulfur brewer's yeast to repel fleas and ticks).

Wysong Institute, 1880 N. Eastman Road, Midland MI 48642-7779. Phone 1-517-631-0009, fax 1-517-631-8801, e-mail wysong@tm.net. Zymase enzyme powder, food grade hydrogen peroxide, Feline Biotic (F-Biotic), Canine Biotic (C-Biotic), Sprout Soak for increasing the mineral content of sprouts, unrefined sea salt, whole food vitamins, probiotic supplements and other products for pets. Extensive information about pet nutrition.

Chapter 4: Herbs for Pets

Recommended Reading

de Bairacli Levy, Juliette. *Cats Naturally.* London: Faber and Faber, 1991. Natural Rearing, raw diet and herbs for cats.

de Bairacli Levy, Juliette. *The Complete Herbal Handbook for the Dog and Cat.* London: Faber and Faber, first published in 1953, most recent revised edition, 1991. The Natural Rearing classic.

Carston, Rachel. *Devil's Claw Root and Other Natural Remedies for Arthritis.* Burnaby, B.C., Canada: Alive Books, 1993.

Christopher, John. *The School of Natural Healing.* Springville, Ut.: Christopher Publications, 1976.

Foster, Steven, and James A. Duke. *Peterson Field Guides: Eastern/Central Medicinal Plants.* Boston: Houghton Mifflin, 1990. Superior field guide with well-documented medicinal uses.

Gladstar, Rosemary. *Herbal Healing for Women.* New York: Simon & Schuster, 1993. Simple remedies, sound advice; much of the general and reproductive information can be applied to pets.

Hancock, Kenneth. *Feverfew: Your Headache May Be Over.* New Canaan, Conn: Keats Publishing, Inc., 1986. Feverfew as an arthritis treatment.

Keville, Kathi. *The Illustrated Herbal Encyclopedia.* New York: Bantam Doubleday, 1992. Recommended.

Lust, John. *The Herb Book.* New York: Bantam Books, 1974. Excellent, inexpensive basic herbal.

Moore, Michael. *Medicinal Plants of the Pacific West.* Santa Fe: Red Crane Books, 1993. Excellent reference.

Mowrey, Daniel B. *Herbal Tonic Therapies.* New Canaan, Conn.: Keats Publishing, Inc., 1993.

Reader's Digest. *Magic and Medicine of Plants.* Pleasantville, N.Y.: Reader's Digest Association, 1986. Good overview, some overly cautious warnings.

Schwartz, Cheryl. *Four Paws, Five Directions: A Guide to Chinese Medicine for Cats and Dogs.* Berkeley, Calif.: Celestial Arts, 1996. Introduction to Oriental medicine as it applies to animals. Herbs.

Theiss, Barbara and Peter. *The Family Herbal.* Rochester, Vt.: Healing Arts Press, 1989. Introduction to European herbalism, recommended.

Tierra, Michael. *The Way of Herbs.* New York: Pocket Books, 1983. Recommended basic herbal.

Treben, Maria. *Health through God's Pharmacy.* Steyr, Austria: Wilhelm Ennsthaler, 1980. European herbal medicine.

Weiss, Rudolf Fritz. *Herbal Medicine.* English translation of the sixth German edition, 1988. Imported by Medicina Biologica, Portland, Ore. Excellent reference.

Magazines and Newsletters

HerbalGram, published by the American Botanical Council, below.

The Herb Companion, published by Interweave Press, below.

Herb Quarterly, P.O. Box 689, San Anselmo, CA 94960. Phone 1-800-371-HERB. General interest herb magazine, published quarterly.

Herbs for Health, published by Interweave Press, below.

Natural Pet, P.O. Box 420234, Palm Coast, FL 32142-0234. Phone 1-800-735-9335. Holistic health care and herbs for pets.

Natural Rearing, published by Ambrican Enterprises, below.

Protocol Journal of Botanical Medicine, P.O. Box 108, Harvard, MA 01451. Phone 1-800-466-5422, fax 1-800-717-1722. Ambitious scholarly journal, published quarterly.

Organizations

American Botanical Council, P.O. Box 201660, Austin, TX 78720. Phone 1-800-373-7105 or phone 1-512-331-8868, fax 1-512-331-1924, online custserv@herbalgram.org, http://www.herbalgram.org. Educational and research organization, publisher of *HerbalGram*, quarterly magazine devoted to herbal medicine. Excellent resource.

American Herb Association, P.O. Box 1673, Nevada City CA 95959. Educational organization, quarterly newsletter.

American Herbalists Guild, P.O. Box 746555, Arvada, CO 80006-6555. Phone 1-303-402-1564, fax 1-303-402-1564. Professional organization, practitioners, referrals, quarterly newsletter.

Herb Research Foundation, 1007 Pearl Street, Suite 200, Boulder, CO 80302. Phone 1-303-449-2265, fax 1-303-449-7849, e-mail info@herbs.org, online http://www.herbs.org. Library of 100,000 scientific articles on the safety and health benefits of herbs. Excellent resource.

International Herb Association, P.O. Box 317, Mundelein, IL 60060. Phone 1-847-949-4372, fax 1-847-949-5896, e-mail ihacathy@aol.com. Association of herb professionals. Newsletter, activities.

Northeast Herbal Association, P.O. Box 479, Milton, NY 12547. Educational, professional organization; publishes journal.

United Plant Savers, P.O. Box 420, East Barre, VT 05549. Phone 1-802-479-9825, fax 1-802-476-3722, e-mail ups@ilhawaii.net. Nonprofit, grass roots organization for restoration and cultivation of environmentally threatened medicinal plants.

Resources

Ambrican Enterprises, Ltd., P.O. Box 1436, Jacksonville, OR 97530. Phone 1-541-899-2080, fax 1-541-899-3414, e-mail ambrican@cdsnet.net. Source of nutritional supplements, including herbal supplements for dogs and cats, publisher of *Natural Rearing* newsletter.

Avena Botanicals, P.O. Box 365, West Rockport, ME 04865. Phone 1-207-594-0694. Herbs and handcrafted herbal products.

Blessed Herbs, 109 Barre Plains Road, Oakham, ME 01068.

California School of Herbal Studies, P.O. Box 39, Forestville CA 95436. Phone 1-707-887-2012, fax 1-707-887-7570. James Green, director. Home of Simplers Botanical Company.

East Earth Trade Winds, P.O. Box 493151, 1620 East Cypress Avenue #8, Redding, CA 96049-3151. Phone 1-800-258-6878, online http://www.snowcrest.net/eetw/. Traditional Chinese herbs.

East Park Research, Inc., 650 Whitney Ranch Drive, Suite 112, Henderson, NV 89014. Phone 1-702-433-9040, fax 1-702-434-8673. Superior quality olive leaf extract at retail and wholesale prices.

Flora Distributors, 7400 Fraser Park Drive, Burnaby BC V5J 5B9, Canada. Phone 1-604-451-8232; P.O. Box 950, Lynden WA 98264. Phone 1-800-446-2110, fax 360/354-5355. Essiac tea and other herbal products.

Frontier Cooperative Herbs, P.O. Box 299, Norway, IA 52318. Large wholesale/retail herb company.

Good Communications, Inc., P.O. Box 10069, Austin, TX 78766. Phone 1-800-968-1738 or 1-512-454-6090, fax 1-512-454-3420, email gooddogmag@aol.dog, online http://www.prodog.com/ dmn/good-dog. Distributes Skin-eze powder and tablets, a blend of Chinese herbs for allergies and skin itching.

Green Terrestrial, P.O. Box 41, Route 9W, Milton, NY 12547. Herbs, supplies.

The Herb Closet, 104 Main Street, Montpelier, VT 05602. Herbs, supplies.

Herb Pharm, P.O. Box 116, Williams, OR 97544. Phone 1-800-348-4372 or 1-800-599-2392, fax 1-800-545-7392. Superior quality herbs, source of alkaloid-free comfrey.

Interweave Press, 201 East Fourth Street, Loveland, CO 80537-5655. Phone 1-970-669-7672. Publishes *Herbs for Health* (quarterly) and *The Herb Companion* (bimonthly), general interest magazines.

Island Herbs, Ryan Drum, Waldron Island, WA 98297. Famous for seaweeds.

Jean's Greens, 119 Sulphur Springs Road, Norway, NY 13416. Phone toll-free 1-888-845-TEAS or 1-315-845-6500 (phone/fax line). Herbs and handcrafted herbal products, including FortiCell, a version of Essiac tea.

L&H Vitamins, 37-10 Crescent Street, Long Island City NY 11101. Phone 1-800-221-1152, fax 1-718-361-1437. Large mail order catalog of herbal products and food supplements.

Mountain Rose Herbs, P.O. Box 2000, Redway, CA 95560. Phone 1-800-879-3337. Teas, herbs and supplies.

Native Essence Herb Company, 216M North Pueblo #301, Taos NM 87571. Phone 1-800-377-4229. Sells different versions of Essiac tea. Free report on alternative cancer therapies.

Norimoor Company, Inc., La Maison Francaise #5222, Fifth Avenue, New York NY 10185-0043, phone 1-212-695-MOOR or 1-212-268-5399, fax 1-212-695-4535. Herbal Melange from Austria.

Richters, Goodwood, Ontario L0C 1A0, Canada. Phone 1-905-640-6677, fax 1-905-640-6641, online orderdesk@richters.com. The most informative catalog, quality plants.

Sage Mountain Herb Products, P.O. Box 420, East Barre, VT 05649. Rosemary Gladstar's company.

Swissette Herb Farm, Clove Road, Salisbury Mills, NY 12577. Phone 1-914-496-7841. Herbs and supplies.

Trinity Herbs, P.O. Box 199, Bodega, CA 94992. Herbs and supplies.

TransPacific Health Products, 3924 Central Avenue, Saint Petersburg, FL 33711. Phone 1-800-336-9636. Traditional Chinese herbs.

Vitamin Shoppe, 4700 Westside Avenue, North Bergen, NJ 07047. Phone 1-800-223-1216 or 1-201-866-7711, fax 1-800-852-7153. Large mail order catalog of herbal products and supplements. Sells most products recommended in this book.

Willner Chemists, 100 Park Avenue, New York NY 10017. Phone 1-800 633-1106 or 1-212-682-2817, fax 1-212-682-6192. Large mail order catalog of herbal products and supplements.

Chapter 5: Aromatherapy

Recommended Reading

Fischer-Rizzi, Susanne. *The Complete Aromatherapy Handbook.* New York: Sterling Publishing, 1990, translated from the German by Elisabeth Reinersmann.

Grosjean, Nelly. *Veterinary Aromatherapy.* Essex, England: C.W. Daniel Co., Ltd., 1994, translated from the French by Joanne Robinson.

Lawless, Julia. *The Encyclopedia of Essential Oils.* Dorset, England and Rockport, Mass.: Element Books Limited, 1992.

Sheppard-Hanger, Sylla. *The Aromatherapy Practitioner Reference Manual.* Two volumes. Tampa, Fla.: Institute of Aromatherapy, 1994.

Tisserand, Maggie, and Monika Juenemann. *The Magic and Power of Lavender.* Wilmot, Wis.: Lotus Light, 1994, translated from the French by Matthias Dehne.

Tisserand, Robert B. *The Art of Aromatherapy.* Rochester, Vt.: Destiny Books, 1977.

Worwood, Valerie Ann. *The Complete Book of Essential Oils & Aromatherapy.* London: Macmillan London Limited, 1990; San Rafael, Calif.: New World Library, 1991.

Resources

American Aromatherapy Association, P.O. Box 3679, South Pasadena CA 91031. Phone 1-818-457-1742.

Aqua Oleium, The Old Convent, Beeches Green, Stroud, Glos GL5 4AD, U.K. Distributed in the U.S. by M. Das Co., 888 Brennan Street, San Francisco, CA 94103. Phone 1-415-626-6166, fax 1-415-626-6812. Essential oils, base oils, aromatherapy products.

Aroma Vera, Inc., P.O. Box 3609, Culver City, CA 90231. Essential oils and supplies.

Aromatherapy Quarterly, Michael Eccles, P.O. Box 421, Inverness, CA 94937-0421. Phone 1-415-663-9519. England's premier aromatherapy publication, now available in the U.S.

Aromatherapy Seminar, 3384 Robertson Place, Los Angeles CA 90034. Aromatherapy courses, education.

Essentially Yours North America. P.O. Box 81866, Bakersfield CA 93380. Essentially Yours Canada, 254 Hart Street, Coquitlam, B.C. Canada V3K 4A6. Aromatherapy products recommended by Valerie Ann Worwood.

Jean's Greens Herbal Tea Works, 119 Sulphur Springs Road, Norway, NY 13416. Phone toll-free 1-888-845-TEAS or 1-315-845-6500. Popular essential oils, herbal supplies.

Joint Adventure, P.O. Box 824, Rogers AR 72757. Phone 1-800-898-9873, fax 1-501-636-3785. Essential oils, aromatherapy supplies.

Laboratoire Aromathérpie Vie 'Arôme la chevêche, petite route du grès, 13690 Graveson-en-Provence, France. Essential oils and hydrosols grown and distilled by Nelly Grosjean, author of *Veterinary Aromatherapy.* Distributed in the U.S. by Aromatherapy International, 3 Seal Harbor Road, Suite 437, Winthrop, MA 02152. Phone 1-617-846-0285, fax 1-617-846-5474, and by SunAire Aromatherapy, Inc., 18681 Halifax Lane, Jordan, MN 55352. Phone 1-612-492-2064, fax 1-612-492-2973.

Liberty Natural Products, 8120 S.E. Stark Street, Portland OR 98714-2356. Phone 1-800-289-8427, fax 1-503-256-1182, e-mail Liberty@teleport.com, online http://www.teleport.com/~liberty. Essential oils, reference books, aromatherapy supplies. My source of opopanax essential oil and water-soluble sulfated castor oil.

NutriBiotic, Lakeport CA 95453. Phone 1-800-225-4345. Jungle Juice insect repellent.

Original Swiss Aromatics, P.O. Box 606, San Rafael CA 94915.

Pacific Institute of Aromatherapy, P.O. Box 606, San Rafael CA 94915. Aromatherapy courses, education.

Chapter 6: Homeopathy for Pets

Recommended Reading

Chambreau, Christina. *Homeopathic First Aid for Pets* (videotape). Video Remedies, PO Box 290855, Davie, FL 33329.

Day, Christopher. *The Homeopathic Treatment of Small Animals.* London: Wigmore Publications Ltd., 1984. Good introduction by a respected English veterinarian.

Dooley, Timothy R. *Homeopathy: Beyond Flat Earth Medicine.* San Diego: Timing Publications, 1995. A family physician explains this medical science.

Hunter, Francis. *Homeopathic First Aid Treatment for Pets.* London: Thorsons/Harper Collins, 1984. A review of 24 homeopathic remedies and their use in common canine and feline conditions.

Macleod, George. *Cats: Homeopathic Remedies.* Saffron Walden, Essex, England: C.W. Daniel Company Ltd., 1990. One of several books by a veterinary surgeon who used homeopathic medicines exclusively.

Macleod, George. *Dogs: Homeopathic Remedies.* Saffron Walden, Essex, England: C.W. Daniel Company Ltd., 1983. The author also wrote guides for the homeopathic treatment of cattle, goats, pigs and horses.

Macleod, George. *A Veterinary Materia Medica and Clinical Repertory with a Materia Medica of the Nosodes.* Saffron Walden, Essex, England: C.W. Daniel Company Ltd., 1983, 1995. Detailed descriptions of 280 individual remedies.

Pitcairn, Richard, and Susan Hubble Pitcairn. *Dr. Pitcairn's Complete Guide to Natural Health for Dogs and Cats.* Emmaus, Penn.: Rodale Books, 1995. All-purpose holistic guide with recommendations for the use of 84 homeopathic remedies in the treatment of different conditions.

Raymonde-Hawkins, M., and George Macleod. *Raystede Handbook of Homeopathic Remedies for Animals.* Collaboration with the founder of a center for animal welfare.

Vithoulkas, George. *Homeopathy — Medicine for the New Man.* New York: Arco Publishing Company, 1980. Good introduction to homeopathy.

Newsletter

Better Health Through Homeopathy, published by Polychrest Publishing, PO Box 3190, Ashland, OR 97520-9020. Phone 1-541-482-2138, fax 1-541-488-4229, e-mail polycrst@mind.net. General interest bimonthly.

Organizations

The following offer information, referrals and, in some cases, classes, workshops, newsletters and other publications. Enclose a self-addressed, stamped reply envelope when requesting information by mail.

Academy of Veterinary Homeopathy, Larry Bernstein, VMD, 751 N.E. 168th Street, North Miami Beach, FL 33162. Phone 1-305-652-5372, fax 1-305-653-7244, e-mail avh@naturalholistic.com, online http://www.holisticvet.com or http://www.acadvethom.org.

American Holistic Veterinary Medical Association, 2214 Old Emmorton Rd., Bel Air, MD 21015. Phone 1-410-569-0795, fax 1-410-569-2346, e-mail 74253,2560@compuserve.com.

Center for Homeopathic Family Education, PO Box 1041, Questa, NM 87556. Phone 1-505-586-1166 or 1-800-484-6683, extension 0600. Workshops and information.

Homeopathic Educational Services, 2124 Kittredge Street, Berkeley, CA, 94704. Phone 1-800-359-9051 or 1-510-649-0294. Books, tapes, remedy kits, information.

Homeopathic Information Resources, Ltd., Oneida River Park Drive, Clay, NY 13041. Phone 1-800-289-4447. Books, tapes, remedy kits.

International Association for Veterinary Homeopathy, Susan Wynn, DVM, 1080 North Cobb Parkway, Marietta, GA 30062. Phone 1-770-424-6303, fax 1-770-426-4257, e-mail swynn@emory.edu.

International Foundation for Homeopathy, 2366 Eastlake Avenue E. #329, Seattle, WA 98102. Phone 1-206-324-8230. One of the leading homeopathy organizations for the general public.

Minimum Price Homeopathic Books, 250 H Street, PO Box 2187, Blaine, WA 98231. Phone 1-800-663-8272.

National Center for Homeopathy, 801 N. Fairfax #306, Alexandria, VA 22314. Phone (703) 548-7790, online http://www.homeopathic.org. One of the leading homeopathy organizations for the general public.

Manufacturers, Distributors

ARNICA, Inc., 144 E. Garry Ave., Santa Ana, CA 92707. Phone 1-714-545-8203. Nosodes and remedies to veterinarians and other licensed healthcare professionals.

Boericke & Tafel, 2381 Circadian Way, Santa Rosa, CA 95407. Phone 1-800-876-9505. America's oldest producer of homeopathic remedies, founded in 1835. Remedies in strengths from 6x to 1M, sold over the counter or by mail; no written prescription necessary, but recommendation from a licensed veterinarian helpful when ordering high potency products. No nosodes.

Boiron, 6 Campus Boulevard, Building A, Newtown Square, PA 19073. Phone 1-800-BLU-TUBE (1-800-258-8823) or 1-610-325-7464, fax 1-610-325-7480. A French corporation, Boiron sells remedies by mail and in health food stores and pharmacies.

Dolisos America, Inc., 3014 Rigel Avenue, Las Vegas, NV 89102. Phone 1-800-365-4767. Full line of remedies in strengths from 6x to 1M and higher, all available by mail without a prescription. Some nosodes.

Homeopathy Overnight, RR1, Box 818, Kingfield, ME 04947. Phone 1-800-ARNICA30 (1-800-276-4223) or 1-207-265-5535, fax 1-207-265-0029, e-mail Rsawyer@somtel.com, online http:// www.som tel.com/homeovernight. Over 550 single remedies in 30c or 200c, most common remedies in strengths from 6x to 1M or 10M. Some nosodes. Special orders at no extra charge, company imports unusual remedies from other countries on request. Mail order retail, no prescription required. Good selection of veterinary titles and other books. Family-owned company, working farm, all animals treated homeopathically.

Luyties Pharmacal Company, PO Box 8080, St Louis MO 63156-8080. Phone 1-800-325-8080 or 1-314-533-9600, fax 1-314-535-9600. Manufactures about 100 single remedies in strengths 6x, 12x and 30x. Some remedies in higher potencies by prescription. No nosodes.

Newton Laboratories, Inc., 2360 Rockaway Industrial Blvd. N.W., Conyers, GA 30207. Phone 1-800-448-7256, 1-770-922-2644, fax 1-800-760-5550 or 1-770-388-7768. About 500 single remedies in 10x, 15x, 30x and 30c plus a limited number of 200c remedies, nothing higher. Some nosodes available to licensed healthcare practitioners. Mail order and retail store distribution.

Standard Homeopathic, 210 West 131st Street, PO Box 61067, Los Angeles, CA 90061. Phone 1-800-624-9659 or 1-310-321-4284, fax 1-310-516-8579. Manufactures hundreds of single remedies in strengths 1c to 200c or 200x and certain remedies in high potencies, such as 1M, 10M, 15M and 500M. Products sold by mail and in retail stores.

Washington Homeopathic Products, 4914 Del Ray Avenue, Bethesda, MD 20814. Phone 1-800-336-1695 or 1-301-656-1695. Manufactures over 1,300 single remedies in potencies from 6x or 6c to 30x or 30c. Some remedies available in strengths up to 50M. Wide range of veterinary nosodes. Most products sold over the counter in stores or by mail; items requiring a prescription sold directly to licensed veterinarians or other healthcare professionals.

Homeopathic Pharmacies

C.O. Bigelow Chemists, 414 Sixth Avenue, New York, NY 10011. Phone 1-800-793-LIFE or 1-212-533-2700, fax 1-212-228-8107.

Estroff Pharmacy, 138 Second Avenue, New York, NY 10003. Phone 1-212-254-7760.

Hahnemann Pharmacy, 828 San Pablo Avenue, Albany, CA 94706. Phone 1-510-527-3003.

Hickey Chemists, Ltd., 888 Second Avenue, New York, NY 10017, Phone 1-800-724-5566 or 1-212-223-6333, fax 1-212-980-1533.

Nutritional Specialties, PO Box 5897, Pittsburgh PA 15209. Phone 1-800-245-1313

P&D Nutrition, PO Box 270, Warrendale PA 15086. Phone 1-800-245-1939

Weleda Apothecary, 6 Red Schoolhouse Road, Chestnut Ridge, NY 10977. Phone 1-914-352-6165, fax 1-914-425-1088. Anthroposophical and homeopathic remedies.

Willner Chemists, 100 Park Avenue, New York NY 10017. Phone 1-800 633-1106 or 1-212-682-2817, fax 1-212-682-6192. Impressive retail catalog.

Chapter 7: Hands-On Therapies

Recommended Reading

Clothier, Suzanne. *Body Posture & Emotions: Shifting Shapes, Shifting Minds.* Stanton, N.J.: Flying Dog Press, 1966. Changing an animal's posture, gently stroking and touching, understanding body language and adopting simple training strategies can transform problem behavior. Highly recommended.

Clothier, Suzanne, and Sue Ann Lesser. *Physical Therapy for the Canine Athlete.* Stanton, N.J.: Flying Dog Press, 1996. Excellent physical therapy booklet.

Clothier, Suzanne, and Sue Ann Lesser. *Your Athletic Dog: A Functional Approach.* Stanton, N.J.: Flying Dog Press, 1995. Video tape and workbook. How to notice, understand and diagnose physical limitations; simple exercises, massage techniques. Very helpful for pet owners, novice competitors, hunters, trainers.

Fox, Michael W. *The Healing Touch.* New York: Newmarket Press, 1990. Well-illustrated step-by-step guide to massaging your dog or cat.

Krieger, Dolores. *Accepting Your Power to Heal: The Personal Practice of Therapeutic Touch.* Santa Fe, N.M.: Bear & Company Publishing, 1993. Therapeutic Touch for everyone.

Krieger, Dolores. *The Therapeutic Touch: How to Use Your Hands to Help or to Heal.* New York: Fireside/Simon & Schuster, 1979. Detailed handbook.

Schoen, Allen M., ed. Veterinary *Acupuncture: Ancient Art to Modern Science.* Goleta, Calif.: American Veterinary Publishers, 1994. Detailed veterinary textbook.

Schoen, Allen M. *Love, Miracles and Animal Healing.* New York: Simon & Schuster, 1995. Great acupuncture stories.

Schwartz, Cheryl. *Four Paws, Five Directions: A Guide to Chinese Medicine for Dogs and Cats.* Berkeley, Calif.: Celestial Arts, 1996. Excellent color photos of dogs and cats marked with meridian lines; traditional Chinese herbs, acupuncture, acupressure and diet applied to common conditions.

Sommer, Marc L. *A Vetrinarian's Guide to Chiropractic Services for Animals.* Wayne, N.J.: Little Critters Chiropractic Service, 1995.

Tellington-Jones, Linda, and Sybil Taylor. *The Tellington TTouch.* New York: Penguin Books, 1992. Revolutionary massage technique for all animals. A "cure all" approach that really works, correcting physical imbalances and changing behavior.

Zidonis, Nancy A., and Marie K. Soderberg. *Canine Acupressure: A Treatment Workbook.* Parker, Colo.: Equine Acupressure Incorporated, 1995. Excellent introduction for the lay reader, clear maps, well-organized. See also Equine Accupressure by the same authors for horses.

Resources

American Veterinary Chiropractic Association, Sharon Willoughby, DVM, DC, 623 Main Street, Hillsdale, IL 61257. Phone 1-309-658-2920.

Equi-Myo, Margie Amster-Herr, 249 Mountain Road, North Granby, CT 06060. Phone 1-800-523-2876 or 1-860-844-8270, fax 1-860-653-4224. Information and referrals to equine and canine myotherapists.

Equine Acupressure, Inc., PO Box 123, Parker, CO 80134. Phone 1-303-841-7211, fax 1-303-841-6939. Publisher of *Canine Acupressure* and *Equine Acupressure* workbooks.

Flying Dog Press, PO Box 290, Stanton, NJ 08885. Phone 1-800-7-FLY-DOG, e-mail clothier@eclipse.net, online http://www.flyingdogpress.com. Publisher of books and videos by Suzanne Clothier.

International Veterinary Acupuncture Society, 268 West 3rd Street, Suite #2, PO Box 2074, Nederland, CO 80466-2074. Phone 1-303-258-3767, fax 1-303-258-0767. Education, certification, quarterly newsletter, referral service, sells *Acupuncture Points and Meridians in the Dog* by Janssens.

Little Critters Chiropractic Service, Marc L. Sommer, D.C., 1825 Route 23, Wayne, NJ 07470. Phone 1-201-696-0006. Publisher of *A Veterinarian's Guide to Chiropractic Services for Animals.*

Therapeutic Touch, Carol Robins, D.C., 25 Plochmann Lane, Woodstock, NY 12498. Phone 1-914-679-1009, e-mail carobin@worldnet.att.net.

TTeam Training U.S.A., Linda Tellington-Jones, PO Box 3793, Santa Fe, NM 87501-0793. Phone 1-800-854-TEAM, fax 1-505-455-7233, e-mail tteamusa@aol.com, 10250.3721@Compuserve.com or tteam-ttouch@horsenet.com, online http://www.horsenet.com/tteam-ttouch. In Canada 5435 Rochdell Road, Vernon, BC V1B 3E8. Phone 1-800-255-2336 or 1-250-545-2336, fax 1-250-545-9116, e-mail rhood@junction.net. Training, practitioners, workshops, videos, books, equipment for Tellington TTouch massage.

Veterinary Institute for Therapeutic Alternatives (VITA), 15 Sunset Terrace, Sherman, CT 06784. Phone 1-860-354-2287, fax 1-860-350-3482. Sponsors weekend introductory seminars on acupuncture and alternative therapies for veterinarians and the public throughout the world. Allen Schoen, D.V.M.

Chapter 8: Flower Essences

Recommended Reading

Barnard, Julian. *Patterns of Life Force.* Hereford, England: Bach Educational Programme, 1987. Review of the life and work of Dr. Edward Bach.

Barnard, Julian and Martine. *The Healing Herbs of Edward Bach.* Bath, England: Ashgrove Press, 1995. Illustrated guide to Dr. Bach's remedies.

Gurudus. *Flower Essences and Vibrational Healing.* Boulder, Colo.: Cassandra Press, 1989.

Howard, Judy. *The Bach Flower Remedies Step by Step.* Saffron Walden, England: C.W. Daniel Company Ltd., 1990. The history of flower essences and guide to prescribing.

Johnson, Steve. *The Essence of Healing.* Homer, Alaska: Alaskan Flower Essence Project, 1996. Guide to Alaskan flower, gem and environmental essences.

Kaminski, Patricia, and Richard Katz. *The Flower Essence Repertory.* Nevada City, Calif.: Flower Essence Society, 1996. Reviews 142 American and English flower essences and their influence.

Kraemer, Dietmar. *New Bach Flower Body Maps.* Rochester, Vt.: Healing Arts Press, 1996. Treatment by topical application.

McIntyre, Ann. *Flower Power.* New York: Henry Holt and Company, 1996. Flower blossoms used in herbalism, homeopathy, aromatherapy and flower essences.

White, Ian. *Bush Flower Essences.* Morrebank, New South Wales, Australia: Transworld Publishers/Bantam, 1991. Guide to Australian flower essences.

Resources

For the most popular flower essences, such as Rescue Remedy, Calming Essence or Five Flower Formula, which are different names for Dr. Bach's emergency formula, check your local health food store or pet supply shop.

Bach, 410 Ocean Avenue, Lynbrook NY 11563. Imports the complete line of Bach remedies.

Ellon USA, Inc., 644 Merrick Road, Lynbrook, NY 11363. Imports English remedies.

Flower Essence Services, PO Box 1769, Nevada City, CA 95959. Phone 1-800-548-0075 or 1-916-265-0258, fax 1-916-265-6467, e-mail info@floweressence.com, online http://www.floweressence.com. Imports English remedies and carries its own full line of North American flower essences, related herbal oils and creams.

The Flower Essence Society, PO Box 459, Nevada City, CA 95959. Phone 1-800-736-9222 or 1-916-265-9163, fax 1-916-265-0584, e-mail info@flowersociety.org, online http://www.flowersociety.org. International organization, information, networking, classes, resources, newsletter.

Flower Remedy Sources, Alaskan Flower Essence Project, PO Box 1369, Homer, AK 99603-1369.

Herbal Essences, Inc., 8524 Whispering Creek Trail, Fort Wort, TX 76134.

The Vitamin Shoppe, 4700 Westside Avenue, North Bergen NJ 07047. Phone 1-800-223-1216, fax 1-800-852-7153. Sells the Bach remedies by mail.

Masteris Flower Essences, 14618 Tyler Foote Road, Nevada City, CA 95959.

Nelson Bach USA, 1007 West Upsal Street, Philadelphia, PA 19119.

Santa Fe Flower Connection, Box 25, Torreon, NM 87061.

The Vitamin Discount Connection, 35 North 8th Street, Indiana PA 15701. Phone 1-800-848-2990, fax 1-412-349-3711. Sells the Bach remedies by mail.

Chapter 9: Healing with Light and Color

Recommended Reading

Burton Goldberg Group. *Alternative Medicine: The Definitive Guide.* Fife, Wash.: Future Medicine Publishing, Inc., 1994. One chapter of this enormous book is devoted to light therapy (p. 319-329) and reviews its modern applications.

Dinshah, Darius. *Let There Be Light.* Malaga, N.J.: Dinshah Health Society, 1996. The tonation bible.

Douglass, William Campbell. *Color Me Healthy.* Atlanta, Ga.: Second Opinion Publishing, Inc., 1995, 1996. Small paperback book of instructions with filters in Dinshah Health Society colors for use with a flashlight.

Liberman, Jacob. *Light, Medicine of the Future.* Santa Fe: Bear & Co. Publishing, 1993. Modern science, color and light therapies.

Light Years Ahead Productions. *Light Years Ahead: The Illustrated Guide to Full Spectrum and Colored Light in Mindbody Healing.* Berkeley, Calif.: Celestial Arts, 1996. Collection of papers given at a Light Years Ahead conference. Traditional and space-age phototherapy.

Ott, John. *Health and Light.* Columbus, Ohio: Ariel Press, 1976. Entertaining adventures by the photobiologist and light expert, fascinating evidence.

Resources

Note: When it comes to full-spectrum light, there is no indoor replacement for natural sunlight. In recent years, "full-spectrum" has become a buzz word among fluorescent tube and incandescent bulb manufacturers. Unfortunately, none of their products is truly full-spectrum. Each has deficiencies or failings, such as the high-energy peaks emitted by all of the standard "full-spectrum" fluorescents, the missing frequencies in neodymium lamps ("full-spectrum" incandescent bulbs) and unnatural dips in the color frequencies of high-efficiency fluorescents. Darius Dinshah of the Dinshah Health Society has used spectroscopic technology to evaluate the deficiencies or weaknesses of different light sources, as documented in *Let There Be Light.* "Fluorescents are short at the red end of the spectrum," Dinshah told me, "while incandescent bulbs have an excess at the red end. Fluorescents can be made to include ultraviolet rays, but incandescents cannot because of technical limitations. I believe that light manufacturers are not aware of the long-term effects their products have on all life forms, and this is why we have not seen the development of an inexpensive, truly full-spectrum light. Also, there is much controversy about the health risks of excessive ultraviolet exposure. I regret that I cannot endorse or recommend any of the products advertised as full-spectrum lights. I hope that your readers will increase their outdoor activities and those of their animals in combination with improved nutrition and other healthful changes of lifestyle." The most effective light for indoor areas inhabited by pets may be a combination of cool-white fluorescent tubes with a single "black-light" ultraviolet tube. This arrangement, which John Ott noticed in a Florida restaurant where the employees were never ill and were known for their happy dispositions, sparked the full-spectrum lighting industry.

College of Syntonic Optometry, 1200 Robeson Street, Falls River, MA 02720-5508. Phone 1-508-672-1251. Members practice optometric phototherapy. For membership and journal subscriptions, contact Dr. Samuel Pesner, Journal Editor, 133 Second Street, Los Altos, CA 94002. Phone 1-415-948-3700.

Dinshah Health Society, P.O. Box 707, Malaga, NJ 08328. Phone 1-609-692-4686. Publishes *Let There Be Light* by Darius Dinshah and instructions for using color filters, building simple projectors and adapting slide projectors, as well as calendars of recommended tonation times. Send self-addressed stamped envelope for information.

Duro-Test Corporation, 9 Law Drive, Fairfield, NJ 07007. Phone 1-800-289-3876. Producers of Vita-Lite full-spectrum fluorescent tubes. Of the many fluorescent and incandescent lights advertised as full-spectrum, this brand, while not a replacement for natural sunlight, may have fewer deficiencies than other fluorescents.

Quantum Herbal Products, 20 DeWitt Drive, Saugerties, NY 12477. Phone 1-800-348-0398 or 1-914-246-1344, e-mail herbs@maine.com, online http://www.maine.com/herbs. Superior quality herbal concentrates infused with color during manufacture.

Samarco, Inc., P.O. Box 153008, Dallas, TX 75315-3008. Phone 1-800-530-4905 or 1-214-421-0757. Source of filters in exact Dinshah Society colors.

Second Opinion, P.O. Box 467939, Atlanta, GA 31146-7939. Phone 1-800-728-2288 or 1-770-399-5617. *Color Me Healthy* book and filter kit.

Chapter 10: The Vaccination Controversy

Recommended Reading

Belfield, Wendell O., and Martin Zucker. *How to Have a Healthier Dog.* New York: Doubleday, 1981.

Coulter, Harris L., and Barbara Loe Fisher. *A Shot in the Dark.* Garden City Park, N.Y.: Avery Publishing Group, 1991. The history of human vaccinations.

Goldstein, Bob and Susan. *Love of Animals* newsletter. Phillips Publishing, 7811 Montrose Road, P.O. Box ⟨illegible⟩ nizations and suggested puppy/kitten guidelines.

McKay, Pat. *Natural Immunity: Why You Should Not Vaccinate.* Pasadena, Calif.: Oscar Publications, 1997. Advice for pet owners.

Pitcairn, Richard. *Natural Health for Dogs and Cats.* Emmaus, Penn.: Rodale Press, 1995. Information about vaccines, homeopathy and nosodes.

Priest, Sandra A. "Homeopathic Nosodes: Holistic Remedies Are Getting a Shot in the Arm." *Dog World,* January 1996, p. 24-27. Review of the scientific literature about vaccinations and the use of nosodes.

Schoen, Allen, and Susan Wynn, editors. *Complementary and Alternative Therapies in Veterinary Medicine: Principles and Practice.* St. Louis, Mo.: Mosby Yearbook, 1997. Comprehensive veterinary textbook.

Yarnall, Celeste. *Cat Care, Naturally.* Boston: Charles E. Tuttle Co., Inc., 1995. The history of vaccinations.

Resources

Academy of Veterinary Homeopathy, Larry Bernstein, V.M.D., 751 N.E. 168th Street, North Miami Beach, FL 33162. Phone 1-305-652-5372, fax 1-305-653-7244, e-mail avh@naturalholistic.com, online http://www.holisticvet.com or http://www.acadvethom.org. Information about homeopathy and nosodes, papers by Richard Pitcairn, a referral service and links to other holistic resources.

For additional information about nosodes, see the resources listed for Chapter 6: Homeopathy.

Ambrican Enterprises Ltd., P.O. Box 1436, Jacksonville, OR 97530. Natural Rearing herbal compound (antiseptic herbs).

National Vaccine Information Center/DPT, 128 Branch Road, Vienna VA 22180. Phone 1-703-938-DPT3. Information about human vaccinations and the vaccine controversy.

Chapter 11: Cancer

Recommended Reading

Several of the following are books about cancer in humans, not animals, but they are excellent sources of information on nutritional and holistic therapies that may save the life of your dog, cat or other pet.

Alternative Medicine Digest, Future Medicine Publishing, PO Box K, Milton, WA 98354. Monthly magazine of holistic therapies.

Alternatives newsletter, David G. Williams, M.D., PO Box 829, Ingram TX 78025. Write for index of back issues.

Clark, Hulda. *The Cure for All Cancers.* San Diego: ProMotion Publishing, 1993.

Fink, John M. *Third Opinion: An International Directory to Alternative Therapy Centers for the Treatment and Prevention of Cancer and Other Degenerative Diseases.* Garden City Park, N.Y.: Avery Publishing Group, Third Edition, 1997.

Fischer, William L. *How to Fight Cancer and Win.* Vancouver, B.C., Canada: Alive Books, 1987.

Jacobsen, Roy M. *Aqua Vitae.* Fargo, N.D.: Christopher Lawrence Communications, 1987. Willard Water's history and uses.

Ley, Beth M. *Dr. John Willard's Catalyst Altered Water.* Fargo, N.D.: Christopher Lawrence Communications, 1990.

Moss, Ralph. W. *Cancer Therapy: The Independent Consumer's Guide to Non-Toxic Treatment & Prevention.* Brooklyn, N.Y.: Equinox Press, 1995.

Robbins, John. *Reclaiming Our Health: Exploding the Medical Myth and Embracing the Source of True Healing.* Tiburon, Calif.: H.J. Kramer, 1996. This informed layman's explanation of American medicine will help you deal with all healthcare professionals, including veterinarians.

Walters, Richard. *Options: The Alternative Cancer Therapy Book.* Garden City Park, N.Y.: Avery Publishing Group, 1992.

Weil, Andrew. *Spontaneous Healing.* Boston: Houghton Mifflin, 1994.

Veterinary References

Schoen, Allen, and Susan Wynn, editors. *Complementary and Alternative Therapies in Veterinary Medicine: Principles and Practice.* Mosby Yearbook, 11830 Westline Industrial Drive, St. Louis, MO 63146, phone 1-800-426-4545 or 1-314-872-8370, fax 1-800-535-9935, online http://www.mosby.com.

Veterinary Institute for Therapeutic Alternatives (VITA), 15 Sunset Terrace, Sherman, CT 06784, phone 1-860-354-2287, fax 1-860-350-3482. Sponsors weekend introductory seminars on alternative therapies for veterinarians and the public throughout the world. Allen Schoen, D.V.M.

Resources

Nutrition Coalition, 2417 12th Avenue South, Moorhead, MN 56560, phone 1-800-447-4793 or 1-218-236-9783, fax 1-218-236-6753. Willard Water extract.

East Earth Trade Winds, P.O. Box 493151, Redding CA 96059-3151. Phone 1-800-258-6878 or 1-916-223-4849, fax 1-916-223-0944. Traditional Chinese herbs, Minor Bupleurum Formula.

East Park Research, Inc., 650 Whitney Ranch Drive, Suite 112, Henderson, NV 89014. Phone 1-702-433-9040, fax 1-702-434-8673. Superior quality olive leaf extract at retail and wholesale prices.

Essiac International, Ecomax Nutrition, 116 West Service Road #177, Champlain NY 12919. Phone 1-800-668-4559.

Flora Distributors, 7400 Fraser Park Drive, Burnaby BC V5J 5B9, Canada. Phone 1-604-451-8232; or P.O. Box 950, Lynden WA 98264. Phone 1-800-446-2110, fax 1-360-354-5355. Essiac (FlorEssence tea).

Health News, 10117 SE Sunnyside Road, Suite F-208, Clackamas, OR 97015. Phone 1-800-370-4057, fax 1-800-370-4457, email testimonial@triple-r.com, info@triple-r.com, online http://www.triple-r.com. Information about noni juice products.

Herb Pharm, P.O. Box 116, Williams, OR 97544. Phone 1-800-348-4372 or 1-800-599-2392, fax 1-800-545-7392. Hoxsey tincture.

Helmut Keller, M.D., Chronic Disease Control and Treatment Center, Am Reuthlein 2, D 8675, Bad Steben, Germany. Phone 011-49-9288-5166, fax 011-49-9288-7815 or Edgar Fischer, Manager, Carnivora-Forschungs-GmbH., Postfach 8, Lobensteiner Strasse 3, D-8646, Nordhalben, Germany. Phone 011-49-9267-1662, fax 011-49-9267-1040. Carnivora.

Herbs for Life, P.O. Box 40082, Sarasota FL 34242. Phone 1-813-349-2095. Essiac (Ojibwa tea).

Jean's Greens Herbal Tea Works, 119 Sulphur Springs Road, Norway, NY 13416. Phone toll-free 1-888-845-TEAS or 1-315-845-6500, fax 1-315-845-6501. Economical source of Essiac (FortiCell tea), antiparasite herbs, bloodroot.

Bea Lydecker's Naturals, Inc., 15443 S. Latourette Road, Oregon City, OR 97045. Phone 1-503-631-8589 or 1-503-631-7389. Source of Hawaiian noni powder, antiparasite herbs, Essiac tea with added chaparral.

Native Essence Herb Company, 216M North Pueblo #301, Taos NM 87571. Phone 1-800-377-4229. Essiac tea, Hoxsey formula, well-done free report on herbal cancer therapies.

NOW, 550 Mitchell Avenue, Glendale Heights, IL 60139. Phone 1-630-545-9000. Economical Ester-C ⟨⟩

Say Yes to Life, P.O. Box 510, Gainsville MO 65655. Phone 1-417-679-4145. Anti-parasite herbs.

Self Health Resource Center, 757 Emory Street #508, Imperial Beach CA 91932. Phone 1-619-429-4408. Anti-parasite herbs.

Tri-Sun International, Inc., Las Vegas, NV 89101. Jason Winters Herbal Tea. Order the blend with chaparral; sold in large containers of dried herb mix or small containers of prebrewed tea. Either can be added directly to pets' food or brewed as tea. Available in health food stores.

Twenty First Century Products, P.O. Box 562, Mineral Wells, TX 76068. Phone 1-817-325-9284 or 1-817-325-9286. Pancreatic enzymes.

Chapter 12: Holistic First Aid

Recommended Reading

Anderson, Nina, and Howard Peiper. *Are You Poisoning Your Pets?* East Canaan, Conn.: Safe Goods, 1995. Good description of household hazards.

Cargill, John, and Susan Thorpe-Vargas. "Avoiding Poison's Perils." *Dog World*, April 1997, p. 24-34. Detailed review of chemicals, plants and other hazards and their treatment.

Pitcairn, Richard, and Susan Hubble Pitcairn. *Natural Health for Dogs and Cats.* Emmaus, Penn.: Rodale Press, 1995. First-aid section emphasizing homeopathy.

Shearer, Tamara S. *Emergency First Aid for Your Dog.* Columbus, Ohio: Ohio Distinctive Publishing, 1996. Comprehensive, well-organized review of conventional veterinary first-aid for numerous conditions. Detailed chapter on toxic plants, good review of chemical poisons. Highly recommended.

Resources

ASPCA National Animal Poison Control Center, 1717 South Philo Road, Suite 36, Urbana, IL 61802. Phone 1-900-680-0000, 1-800-548-2423 or 1-217-337-5030.

The first number bills your telephone automatically; the third is for credit card or automatic phone billing. In 1997, fees averaged $30 per case. Fees are described at the beginning of each call. The National Animal Poison Control Center handles over 200 calls per day from veterinarians, pet owners and farmers, especially during summer months. Most involve plant ingestion, the ingestion of human medicines or pesticide exposure by farm animals, birds, dogs, cats and other animals.

National Pesticide Telecommunications Network (NPTN), phone 1-800-858-7378, fax 1-541-737-0761, e-mail nptn@ace.orst.edu, online http://ace.orst.edu/info/nptn/.

NPTN receives more than 2,000 phone calls per month regarding pesticides; objective information regarding pesticide products, poisonings, toxicology and environmental chemistry. Sponsored by Oregon State University and the U.S. Environmental Protection Agency. No fee. Weekdays and weekends, 6:30 a.m. to 4:30 p.m. Pacific Time, excluding holidays.

Chapter 14: Volunteering with Your Pet

Recommended Reading

Arkow, Phil, editor. *The Loving Bond.* Saratoga, Calif.: R&E Publishers, Inc., 1987.

Beck, Alan, and Aaron Katcher. *Between Pets and People: The Importance of Animal Companionship.* New York: G.P. Putnam's Sons, 1983.

Burch, Mary R. *Volunteering with Your Pet: How to Get Involved in Animal-Assisted Therapy with Any Kind of Pet.* New York: Howell Book House, McMillan, 1996.

Davis, Kathy Diamond. *Therapy Dogs: Training Your Dog to Reach Others.* New York: Howell Book House, McMillan, 1992.

Palika, Liz. *Love on a Leash: Giving Joy to Others through Pet Therapy.* Loveland, Colo.: Alpine Blue Ribbon Books, 1996.

Resources

The following national organizations promote Animal-Assisted Therapy and Animal-Assisted Activity.

Delta Society, 289 Perimeter Road East, Renton, WA 98055-1329. Pet Partners Program Director: Maureen Frederickson. Phone 1-800-869-6898 or 1-206-226-7357, TTD 1-800-809-2714, 1-206-235-1076, e-mail deltasociety@cis.compuserve.com. Offers training by home study course and regional workshops followed by pet and handler team testing and a comprehensive veterinary exam following Delta Society medical form. Excellent training materials, videos and guidelines. Delta Society is an important source of information regarding service dogs and bereavement counseling as well as volunteer activities. Membership is open to all domestic animals.

Therapy Dogs Incorporated, 2416 East Fox Farm Road, Cheyenne, WY 82007. Director: Ann Buttrick. Phone 1-307-638-3223. Prospective members make three consecutive visitations to a nursing home or other facility with a TDInc evaluator, who tests the dog and observes dog and handler. Of the organizations listed here, TDInc is unique in offering primary liability insurance coverage; all the others offer secondary insurance, which pays in event of a lawsuit only after the member's household insurance and other carriers have paid in full. Membership limited to dogs.

Therapy Dogs International, 88 Bartley Road, Flanders, NJ 07836. Phone 1-973-252-9800, fax 1-973-252-7171. E-mail tdi@gti.net. Director: Ursula A. Kempe. The oldest American therapy pet organization. Evaluators give a modified version of the American Kennel Club's Canine Good Citizen test. Comprehensive veterinary examination. All national therapy dog organizations require proof of rabies vaccination; only TDI requires proof of multiple vaccinations regardless of veterinarian's recommendations. Documented titer counts can replace annual revaccination. No training workshops.

Foundation for Pet Provided Therapy, Love on a Leash Therapy Dogs, 3809 Plaza Drive No. 107-309, Oceanside, CA 92056. President: Liz Palika. Phone/Fax 1-619-630-4824. The newest therapy organization, most active on the West Coast but growing nationwide. Excellent training handbook.

Alpha Affiliates, Inc., 103 Washington Street, Suite 362, Morristown, NJ 07960. President: Barbara R. Irwin. Phone 1-201-539-2770, fax 1-201-644-0610. Not a therapy pet organization but a volunteer organization that promotes human-animal interaction. Its newsletter, *Alpha Bits,* reviews events and literature related to this theme. The organization provides educational programs, resource lists, literature, videos and other information of interest to everyone involved with pet visitations.

Index